Gendering the Fertility Decline in the Western World

Population, Family, and Society
Population, Famille et Société

Volume 7

Edited by / Edité par
Michel Oris

PETER LANG
Bern • Berlin • Bruxelles • Frankfurt am Main • New York • Oxford • Wien

Angélique Janssens (Ed.)

Gendering the Fertility Decline in the Western World

PETER LANG
Bern • Berlin • Bruxelles • Frankfurt am Main • New York • Oxford • Wien

Bibliographic information published by Die Deutsche Bibliothek
Die Deutsche Bibliothek lists this publication in the Deutsche Nationalbibliografie; detailed bibliographic data is available on the Internet at ‹http://dnb.ddb.de›.

British Library Cataloguing-in-Publication Data: A catalogue record for this book is available from *The British Library*, Great Britain

Cover Illustration: Motif of a postcard. Collection Library of the University of Bergen.

ISSN 1660-6043
ISBN 978-3-03911-311-8

Hochfeldstrasse 32, Postfach 746, CH-3000 Bern 9, Switzerland
info@peterlang.com, www.peterlang.com, www.peterlang.net

Printed in Germany

Contents

List of Contributors

Pau BAIZÁN, ICREA and Universitat Pompeu Fabra, Barcelona, Spain

Caz BATSON, University of South Australia, Australia

Ida BLOM, University of Bergen, Norway

Enriqueta CAMPS, Universitat Pompeu Fabra, Barcelona, Spain

Fernando GIL ALONSO, Centre d'Estudis Demogràfics, Universitat Autònoma de Barcelona, Spain

Jane HUMPHRIES, All Souls College, Oxford University, Great Britain

Angélique JANSSENS, Radboud University Nijmegen, The Netherlands

Sofia KLING, Umeå University, Sweden

Alison MACKINNON, University of South Australia, Australia

Christa MATTHYS, Ghent University, Belgium

Rita MÜLLER, Sächsisches Industriemuseum, Chemnitz, Germany

Anne-Françoise PRAZ, Unité Etudes Genre, Université de Genève, Switzerland

Sylvia SCHRAUT, Universität der Bundeswehr, München, Germany

Jutta SCHWARZKOPF, Universität Hannover, Germany

Eric VANHAUTE, Ghent University, Belgium

Gendering the Fertility Decline in the Western World

Angélique Janssens

Introduction

In 1993 Susan Cotts Watkins published an article under the provocative title 'If All We Knew About Women Was What We Read in *Demography*, What Would We Know'. In her contribution Watkins reviews all articles on marriage, family and fertility published in this influential demographic journal from 1964 onwards to see what demographers tell us, not only about women but also about gender, meaning the relationships between men and women. Her conclusions are almost hilarious. If we would only have *Demography* as our main guide in the world, this is what we would know about women. Women are creatures who are primarily producers of children, and they do this without the assistance of men. But the typical demographer's assumption is that whenever and wherever women perceive a way out, through higher education or paid labour, they will turn their back on marriage and avoid having children. About men however we would know even less than that, although the suggestion is that 'he' is hiding behind such variables as 'household demand'. On the pages of *Demography* children appear as the products of immaculate conceptions and sexuality as a topic is avoided or at best neutralized, so that the role of men in the production of population remains completely obscure. Watkins also concludes that power relations between the sexes, or between husbands and wives are largely ignored. Family and fertility behaviour are simply presented as the results of macro-level and above all impersonal forces.

However, compared to the work by historical demographers who are involved in the attempt to (re)construct the development, the causes and the mechanisms of the first demographic transition in the western world, *Demography* is not doing all that bad at all. Demographers are at least aware of the need to take women's characteristics such as education and labour force participation into account when studying family and fertility. Of course, demographers have an easy job here. As they are studying contemporary societies, their datasets – mainly consisting of surveys – can relatively easily be made to fit these research requirements. The work of historical demographers came under feminist scrutiny only two years later in 1995, when Alison Mackinnon asked an even more provocative question, namely 'Were Women Present at the Demographic Transition?'. Mackinnon argues that mainstream historical demography does not portray women as decision-makers where it concerns marriage, fertility and family formation. In historical demography women 'appear' at best under demographic variables such as 'woman's age at marriage', or in more macro-level work under variables such as 'percentage of women in agriculture' which are intended to indicate levels of modernisation. Because women's agency is completely left out of the picture of the demographic transition, they are perceived as undergoing rather that (co-)constructing social change. Mackinnon's main point however is – and here she is siding squarely with Watkins – that the issue of power relations between the sexes should take a central place in discussions on the fertility decline.

One of the problems of much of the older work on the first demographic transition is that it made use of large scale databases, modelling demographic behaviour on a regional, provincial or even a national level. The important work done by the researchers of the Princeton European Fertility Project is a good case in point here, assembling and analyzing aggregate statistics for 700 provinces and regions (Coale, Watkins, 1986). These huge macro-statistical approaches have the negative tendency to completely hide any individual agency, whether of women or of men. Or as David Levine summarized the Princeton Project's most important shortcoming: 'One is bound to ask whether couples or regions, as it were, had babies.' He concludes that the Princeton Project by its method of analysis suggests that 'regions had babies' (Levine, 1992). However, Levine here constructs a misleading assumption of his own, namely that babies are the result of a harmonious and neutral decision-making unit called the 'couple' or 'parents'. Again, the possibility of spousal conflict or opposition in relation to fertility decisions is ignored. It is implied that women and men have mutual interests. This may be the case, depending upon historical circumstances, but it should be demonstrated rather than assumed a priory.

This volume aims to provide a coherent contribution towards answering the question whether women have been present at the demographic transition. All chapters are based on papers presented at a conference held in 2005 at the Radboud University Nijmegen in the Netherlands under the title *Were Women Present at the Demographic Transition?*. They are devoted to the attempt of gendering the fertility decline that took place in the western world between roughly 1830 and 1960 by asking precise questions about the role women played as innovators or social diffusers, and the circumstances which may have enhanced or hindered these roles. As a collection these articles have the pretension to offer some important evidence and insights on issues which play a central role in the debate on female agency in the fertility decline. By doing so it may contribute to a methodological and substantive revitalisation of the field of historical demography which historians and anthropologists have been calling for since the 1990s. For instance, the American anthropologist Susan Greenhalgh (1995) has pointed out the need to construct 'whole demographies'. By this she denotes an approach which situates fertility, that is to say an approach which attempts to show how fertility behaviour makes sense given the social and economic, the cultural as well as the political context in which it is embedded. By constructing 'whole demographies' in this sense we will also be able to bring the economy back in – after its expulsion following the disappointing results of the Princeton project on the relevance of economic variables for demographic change – and link it up with social and cultural explanations in complex models which are sensitive to diversity, to historical context, and to contingency. However, as Greenhalgh underlines, crucial to the approach of 'whole demographies' is the need to incorporate the analytical tool of gender.

What does that entail? Incorporating the analytical tool of gender in research on the fertility decline requires much more than just adding a few variables related to women. Rather 'doing gender' involves what Greenhalgh calls a feminist transformation of demographic knowledge. This means, to begin with, that historical demographic research should study men as well as women. It should recognise the fact that reproduction is a social process in which power differentials between men and women and sex-related ideologies come into play, as well as material inequalities or differential social positions. Questions should therefore also include to what extent women and men shared similar interests in children and in the limitation of their families, or where and how these interests may have changed as a result of historical contigencies and shifts in the power relations between men and women. Gender is thus above all a relational category of analysis so that the study of men or women in isolation does not necessarily come up with meaningful results (Scott, 1988). Gendering the fertility decline certainly precludes a perspective whereby women are merely reduced to biological variables, and men are assigned the social and economic variables. This contributes to a construction of the male as an agent of modernisation despite the fact that the role of men *as men* is almost never focused upon explicitly. Secondly, applying gender in social historical research assumes agency. Neither women nor men should be portrayed as passively undergoing change or passively submitting to authority or cultural values. Even when faced by oppressing patriarchal structures, women should not be portrayed as only passive victims. Men and women are also active agents negotiating and challenging these structures.

Greenhalgh here applies insights developed in gender studies in the 1980s. These developments however have been slow to influence the work of historical demographers. For this not only historical demographers themselves are to blame. Feminist scholars have not been very eager to contribute to the field. This is remarkable of course as feminist scholars have always had a particular interest in the topic of motherhood and not in the least also because women's lives have been so much transformed by the demographic transition itself.

Brief Overview of the Field

The question whether women have been present at the demographic transition is certainly long overdue. That is not to say however that so far nothing has been achieved in this field. Indeed, a number of important studies have been published over recent years, such as the volume published by Nora Federici and her co-editors titled *Women's Position and Demographic Change* (1993). The contributions in this volume place women squarely in the middle of demographic investigation. However, for historians researching the demographic transition in the 'old' world only few chapters are of direct interest, as many contributions are devoted to contemporary demographic change in the less developed countries in the Third World. Those that remain are to some part devoted to issues not directly related to the demographic transition, such as one chapter on the late twentieth-century changes in gendered mortality patterns, or for the other part remain too far removed from a proper empirical investigation of the gendered nature of the demographic transition, such as the chapter by Julémont on the issue of the complementarity or competition between women and their children. Thus women's and men's roles in the demographic transition of the First World still remain largely obscure. Nevertheless, various chapters of this volume offer intriguing ideas which may be useful in further studies.

Other studies have likewise placed women's lives during periods of demographic change in the centre stage, such as George Alter's work on the women of Verviers (1988). Based on a sophisticated analysis Alter is able to produce important results concerning the changing marriage and fertility patterns of different cohorts of women during the Belgium fertility decline. These results are also relevant when viewed from a gender perspective, for instance when he demonstrates the strong obligations binding daughters rather than sons to their families of origin, in particular where there was only one surviving parent left, namely the widowed mother. However, in his treatment of fertility patterns Alter does not step beyond the usual demographer's repertoire with an analysis which is primarily aimed at 'couples' deciding within the framework of their family economy – a model which he has made dependent upon the occupation of the husband – whether or not to have additional children. The Verviers women themselves and their possibly gendered motives and interests have clearly disappeared from view here, as have the interests of their husbands.

The idea that gender cannot be ignored in studies of the 'quiet revolution' also speaks from the valuable collection of chapters brought together by John Gillis and his co-editors (1992) with 5 contributions grouped under the heading 'family and gender'. Here the changing relations between the spouses and the changing position of women are moved to the forefront of the discussion on the fertility decline. For instance, Seccombe argues that women were 'the driving force behind family limitation' but that men were not ready to refrain from imposing their 'marital rights' upon their wives until breadwinner responsibilities began to weigh heavily from about the end of the nineteenth century onwards. Similarly, Angus McLaren relates the use of abortion as a means of birth control to class-based gender cultures and argues that spousal relations and conflicts were crucial in women's decision-making process whether and above all *how* to control her fertility.

Class-based gender cultures are also central in the work done by Simon Szreter on the English fertility decline (1996). Szreter skilfully demolished the idea that the fertility decline should be viewed as a single and unitary transition and he carefully breaks that transition down into a large number of transitions followed by different socio-economic groups along different paths and for different reasons and motives. Gender relations, he argues, are central to an understanding of the various transitions taking place. Indeed, it is only with the construction of separate spheres and related conceptions of masculinity and feminity that at least in the middle classes the required 'culture of abstinence' within marriage – abstinence being the only 'respectable' form of birth control – was at all feasible. Causality however, for the various separate fertility declines Szreter primarily locates elsewhere, for instance in the gender and age wage discrimination in various local labour markets. Still, despite the richness of Szreter's study, or perhaps because of it, one is left wondering about the question to what extent wives and husbands in the various occupational and social status groups were harmoniously moving forward in the creation of their own culture of abstinence in marriage. What were men and women's separate contributions to all these fertility transitions going on? To what extent did men and women perceive the relative costs of children – Szreter's central explanatory concept – in different ways? Nevertheless, Szreter's study is an important step forward in integrating gender into historical accounts of the western fertility decline which is also evident from the way in which various studies presented in this volume are taking up from where he left off.

The above brief overview is not intended to be exhaustive. Others have called for a more gendered approach to the study of the fertility decline. For instance, as early as 1983 Nancy Folbre signalled the need for feminist scholars to offer a distinctive contribution to the explanation of fertility decline. And others have contributed to it through empirical work to a greater or lesser extent, such as Diana Gittins with her early work (1982) on the fertility decline amongst the English working classes. Gittins argued that contraceptive knowledge amongst nineteenth- and early twentieth-century working-class women was acquired and exchanged on shop floors and within factory walls. Unlike other women, more specifically those who did not have the opportunities for this type of intimate female exchanges before marriage, women working in industrial occupations would ultimately have smaller families. In addition, Gittins suggested that industrial work bolstered women's bargaining power vis-à-vis their husbands. Industrial occupations mostly brought women not only relatively high earnings but also the experience of working side by side with men. Thus, the absence of rigid gender divisions in the labour process would not only ensure a greater intimate bargaining power of women in marital relationships, but also engender the emergence of common goals and a common language between husbands and wives where it concerned family formation and the desired number of children. Women working in isolated occupations, for example domestic servants, or women who did not have any experience in waged work, would thus remain not only ignorant of the means and methods to control fertility, they also would remain dependent upon their husbands' initiatives in this matter.

The Gittins thesis was based on the very low fertility levels found amongst the female textile workers in the north of England. Indeed, her findings were confirmed by Szreter (1996) in his work on the 1911 English census. The particular age and gender structure of the textile industry, with relatively high wages for adult females compared to adult male and children's wage rates, favoured high participation of both married and single women. The perceived costs of childbearing and childrearing therefore were relatively high, in the form of women's opportunity costs as well as in the form of modest children's earnings which could not offset the loss of their mother's time in market work. This prompted female textile workers to reduce the number of their births.

This overview of some of the major work done so far on the role of gender in the first fertility decline of the 'old' world sufficiently underlines the need for systematic research in this field. In the following I will briefly present the various contributions incorporated in this volume, and discuss the way in which they fit in with the major topics in the field under study. Various papers focus upon the different structural ways which may have influenced women's fertility options, their choices and their ability to determine their own fertility outcomes. Here we are dealing with industrial labour market experiences, female domestic work cultures, the effects of levels of education, the role of class-based gender models as well as the constraints posed by specific religious cultures. However, several papers also contribute to the discussion on men and women's motivation for smaller or larger families, as well as on men and women's role in sexuality and contraception. I will close off with a discussion of the various issues still awaiting proper investigation.

The Industrial Labour Market and Women's Bargaining Power

One important field on which discussions about the gendered nature of the fertility decline have centred is the aspect of women's gainful employment and their involvement in the modern or industrial labour market. Of course, this tendency is reinforced by contemporary analyses of the relationships between fertility patterns and women's work experiences in the western world (Janssens, 2003). Likewise, in contemporary work on non-western countries women's paid employment is often seen as an important source of women's empowerment: a crucial factor in the introduction of family planning. However, the relationship between women's employment and higher/lower levels of fertility is also seen as controversial (Mason, 1997). On the one hand, mother's in paid employment have less time to spend on child care, resulting in higher child mortality, and through mortality there is higher fertility. On the other hand, however, employment may also give women resources with which to improve child survival, through better nutrition or better medical care. But then again, this latter effect is dependent upon patriarchal structures: if women are obliged to hand over their earned resources to their parents or husbands, the effect will be minimised at best.

That there is no easy and simple mechanistic relationship between large numbers of women in paid employment and low or declining levels of fertility can be nicely demonstrated by way of nineteenth-century Netherlands. Fertility levels remained very high in this country, primarily in the east and south of the country, which were also the regions where women participated in paid labour in larger numbers than in the west and north of the country. Industrialisation, which came late to the Netherlands, was limited to specific towns in the south and the east of the country. Even compared to the rural areas in the western and northern parts, the industrial towns in the south and east produced far higher birth rates right up to the sixties of the last century.

My own research, presented in this volume, into the fertility levels of textile weavers in Enschede, an industrial cotton town in the east of the country, indeed shows that the Gittins thesis (see above) cannot simply be transferred to other historical contexts. The Enschede female weavers, much like the ones in Lancashire working side by side with men, and often continuing their paid employment after their marriage, were maintaining very high fertility levels right through to the first decades of the twentieth century. Instead of limiting their fertility, they seemed to be maximising the numbers of their children. Of course female wage levels in textiles were lower than those of male workers, but still adult women's earnings were considerably higher than those of their thirteen- to eighteen-year old children. The suggestion nevertheless remains that these female textile workers were maximising the number of child workers during the period in which the textile factories still had ample employment for children. It may well have been the case that in the face of insecure male employment, for which there is sufficient evidence, women felt they needed to rely on the labour of their children. Indeed, despite the risks and burdens large families held for women, they may have had their own reasons not to want to resist high fertility levels. This is an issue to which I will return later on.

Evidence suggests that the relationship between paid employment of women and fertility is largely the combined result of household economics and gendered local labour market opportunities. If women are able to continue in paid employment after their marriage, given local community market opportunities as well as norms and values, opportunity costs will prevent them from having too many children. However, it would be wrong to focus solely on the issue of household economics where it concerns the relationship between fertility and women's industrial work. Gendered experiences of the work process and particular gendered work cultures may also generate constructions of masculinity and feminity that are more or less conducive to an early adoption of birth control. This is demonstrated in this volume by Jutta Schwarzkopf who investigates the gendered work cultures of the Lancashire cotton weavers. The large numbers of women working in these factories created a female work culture in which information about 'the facts of life' were easily exchanged and mutual support in work and family was central to female labour relations. Moreover, the weaving factories evolved their own notions of masculinity and femininity, resulting in shifts of power in spousal relations which made it easier for husbands and wives to actively discuss and carry out strategies to limit fertility. This was all the more important in a context in which all means of birth control available to working-class couples were heavily dependent upon male cooperation. Thus, reproduction and sexuality were embedded in local gender cultures in which women's heavy involvement in the labour market, shared breadwinning and spousal cooperation in the limitation of family size were not viewed as problematic. In this context fertility could decline to very low levels indeed.

The Debate on Domestic Servants

Whereas traditional historiography sketched out a modernising role for female industrial workers, female domestics were often relegated to the traditional world. Female domestic workers were believed to be isolated in their work roles – the Gittins hypothesis – or they were deemed not very likely to have played a part in the diffusion of new reproductive ideals or behaviour. This is more or less the argument advanced by Szreter who points out that a large proportion of domestic servants in England were employed in working-class households, and that anyway social distance ensured that few opportunities were available for intimate communication between masters and servants.

Building on the extensive literature in this field, Eric Vanhaute and Christa Matthys offer a complex life course analysis of the role female domestics may have played in the diffusion of birth control behaviour in Belgium. Vanhaute and Matthys make use of the concept of 'social learning' to assume that domestic servants may have been able to 'learn' from their masters about reproductive norms and behaviour not so much through communication, but rather through observation only. After an intricate analysis – first establishing the numerical importance of domestic servants, their employment in mainly middle-class households, and their considerable mobility between rural and urban areas – they come up with some striking results. Considerable differences in fertility patterns existed between various groups of servants, and between servants and non-servants. Specific groups of domestic servants around the late nineteenth and the early twentieth century even seem to have been practicing stopping behaviour. If indeed domestic servants were adopting middle-class reproductive behaviour, the interesting question then becomes to what extent reduced family size was instrumental towards social mobility, either for themselves or for their children.

My own work presented in this volume confirms the innovative role of domestic servants in the fertility decline. Domestic servants, as well as seamstresses, were showing great demographic restraint because apart from spacing births, they were also the ones limiting their fertility through late ages at first marriage and abstinence before marriage. Other evidence on the innovative role of domestic servants comes from Jan Van Bavel (2002: 339) in his study of Leuven, in Belgium. Thus, sufficient evidence is now available to re-open the debate about the innovative role of female domestics as social diffusers in the fertility decline.

Class-based Gender Models

Generally it is assumed that fertility control and the limitation of family size appeared first in higher social groups, and began to be introduced amongst the working population at a later date. This is also the picture which emerges from Szreter's study. Albeit for different reasons, upper-class entrepreneurial and professional groups as well as clerical and white-collar workers had lower fertility levels than various working-class groups. In particular the social group of medical, commercial and financial professionals, who were heavily entrenched in what Szreter calls a status war of domestic consumption, was strongly motivated to limit the size of their family so that enhanced conspicuous consumption was possible. This family model was strongly supported by a gendered culture of masculine self-control and independence and a femininity defined by active mothering.

Likewise in their chapter on the demographic transition in the German city of Stuttgart, Müller and Schraut demonstrate that the earliest adoption of fertility control within marriage was supported by the specific gender and family model found amongst the many white-collar employees and civil servants in this administrative centre. Together with the entrepreneurial upper classes they were 'leaders' in the city's fertility decline, employing not only spacing techniques, but also stopping as a means to limit fertility. Although the specific economic and social circumstances of these nineteenth-century Wurttemberg civil servants may have been different in important respects as compared to the English professional middle classes, their problems may have been similar to a certain extent. Undoubtedly, they will have been faced by the necessity for higher education for their sons in order for them to qualify for civil service positions in the *Länder* government – for which opportunities will have been few – while maintaining unemployed daughters until they could be married off in the proper way.

Müller and Schraut are however taking an important next step in their gender analysis of Stuttgart's fertility patterns. They offer us some insight into spousal relations and are able to show that men and women made different contributions towards these particular family models. These issues are notoriously difficult to investigate. We are allowed a small insight into spousal relations amongst Stuttgart couples through an analysis of the effects on fertility of the social background of the wives. It appeared that above all white-collar and civil-servant daughters had a decisive effect on the ultimate fertility levels of husbands from all social groups, except the winegrowers. Thus, if a white-collar daughter married a blue-collar worker, they would have lower fertility levels than all-blue-collar couples. Likewise, a white-collar worker's fertility would be much lower when married to a white-collar daughter, compared to other white-collar workers. The winegrowers' families were different in that this group was clearly maintaining a high fertility regime. In this clearly separate fertility culture women's familial background did not make a difference. However, in the other social and occupational groups wives appear to have been a driving force behind lower levels of fertility, and thus a driving force behind family models which increasingly removed them from the public sphere and limited their opportunities for economic independence. Perhaps the enhancement of motherhood, which was an essential part of this new family model, may have taken the sharp edges off these disadvantages.

Education

In bringing down fertility levels, prime importance is attached to the effect of education on the propensity for women to limit the size of their families. The effect is well-known for late twentieth-century women: women with higher level educational attainment are the ones postponing child birth, they have smaller families and they are more often childless than women with lower level educational attainment (Janssens, 2003). The effect is also well-known for developing countries in the twentieth century where generally more education for men will help to increase fertility whilst more education for women will lower fertility (Schultz, 1997).

The effect of education can be twofold. Firstly, more education increases women's earning power in the paid labour market and the opportunity costs of women's time, and thus the costs of caring for children. In other words, with more education women give up more wage income when they care for children. In this model it is assumed that married women are allowed to engage in paid labour but that they give up working when they have children. Secondly, if women's educational levels increase relative to those of men, this will reduce their dependency on men and will further their emancipation. This will reinforce their position in the family and increase their bargaining power in marital relations. Note that when women's educational attainment increases in step with men's, the effect on fertility may be absent. Robert Allen has demonstrated the effect of this relative increase in female education for the rapid fertility decline in the Soviet Union in the twentieth century (Allen, 2003: 123–131). His study also showed that the effect of education decreased as educational levels increased further. Thus, giving all women primary education was highly effective in reducing the Soviet birth rate.

The effect of education on fertility in historical populations is difficult to examine because sources carefully indicating the length and type of education which may be linked on an individual level with vital data are extremely scarce. In their contribution to this volume Alison Mackinnon, Caz Batson and Julie Petersen-Gray present an analysis based on rich and detailed information of the effect on fertility of education for girls in late nineteenth- or early twentieth-century Australia. It appears that education first of all influences fertility through delayed marriage, although it is still unclear in what way this effect was produced. Did these young women remain in the workforce longer than their counterparts with less education because they were better prepared and had been able to acquire better-paid jobs as a result? Or had young women through their increased education acquired a different mental outlook on life favouring options other than marriage and childbearing? But there were other effects as well. It appeared that not so much the effective grade the girl had acquired was significant, but that above all the average duration of schooling was important in making a difference in fertility patterns, independent of age at marriage. Girls who had spent more years in school, a measure called 'depth of education', were more likely to control their fertility than girls with fewer years of schooling. This ties in with other evidence reported by John and Pat Caldwell (1997) that women at the beginning of the Australian fertility decline described their wish to have smaller families almost entirely in terms related to the changes brought about by universal schooling.

Remarkable evidence on the relationship between women's education and fertility levels comes from Spain. In a sophisticated analysis presented in this volume of a large database of women born between 1901 and 1950 Baizán and Camps identify women's education 'as the main driving force' behind their model of low fertility. Moreover they are also able to show the working of what I would like to call the 'grandmother effect'. Increased levels of education of grandmothers have a positive effect on the educational level of their daughters and a negative effect on their daughters' fertility. The educational level of fathers and grandfathers on the other hand was irrelevant. Thus, one could say that educated women raise educated children, and moreover that educated women pass on certain reproductive ideals and behaviours to their educated daughters. Baizán and Camps interpret this result as the effect of greater female human capital formation, which also influences the value of their market work, although this latter variable did not have an independent statistical effect comparable to the educational variable. Their work clearly makes an important and convincing case for women's education as a central issue in demographic change.

The strong connection between women's position and demographic behaviour in Spain is further strengthened by Fernando Gil's contribution on the regional distribution of fertility decline and birth control behaviour in the early twentieth century. He is able to show that those regions where women's position had changed most remarkably through education and non-agrarian labour force participation, the three Catalan provinces of Barcelona, Tarragona and Gerona, were the early pioneers in Spain's fertility decline. At the other end of the distribution of fertility levels were regions with large proportions of women in agricultural labour, most notably in central and southern Spain. Whilst women in these latter provinces were still following 'natural fertility' patterns, women in the Catalan region were already applying stopping methods as early as the 1930s.

Religious Cultures

Religious ideologies are seldom gender neutral and what is more, they mostly explicitly formulate rules and values concerning sexuality and reproduction. Religion therefore may be an important variable affecting the relationship gender and fertility. Many studies are available showing that indeed traditional religious denominations such as Catholicism or the more dogmatic Calvinist churches favoured high reproduction rates in most European societies until well into the twentieth century. Usually, these patterns are explained by referring to the traditional outlook on life in general which prevented the adoption of modern ideas regarding family size and procreation. The precise way in which the connection between religion and fertility works, and in particular the way gender operates in this connection, remains largely obscure. The contribution by Anne-Françoise Praz in this volume, with detailed work on two Swiss cantons in the second half of the nineteenth century, demonstrates two distinct ways in which religiously based gender models operate to influence fertility levels.

As we would expect, both state and church authorities in the Catholic cultures examined by Praz tried to repress all information on matters regarding sexuality and birth control, whilst pronatalist church discourse glorified families with numerous children. But the 'Catholic cultural software of fertility', as Praz so nicely calls it, also supported gendered codes of sexual behaviour allowing husbands unlimited rights to marital sexuality and frequent sexual intercourse, and thereby sustaining high levels of fertility. In Protestant communities a man's rights were at least moderated by an emphasis on his obligations towards the wellbeing of his family members. Protestant husbands were expected to exercise self-restraint and to avoid the poverty connected with large families. However, quite some agreement consisted between both religions where it concerned the construction of femininity. Both Catholic priests and Protestant ministers were adamant that access to and use of contraceptive means were unthinkable for women of all classes and all categories. Women had to remain ignorant in matters of sexuality and birth control.

In the Catholic pronatalist and repressive climate some circumstances effectively improved women's autonomy and bargaining position in sexual matters. Paid industrial employment appeared to be one such circumstance. If Catholic women continued their work in the local chocolate factory after their marriage, this significantly reduced their fertility level compared to all other married women (whose occupations remained unknown). This is a nice result, which Praz links up with the increased bargaining power of these female factory workers and their greater access to birth control information for which factory work offered ample opportunities. According to oral history testimonies, contacts with other women in the factory were the only way for working-class women to gather information about birth control. However, the employment factor must also have increased the opportunity costs of children: with large numbers of children to raise, female factory workers would have been forced to leave the labour market.

But Praz also argues that traditional religious orientations produce gender-differentiated perspectives on the value of children, thereby affecting the perceived relative costs of childbearing. In Swiss Catholic families parents were not willing, or only to a lesser extent, to invest in the education of girls as compared to boys. In Catholic families large and significant differences between boys and girls existed in terms of school enrolment and in terms of age at leaving school. Birth control was therefore less of an imperative for Catholic parents who could afford relatively large families even at a time when educational costs for children were rising. Thus, the gendered effect of traditional religions is not restricted to the working of specific doctrines on morality.

Male versus Female Motivation for Smaller Families

As mentioned earlier, the implicit assumption in most studies is that women have always wanted fewer children whilst men were mostly not prepared to give up their rights to unrestricted marital intercourse. This antagonistic situation gave rise to what Wally Seccombe (1992) described as 'a simmering tension, if not open conflict, between spouses over the terms and conditions of intercourse' in most nineteenth-century working-class families. According to Seccombe it was only with the arrival of the male breadwinner family in the final quarter of the nineteenth century that men's reproductive interests were brought increasingly into line with those of their spouses. This shift in the family economy had the effect of 'moving men's reproductive interests increasingly into line with those of their spouses'.

However, based on a large collection of nineteenth-century autobiographies Jane Humphries argues in this volume that long before the British fertility decline set in amongst the working classes men had already become burdened by the pressures of breadwinning. These breadwinnig activities took them away from their homes for long hours and extended periods of time. The autobiographies describe them as figures who were distant and aloof, and in every sense far removed from the difficulties women had in stretching the male breadwinner's wage to cover their family's needs. The burden of additional children was little felt by men who were used to take their breadwinner's levy off their weekly pay package to be spent on personal needs such as drink or tobacco. Indeed, Humphries carefully outlines the negative effects of increased family size for existing children's social, economic and educational outcomes. The autobiographies she uses also make clear that mothers were very much aware of the costs new babies meant for existing children.

So why did mothers accept, or perhaps refrain from resisting, these high fertility regimes? Why were they prepared to continue making these 'Sophie's choices' – a metaphor used by Humphries – in the distribution of high fertility costs amongst their existing children? Humphries argues that while fathers were clearly the family's economic mainstays, sons in particular were a much more reliable source of economic support, albeit a secondary source, for their mothers. This may have been a factor for women not to restrict fertility despite the toll this exacted, not only from themselves but also from their existing children. This may be part of the explanation why at least some nineteenth-century working-class women went along with high fertility regimes. Faced by recurring economic insecurities of men's jobs and male breadwinner's prerogatives women were relying on child workers to cover family needs.

The evidence from the autobiographies nicely ties in with the argument made by Nancy Folbre (1983) that patriarchal control over women clearly enhanced men's ability to shift a significant proportion of the cost of children unto individual mothers. But these high fertility regimes were also dependent upon parents' ability to extract economic resources from their adolescent and young adult children. However, although mothers played a central role in this process of extraction, it is also clear that this role was predicated upon the existence of patriarchal control over women and children. Clearly, the relationships between parents and children are thus highly intertwined with those between men and women.

Two other contributions in this volume, by Ida Blom and Sofia Kling on Norway and Sweden respectively, confirm the central economic role working-class women held in their families. Even in the 1930s women, not men, were the ones to advance economic arguments as the main motive for wanting smaller families in their letters to a national organisation for sexual education. In both the Norwegian and the Swedish case, mothers were especially worried about present and future welfare conditions of their existing children.

Mother's health was another important motive justifying requests for birth control measures advanced by both men and women. Justification for these claims women may have derived from the role played by medical men. From the opening decades of the twentieth century doctors were increasingly telling women to stop childbearing when their health became affected. In most countries medical discourse strongly underlined that if the nation as a whole was to survive women's health should be improved, as well as the health of their children. Health had become an important issue in every way. Moreover, the growth of the women's movement and its achievements may have given some women the confidence to come forward with their experiences and their requests for birth control, both towards their husbands and towards public organisations. As Ida Blom demonstrates, in particular the younger generation of middle-class women already around 1900 began to connect fertility limitation with women's rights and women's emancipation.

Gender, Sexuality and Contraception

If indeed working-class fathers in the nineteenth century were far removed from the pressures of high fertility, as portrayed by Jane Humphries, what did bring them around to take an interest in the limitation of their family's size? This issue is all the more important given that at least until the 1960s all methods to regulate births available to working-class couples, such as withdrawal or temporary abstinence, were heavily dependent upon male cooperation. The reduction in family size can thus not have been brought about without male cooperation. However, the question is to what extent sexuality and birth control were exclusively male prerogatives whilst women – if they wanted to belong to the respectable part of the population – had to comply with constructions of femininity in which ignorance of sexual matters was a vital element. In recent years a lively debate has opened up to which several of the authors in this volume are making a contribution (Fisher, 2000).

Müller and Schraut for instance argue that before and during World War I German women were often the driving force behind attempts to seek contraceptive advice from doctors and clinics. They also report of the conflicts between husbands and wives around the issue of birth control suggesting that in the first two decades of the twentieth century not all men had accepted the need to control fertility and adopt some means of contraception. Jutta Schwarzkopf likewise makes a case for an active role of the Lancashire female textile workers in sexuality. Indeed, as Angus McLaren (1992) argues, women had a far from passive role where it concerned their own fertility. They were even prepared to run great risks if necessary by having illegal abortions, which they saw as the only solution if they failed to get their husbands' cooperation for other more male-oriented methods of fertility control.

In their contributions both Blom and Kling demonstrate the initiating role of women in the adoption of birth control which is evident in the many examples of women writing to local or national agencies working in the field of birth control and sexuality in the first decades of the twentieth century. For example, in Sweden in the 1930s a national organisation for sexual education, affiliated to working-class organisations, received hundreds of letters seeking help and advice on sexual matters and birth control. Correspondents were from working-class backgrounds and about 66 percent of the letter writers were women.

Nevertheless, Kling makes a case of underlining men's control in sexuality and women's imposed restraint regarding sexual matters. How are we to reconcile this position with the active role women played in writing to these national agencies? To solve this problem it is helpful to look more closely at the problems men and women presented in their letters. As Kling explains, men and women wrote about different matters. Men were more interested in sexual matters and the technological aspects of contraceptive devices; women on the other hand were first and foremost interested in avoiding pregnancies at all costs. This demonstrates the necessity to distinguish *aims* of sexual behaviour from *control* of sexuality (Cook, 2004). Indeed, it is not unlikely that working-class masculinity well into the 1960s and 1970s hinged on the leading role in sexuality, if even only on the illusion of such a position. But what women were increasingly doing from the final decades of the nineteenth century onwards was to express their particularly strong motivation for fertility decline, and quite clearly fewer social obstacles separated them from expressing this specific *aim* of sexual behaviour. And, as is evident from Blom and Kling, by the 1930s most men in Norway and Sweden had converged with their wives' wishes regarding sexual aims in marriage, making it even less of a problem for their wives to come forward with their wish for smaller families.

When trying to determine to what extent women's role in sexuality was characterised by ignorance or passivity, problems of interpretation easily crop up. How are we to interpret women's narratives about their sexual lives? Although many women born in the first half of the twentieth century – often proudly – state that they were totally ignorant about sexuality and birth control, it is likely that they were above all reflecting prevailing taboos on speaking about sexuality and reproduction. Indeed Alison Mackinnon shows us how the complicated mix of actual historical experiences of fertility and the dominant gendered discourses on sexuality may lead to complex contradictions in women's own narratives on childbirth and sexuality. And even if men were not very inclined to share control with their wives over the decision whether or not to apply birth control, it does not necessarily mean that women were powerless. If necessary women resorted to a variety of strategies to avoid or discourage sexual contact with their husbands ranging from staying up late, sharing beds with children or stripping the sexual act from all erotic excitement (Cook, 2004). And, as this volume shows, women took good advantage of possibilities to acquire and exchange information on sexuality and birth control in order that they might pursue their aim of regulating the number of their offspring.

Conclusions

The papers in this volume provide considerable support for the central role women have played in the fertility decline in the western world. Women have indeed been present at the fertility decline in various ways, they have often played a strong role either as innovators or as diffusers of new reproductive ideals and behavioural patterns. The important effect found in nineteenth-century Stuttgart of the woman's social background in the shape of family models and the number of her children is suggestive of this driving force. The strong role of women in limiting the family's size is also evident from the Spanish case where the educational levels of both mothers and grandmothers were most decisive for the fertility levels of successive birth cohorts of women. Issues connected to the gendered structuring of the labour and wage system are important for fertility outcomes and for specific patterns in the decline of fertility. If married women could and did work this appeared to affect the number of children they ultimately had. If rural women acquired reproductive knowledge through domestic work in urban middle-class households they could and did act as diffusers, copying middle-class fertility behaviour and introducing these new behavioural patterns into their native villages. Women were also actively trying to gain information on how to regulate fertility or how to prevent additional births. However, harsh nineteenth-century working-class realities could also lead women to accept high fertility despite the high costs involved. Thus, all papers in this volume are restoring agency to women during the 'quiet revolution'.

However, reproduction is a socially constructed phenomenon, strongly embedded in local – or even sub-local – and regional cultures; hence the great variety of reproductive regimes that we have seen also in this volume. The mere fact that women participated in large-scale factory work before or during marriage does not necessarily mean they also had reduced fertility levels. Likewise, increased levels of female education do not always lead to smaller numbers of babies being born. Fertility takes shape in local and regional cultures and some of these cultures have 'institutional endowments [...] which appear to allow a relatively easy path to low fertility', to use insights from institutional approaches to fertility (McNicoll, 1994: 211). Such a local and regional culture can for instance be found amongst the Lancashire weavers where gendered economic and social institutions combined to enable historical actors to make radically different reproductive choices from their male and female colleagues in for instance the textile towns of the Netherlands or the Catholic communities in Switzerland. In these latter cases religiously based gender models promoted and facilitated local cultures characterised by high fertility regimes.

Finally, these papers make clear that introducing gender in historical demography provides complexity to historical explanations. Reproductive behaviour and fertility outcomes are seen as the result of both structural and institutional factors and individual motives and behaviour within the context of relations between men and women. And moreover, introducing gender facilitates explanations which connect social, economic and cultural aspects, rather than treating them separately. This is no doubt connected to the fact that gender itself as a analytical category refers to a social-cultural construction and is therefore related to the economic, the social, the cultural as well as the political realm.

Clearly, gendering the first fertility decline is a fruitful approach and a necessary prerequisite for a better understanding of this fundamental transformation of families and societies. The volume suggests ample routes for further investigations of the gendered nature of the fertility decline. But what we need above all is more extensive research into the decision-making process between husbands and wives, and their respective roles and motives for larger or smaller families. Have women indeed always wanted smaller families, whilst men were distant and aloof, or alternatively, wanted large numbers of children to indicate their status and masculinity? And what made them change in favour of smaller families? Indeed, the role of men in the decline of fertility still remains in considerable shadow.

References

Allen, Robert C. (2003), *Farm to Factory. A Reinterpretation of the Soviet Industrial Revolution*, Princeton, Princeton University Press.

Alter, George (1988), *Family and the Female Life Course. The Women of Verviers, Belgium, 1849–1880*, Madison, Wisconsin, University of Wisconsin Press.

Caldwell, John and Caldwell, Pat (1997), 'What Do We Now Know about Fertility Transition?' in Jones, G. W. et al. (eds), *The Continuing Demographic Transition*, Oxford, Clarendon Press, 15–25.

Coale, Ansley J. and Watkins, Susan Cotts (eds) (1986), *The Decline of Fertility in Europe*, Princeton, Princeton University Press.

Cook, Hera (2004), *The Long Sexual Revolution. English Women, Sex, and Contraception 1800–1975*, Oxford, Oxford University Press.

Federici, Nora, Mason, Karen Oppenheim and Sogner, Sølvi (eds) (1993), *Women's Position and Demographic Change*, Oxford, Clarendon Press.

Fisher, Kate (2000), '"She Was Quite Statisfied with the Arrangements I Made": Gender and Birth Control in Britain 1920–1950', *Past and Present*, 169, 161–193.

Folbre, Nancy (1983), 'Of Patriarchy Born: The Political Economy of Fertility Decisions', *Feminist Studies*, 9, 261–284.

Gillis, John R., Tilly, Louise A. and Levine, David (eds) (1992), *The European Experience of Declining Fertility. A Quiet Revolution 1850–1970*, Oxford, Blackwell.

Gittins, Diana (1982), *Fair Sex: Family Size and Structure 1900–1939*, London, Hutchinson.

Greenhalgh, Susan (1995), 'Anthropology Theorizes Reproduction: Integrating Practice, Political Economic and Feminist Perspectives', in Idem (ed.), *Situating Fertility. Anthropology and Demographic Enquiry*, Cambridge, Cambridge University Press, 3–28.

Janssens, Angélique (2003), 'Economic Transformation, Women's Work and Family Life', in Kertzer, David I. and Barbagli, Marzio (eds), *The History of the European Family, Family Life in the Twentieth Century*, vol. 3, New Haven/London, Yale University Press, 55–110.

Levine, David (1992), 'Moments in Time: A Historian's Context of Declining Fertility', in Gillis, John R., Tilly, Louise A. and Levine, David (eds), *The European Experience of Declining Fertility. A Quiet Revolution 1850–1970*, Oxford, Blackwell, 85–100.

Mackinnon, Alison (1995), 'Were Women Present at the Demographic Transition? Questions from a Feminist Historian to Historical Demographers', *Gender&History*, 7, 222–240.

Mason, Karen Oppenheim (1997), 'Gender and Demographic Change: What Do We Know?', in Jones, G. W. et al. (eds), *The Continuing Demographic Transition*, Oxford, Clarendon Press, 159–182.

McLaren, Angus (1992), 'The Sexual Politics of Reproduction in Britain', in Gillis, John R., Tilly, Louise A. and Levine, David (eds), *The European Experience of Declining Fertility. A Quiet Revolution 1850–1970*, Oxford, Blackwell, 85–100.

McNicoll, Geoffrey (1994), 'Institutional Analysis of Fertility', in Lindahl-Kiessling, Kerstin and Landberg, Hans (eds), *Population, Economic Development, and the Environment*, Oxford, Oxford University Press, 199–230.

Schultz, T. Paul (1997), 'Demand for Children in Low Income Countries', in Rosenzweig, Mark R. and Stark, Oded (eds), *Handbook of Population and Family Economics*, Amsterdam, Elsevier, 349–430.

Scott, Joan Wallach (1988), *Gender and the Politics of History*, New York, Columbia University Press.

Seccombe, Wally (1992), 'Men's "Marital Rights" and Women's "Wifely Duties": Changing Conjugal Relations in the Fertility Decline', in Gillis, John R., Tilly, Louise A. and Levine, David (eds), *The European Experience of Declining Fertility. A Quiet Revolution 1850–1970*, Oxford, Blackwell, 66–84.

Szreter, Simon (1996), *Fertility, Class, and Gender in Britain 1860–1940*, Cambridge, Cambridge University Press.

Van Bavel, Jan (2002), *Van Natuurlijke naar Gecontroleerde Vruchtbaarheid? Geboortebeperking in Leuven, 1846–1910*, Leuven, Leuven University Press.

Watkins, Susan Cotts (1993), 'If All We Knew About Women Was What We Read In *Demography*, What Would We Know', *Demography*, 30, 551–577.

The Impact of Women's Educational and Economic Resources on Fertility. Spanish Birth Cohorts 1901–1950*

PAU BAIZÁN and ENRIQUETA CAMPS

Introduction

In this chapter we wish to take a step forward in the deepening and broadening of our understanding of the Spanish demographic transition. We aim to provide information on the economic condition of mothers (both educationally and professionally) and the impact it had on fertility patterns. Since the economic and social condition of women has been the missing value in the analysis of the vital events relating to the demographic transition[1], in our case study we seek to give the necessary centrality to the transformation of women's lives coupled with the diffusion of fertility control.[2] Furthermore, we shall

* An earlier version of this paper was presented at the Conference 'Were Women Present at the Demographic Transition?', organised by Angélique Janssens, Radboud University Nijmegen, The Netherlands, 20–21 May 2005. We thank the participants at the conference for their very useful suggestions and comments. Pau Baizán's contribution was part of the project SEC2003-02699 financed by the Ministry of Science and Technology of Spain. Enriqueta Camps's contribution benefited from financial support of the project BEC 2003-00190 by the Ministry of Science and Technology of Spain. Her contribution has been written while being an academic visitor of the Economics Department of Harvard University. She wants to express her gratitude to Generalitat de Catalunya who sponsored her visit to Harvard. We also want to acknowledge comments by Jeff Williamson, Robert A. Margo and Angelique Janssens that hopefully have improved the final quality of the paper. However remaining mistakes if any are of the authors own.

1 Because of a problem of underregistration in the sources. This is not particular to the Spanish case and can be found in most analyses of the demographic transition.

2 See F. Gil, this volume.

see that in fact the analysis of women's economic condition in motherhood deserves a central part in the analysis of the demographic transition.

Our case study is based on the female birth cohorts from 1901 to 1950 in Spain. The demographic transition in Spain was a long process that spread over the entire twentieth century with the exception of some regions like Catalonia that witnessed fertility control already in the second half of the nineteenth century.[3] Out of the various aspects of the demographic transition we shall concentrate on fertility and human capital patterns. The cohorts under study place our analysis on population dynamics during the second stage of the demographic transition, between the years 1915 and 1980, for which the number of children (completed fertility) per woman was already low, between 3.3 in the birth cohorts born in 1901 and 2.2 for women born in 1950 (Fernández Cordón, 1986). Therefore, the broader question we shall answer is why women (and couples more generically) controlled their fertility in the specific historical context of Spain in the aforementioned years.

The time span from the years 1936–1939 until 1980 covers the whole of the Franco period, and historical events during these years did not foster low levels of fertility or intentional fertility control. With the advent of Francoism in 1939 all the religious values concerning the traditional gender roles of the family and the virtues of large numbers of children (including economic subsidies) were part of the regime's discourse and ideology. Other factors leading to fertility control elsewhere, like the diffusion of the pill[4] and other contraceptive methods, were forbidden in Spain. Moreover, during the 1940s and early 1950s Spain diverged more than ever from the European pattern of economic growth.[5] Other factors also fostering modern fertility patterns were temporarily absent. Living standards worsened in absolute terms, especially in the period 1940–1955, while the urban network lost density and the country experienced a trend towards ruralisation during the same years. Nonetheless, fertility levels remained low and according to our results they maintained a downward tendency: completed fertility was 3.1 for the 1901–1910 cohort, 2.7 for the central cohorts of 1911–1940 and 2.5 for the 1941–1950 cohort. Yet neither ideology nor the macroeconomic circumstances were prone to modern fertility patterns.

3 See Cabré (1999) and Nicolau Nos (1991).

4 See Goldin and Katz (2002).

5 See Carreras and Tafunell (2003).

Given that the overall context was so adverse to the demographic transition, other factors must have had the opposite effect in order for levels of fertility to remain low. One factor leading to fertility decline we already know is the drop in infant mortality during the same period.[6] From levels of mortality of 185 per thousand in 1900 it diminished to 120 per thousand in 1940, 40 per thousand in 1960 and 15 per thousand in 1970.[7] Therefore, the probability of survival of newborns continuously improved over this period. The size of the surviving offspring could remain constant with a lower number of births, along with the normal delay this process of adjustment takes in most demographic transitions. Exogenous human capital health improvements causing a decrease in infant mortality[8] were therefore leading to a decline in the desired number of children by families.

However, in this chapter we shall focus our analysis on the role of women's social and economic position, rather than exogenous factors, in the fertility decline. We shall stress the role of education of women, their social family backgrounds and levels of participation of mothers in the paid labour force. In Section 2 we present the source and the methodology. In Section 3 we proceed to analyse the effects of female education on fertility patterns. In Section 4 we see that female human capital investment had consequences on the occupational profiles of women and therefore also on their reproductive pattern. In Section 5 we present our conclusions.

Data and Techniques

Data Source

Our analyses will be based on the Spanish Sociodemographic Survey (ES), conducted in the second half of 1991 by the National Institute of Statistics (INE, 1993a). This survey collected information on the life histories of the respondents, in particular on their education, social background, work, migration and family formation. The focus was on the timing of relatively objective

6 See Nicolau Nos (1989).

7 See Nicolau Nos (1989), Reher and Sanz-Gimeno (2000).

8 As a consequence of medical innovations and improvements in health care.

events, and thus it provides no information on values, attitudes and religious beliefs. The sample comprises 158,264 individuals resident in private households in Spain, aged 10 years or over on the date of interview, and representative of the Spanish population at that time. For the present analysis we restrict ourselves to a sub-sample of 45,565 women born between 1901 and 1950, for whom complete fertility histories are available. The ES survey has been the basis of several studies that focus mostly on the postwar birth cohorts, while previous birth cohorts have been comparatively neglected. We have not made a detailed evaluation of this data source. However, the results obtained previously by several authors and the results presented here are generally consistent with those obtained by other data sources (see below). A detailed description of the survey, data editing, data checks, as well as some data quality evaluations are given by various publications of the National Institute of Statistics (INE, 1993a and 1993b).

Table 1. Number of Individuals Selected for the Analyses. Spanish Sociodemographic Survey 1991

	1901–1910	1911–1920	1921–1930	1931–1940	1941–1950	Total
Men	2,075	5,876	10,488	9,151	8,998	36,588
Women	4,106	9,889	12,856	10,243	8,471	45,565
Total	6,181	15,765	23,344	19,394	17,469	82,153

The use of a retrospective survey immediately raises the issue of the selectivity of the interviewed population with respect to the variables studied (Auriat, 1996). It is clear that the combined effects of mortality and international migration will increasingly affect our sample the earlier the cohort was born. Their effects may bias the sample to the extent that they are selective with respect to the variables we study.[9] However, with the existing evidence it is

9 For instance, a selection effect could arise if the individuals belonging to the birth-cohorts studied who have died before the date of the survey had had a higher level of fertility. If such were the case, our measures would underestimate the fertility levels of the birth-cohorts.

not possible to know in detail, and *a fortiori* to correct, the diversity of selection sources that have depleted the original members of each birth cohort. Therefore, the strategy followed in this chapter is to base the analyses on multivariate regressions in which the main known sources of selectivity are controlled as independent variables.[10] The focus is primarily on the effects of variables between each other across the life course, which should minimize that type of biases (Blossfeld and Rohwer, 1995; Courgeau and Lelièvre, 1992). We will also present several descriptive tables and graphics, essentially for illustrative purposes, and whenever possible compare the results with other sources of data.[11] Although studies on international migration and mortality in Spain covering the twentieth century are not scarce, there is much less individual-level evidence on the impact of variables affecting them. It is clear, however, that there have been great differentials in mortality according to geographical location, education, and social class/occupation (e.g. Trifiró, 1991; Gómez Redondo, 1989 and 1990; Regidor Poyatos and González Enríquez, 1989; Ramiro Fariñas and Sanz Gimeno, 2000; Reher and Sanz-Gimeno, 2000). Unfortunately, we lack studies on a potentially important source of bias, namely social differentials in delivery-related mortality. Existing information concerning international migration mainly refer to geographical origin of emigrants.[12]

Variables

Complete fertility histories can be obtained from the ES, including the age of the women at each birth. In table 2 we present the distribution of women by parity and the average number of children per woman. Our results are

10 For instance, a low educational level is related to both higher levels of mortality and higher fertility. Once we control for education in a multivariate model, probably most of the effect of mortality on fertility would disappear. Obviously, heterogeneity arising from variables not included in the survey cannot be taken into account.

11 Of course, these other sources of data (census, labour force surveys, civil registration), are also affected to some extent by biases and quality problems. A thorough discussion of these issues is beyond the scope of this work.

12 Immigration played a relatively minor role in the period studied. The existing studies relating to *internal* migration provide evidence of a strong selectivity of migration according to occupation, educational level, and household and family situation (Baizán, 2002).

Table 2. Completed Fertility: Distribution of Women by Parity. Spanish Birth Cohorts 1901–1950

Parity	1901–1910	1911–1920	1921–1930	1931–1940	1941–1950
0	15.9	18.1	15.2	10.4	9.5
1	11.8	13.9	12.9	10.9	10.1
2	18.5	22.2	25.9	30.2	37.3
3	15.3	16.7	19.1	22.9	25.2
4+	38.5	29.1	26.9	25.6	17.9
Average	3.1	2.7	2.7	2.7	2.5

Source: Sociodemographic Survey 1991. Weighted data[13]. These data are slightly different from those published by INE, 1993b, p. 409.

remarkably similar to those obtained from civil registration and census data (Fernández Cordón, 1986).

Full educational trajectories were requested, including information on informal studies. For our present purposes, only studies taken in the official system of education were taken into account. Given the crucial role of education, we included a multivariate analysis in which the dependent variable is the women's highest educational attainment (see table 6 in the appendix to this chapter). The purpose of this analysis was to measure the impact of several background variables on the accumulation of this form of human capital. The Kaplan-Maier estimate depicts age at end of educational enrolment, i.e. the age at which the individual left the educational system for the last time (although only periods of enrolment beginning before age 25 are included), irrespective of the possible discontinuities of enrolment (see figure 3 on p. 45). Changes in educational level over the life course are directly estimated from

13 The National Institute of Statistics provides weights that mainly control for the region of residence and type of settlement composition (rural/urban), in addition to age and sex (INE, 1993a).

the data, since the year that the person obtained the corresponding diploma is available in the dataset. The time-varying covariate 'educational level' reflects the progression in the level attained at each age. Note that the ES does not allow an exact measure of the number of illiterate individuals, as the question 'can you read and write?' is only asked to those individuals that never went to school. Table 3 shows the highest educational level attained by individuals at the time of the survey.[14]

Table 3. Distribution of Women and Men by Highest Educational Level Attained. Spanish Birth Cohorts 1901–1950

	1901–1910		1911–1920		1921–1930		1931–1940		1941–1950	
	Wom	Men	Wom	Men	Wom	Men	Wom	Men	Wom	Men
Illiterate (never went to school)	25.0	11.6	18.3	8.2	12.3	6.2	9.3	4.2	3.1	1.4
Literate (never went to school)	10.6	15.6	9.1	10.6	8.0	9.5	8.2	9.5	4.1	4.3
Primary school not completed	27.0	31.4	27.9	29.2	29.5	29.6	26.4	24.7	21.2	15.8
Primary school completed	34.4	33.2	40.7	41.6	44.5	43.6	47.6	45.3	50.8	47.6
Lower secondary	1.1	2.9	2.0	4.3	2.8	4.5	3.6	5.1	7.7	8.8
Upper secondary	0.3	0.8	0.4	1.5	0.5	1.5	1.8	4.2	5.6	10.5
Tertiary	1.6	4.5	1.6	4.5	2.4	5.1	3.2	7.0	7.5	11.5
	100.0	100.0	100.0	100.0	100.0	100.0	100.0	100.0	100.0	100.0

Source: Sociodemographic Survey 1991. Weighted data.

14 These data confirm our suspicions that the ES overrepresents highly educated groups (see Núñez, 2005).

The information concerning labour market trajectories was not as complete as that of the educational career. It was nevertheless possible to compute the age at which the individual started her first 'stable' employment (i.e. lasting more than six months). The Sociodemographic Survey provides information on periods of labour force participation that are interrupted for no more than twelve months, i.e. short interruptions of work or short spells of unemployment are not recorded. This should result in some over-estimation of participation, although its relevance for our purposes is not great. Furthermore, seasonal jobs (very widespread in the agricultural sector) as well as part time jobs (irrespective of the number of hours worked) are counted as participation in the labour market. The survey also asks for the type of job and the status of the individual that predominates (i.e. the longest) in each of these labour force spells. We have classified spells according to seven categories that take into account the profession[15] and power relationships.[16] Thus, the category 'High' includes individuals that are employers (family employees are not counted) or employees in the most prestigious occupations (e.g. managers of large or medium enterprises, high and middle level technicians, lawyers, teachers, nurses). 'Middle' occupations include employees in 'non-manual' occupations (e.g. administrative employees, salespeople, waiters, cooks, hairdressers, postwomen). The category 'self-employed' includes agricultural and non-agricultural heads of enterprises with no employees (excluding family employees); this category includes individuals working in a family enterprise, even if unpaid. The rest of employees are classified according to the sector in which they work, i.e. agricultural workers, domestic service and 'other workers' (including factory workers and occupations in services such as washerwomen, cleaners). Finally, a residual category comprises individuals outside the labour force.

In some of the models we also include age at union formation. The date of the first union formation given in the survey refers to the year when actual coresidence between partners began, not necessarily to the date of legal marriage

15 This is based on the National Classification of Occupations provided by the National Institute of Statistics (INE, 1993a).

16 This classification is adapted from Erikson and Goldthorpe (1993).

17 Unmarried cohabitation was very uncommon in Spain until the 1990s (Delgado and Castro Martín, 1998).

(if it had occurred).[17] This is an ordinal variable, measuring the completed age at union formation. As we focus in this study on the fertility effects of the availability of own resources by women, we restrict the analysis to age at marriage, and we do not make any analysis including partner's characteristics. Furthermore, the timing and intensity of union formation and especially the characteristics of partners are likely to be a consequence of the factors we are interested in.[18] Union formation takes place relatively late in the life course of Spanish women born in the first half of the twentieth century, when they had progressed a great deal in their transition to adulthood (Baizán, 1998 and 2001).

Finally, we include in the analysis several indicators of the individual's social background and an indicator of the cultural and economic regional context in which the person grew up. The parents' socioeconomic status and their educational level refer to the father's and mother's situation when the child was 16 years old. They are constructed in a similar way to the variables concerning the women studied (see above). The 'region' of birth comprises four groups of 'autonomous communities': 'Centre' (Madrid, Castilla-León, Castilla-La Mancha, La Rioja), 'North' (Galicia, Asturias, Cantabria, País Vasco, Navarra), 'South' (Andalucía, Extremadura, Canarias, Murcia, Ceuta, Melilla), and 'East' (Aragón, Cataluña, Valencia, Baleares). The grouping of these regions is based on the timing of the fertility transition, regional household composition and nuptiality patterns (Solsona and Treviño, 1990; Pujadas and Solsona, 1988). Furthermore, given the relatively low levels of interregional migration during childhood and adolescence for these birth cohorts (Baizán, 2002), this indicator can approximate the conditions experienced by the individual during those stages.

Techniques

In this chapter we apply two complementary techniques of analysis: event history analysis and ordered logit regression. The first type of technique focuses on the effects of several variables on the age of women at conception of their

18 Marital homogamy in Spain has been studied by González (2003) using the Sociodemographic Survey 1991.

19 We also calculated models for second and third birth, that we do not present here for reasons of space and because the effects of most variables are essentially similar to those provided by the logit regressions.

first child (table 4 in the appendix).[19] The dependent variable is age at birth of first child minus 9 months, i.e. conception time, in order to avoid reverse causation.[20] Event history models make it possible to include variables that change in time, facilitating the interpretation of their (causal) effects on the dependent variable. For example, in the model applied in table 4, we include time-invariant variables, such as birth cohort and father's educational level, as well as time-changing variables, such as educational enrolment (enrolled versus not enrolled at a school), educational level, employment status, and historical period, thus measuring the effect of changes over time in the categories of these variables for a given individual. The multivariate event history model applied here is the piecewise constant exponential, a particularly flexible model that does not need any *a priori* knowledge of time dependency of the risk (Blossfeld and Rohwer, 1995).[21] In this model the time axis (baseline) is divided into a number of intervals and it is assumed that the transition rates are constant in each of these intervals but can change between them.[22]

In order to evaluate the consequences of several explanatory variables on completed fertility, we have applied a maximum-likelihood ordered logit regression model. This is a cross-sectional technique, that measures at age 40, i.e. near the end of the childbearing period, the effects of a number of fixed variables, on the one hand, on the educational level attained by the women at that age (model 6), and on the other hand, on the total number of children she has had up to that age (models 7 and 8). The categories included in the models for completed fertility are: 0 children, 1 child, 2, 3, 4, and 5 children and over. Here we have included women with no children, and we have grouped parities five and over, that is, parities five and over are considered as equivalent. Estimated parameters will then be interpreted in terms of log-odds of parity

20 Reverse causation would take place, for instance, in the case of a particular woman whose labour force status changes as a consequence of her pregnancy. In such a situation, if we measure her labour force status at the moment of birth, we would erroneously interpret that change as a cause of the birth. Measuring the dependent variable at conception time overcomes that error.

21 Event history models make the risk of experiencing an event dependent upon the duration a given individual has been exposed to that risk (in addition to other covariates). The impact of duration dependence may be specified in several ways. For instance, the risk may be considered constant (exponential model), or the transition rate may decrease monotonically with time (Gompertz distribution), among other possibilities.

22 The baseline is split in three-year time periods between age 13 to 45.

progression, that is, of having an additional child, for women with a given number of children (Billari and Rosina, 2004). In the model on educational attainment, the categories are: illiterate (never went to school), can read and write (never went to school), primary school not completed, primary school completed, lower secondary, upper secondary, higher education. Analogously, the results should be interpreted as the probability of attaining an immediately higher level of education for women with a given level. Additionally, we have presented the results of the analyses in terms of relative risks, in order to facilitate their interpretation.

Women's Family Background and the Role of Women's Education

Before considering the educational results attained by the women in our sample it is important to stress that Spanish authors dealing with education regard the Civil War of 1936–1939 as a major setback that clearly slowed the improvement of education levels during the decades that followed it.[23] In fact we cannot know the educational supply during the years of the war, but we can infer that the completion of studies was hindered from the cohort of 1922 (aged 14 in 1936 and therefore finishing basic secondary school) to the cohort of 1939, with the end of the armed conflict. In the postwar years the Spanish economy and with it the supply of schooling had to recover from the destruction of the war and it can be estimated that until the 1950s schools had not reached normality.[24] Postwar economic strangulation affected all spheres of economic activity[25] including the supply of schooling for children.

As we said earlier in the methodological section the results we obtain on the basis of our source are merely representative of a sample of survivors and not necessarily of the whole population. The rates of illiteracy of the overall

23 See Núñez (2005).
24 See Núñez (2005).
25 See Catalán (1995).

population according to the census returns are higher than those provided by our sample and presented in table 3.[26] It is obvious that longevity is positively correlated with education, and therefore in a retrospective survey such as the ES educated people should be overrepresented.

Table 3 and figure 3 show that the supply of schooling was very poor at the beginning of the period (among the cohorts born before the war, during the years of Primo de Rivera's dictatorship and the Second Republic). With the advent of democracy during the Second Republic (1932–1936) the state improved the public supply of education by increasing the shares of public expenditure financing education. Indeed, this was a pressing need. Notice in the table the very low levels of education of the first cohort under study, 1901–10, with 25 percent illiteracy for women and 11.6 percent for men.[27] Notice also in the same table how households reacted to the scarce and scanty investments in education by providing literacy at home (10.6 percent of women and 15.6 percent of men). These very basic levels of education are important because they show the adaptive family strategies to provide a scarce service in the Spanish context of the beginning of the century. From the table we can also see that despite the dramatic events that brought the democratic years to a close, the generous educational policy of the Republican governments helped to mitigate the negative effects of the war and postwar period. The levels of education of the cohorts under study continuously improved, albeit on a modest scale. Among the 1941–1950 birth cohort illiteracy and the educational gender gap were nearly overcome. We know that the educational improvement of the overall Spanish population was in line with the trend observed in the table, despite the fact that literacy and education are somewhat overestimated by our data, as mentioned in Section 2.[28]

The general improvement in levels of education among women has been considered as an important factor fostering a fertility decline and also the human capital quality of their children. Education raises the price of women's time for performing domestic chores and also the opportunity cost of time

26 The rates of female literacy according to the census returns are: 41 percent (1910), 51 percent (1920), 63 percent (1930), 76 percent (1940), 83 percent (1950), 87 percent (1960). These are cross-section results and not dynamic as those presented in our analysis. See Núñez (2005).

27 These results are lower than those provided by the census returns. See footnote 26.

28 See footnote 26.

devoted to child bearing and child rearing. Furthermore, educated women are usually more free to decide on their sexual and procreative life. And a third important factor is that women who had attended school and are competent in written and oral language are in a better position to educate their children and to make use of distant health services.[29] This is why couples with educated mothers usually have less quantity and more quality of children.[30]

If we look at the social background of educated mothers we see in table 5 (in the appendix) that they belong to the wealthiest families in society, and that their parents were also highly educated. Both the father and the mother of educated women were also educated and belonging to the middle-high social strata of society (see tables 5 and 6 in the appendix). On the other hand, in table 6 we can observe that the impact of the education of the mother of the woman interviewed is much more influential in her final educational achievements than the educational background of her father. This result is in line with the conclusions of the chapter by Jane Humphries in this volume.[31] According to this author while women constituted the emotional basis for the education and socialization of children (in our case girls), men made the bridge towards the external economic world. An obvious outcome of this particular male breadwinning model of gender roles is that women were at their strongest in the transmission of education while men were providing the income foundations of the household. The conclusion of table 6 is not that the role of men in the transmission of education was nil. But it was much less influential than the role of the mother's education. This result sheds some light on a mechanism of amplified transmission of education from mother to daughter which had as a final result increasing levels of education of women before conception. Or to put it in other words, once the mother attained a certain level of education, being the emotional and educational basis of the family, she was in turn the responsible agent in the decision-making on the education children had to achieve and also on the economic resources the family could invest in this

29 See Caldwell (1982), Cochrane (1979), Inkeles and Holsinger (1974), Galor and Weil (1996), Hazan and Berdugo (2004), Le Vine, Le Vine, Richman, Medrado, Correa, and Millar, (1991).

30 See Mackinnon, this volume, and Becker (1981).

31 See Humphries in this volume.

32 See Humphries in this volume.

education.[32] Therefore the final number (and the final features) of the children the couple decided to raise was also an endogenous variable to the levels of education attained by mothers before conception in the aforementioned model of male breadwinning.

In table 7 in the appendix (models 6 and 7) we can see the correlated effects the increase in women's education levels had on the future reduction of fertility. The event history results in table 4 are similar and make explicit that the education of the mother was one of the most significant variables shaping low levels of fertility. For instance, according to model 6 in table 7 the probability of an illiterate mother bearing an additional child was double that of a woman with secondary schooling. The amplified mechanism of transmission of education from mother to daughter just presented thus has further consequences in the reduction of the size of the completed offspring.

At least among the first cohorts (see table 8 in the appendix) in the beginning of the century the main differences when explaining fertility patterns can be found in the gap between literate and illiterate mothers. At very modest levels such as 'can read and write' (not having attended school), education has a noticeable influence on the size of the offspring or the time at risk before the birth of the first child. As we have already mentioned, education at home may have been caused and amplified by the effects of economic backwardness in the decades of the beginning of the century and the Civil War after 1936. In this period the influence of the education of the parents of the woman studied was negligible, since from figure 3 we can infer that educational attendance of the cohorts before 1900 reached very low levels. Therefore, here we are faced with another kind of education, mainly training in industrial activities offered by trade schools during the second industrial revolution in the areas of Spain where the adoption of these new technologies succeeded.

As a general result we can stress, both from the event history analysis model and the parity progression ratios model, that the education of the woman and also of her mother – having as an outcome the revaluing of the time of women – had a direct effect on the lower demand of children.[33] The revaluation of women's time implied by education, and also the need to educate children by literate and educated mothers, were factors leading to the decision to

33 A similar result is obtained by Brown and Guinnane (2002).

34 See Becker (1991).

have fewer children who were more expensive to raise.[34] This process was led by women from the highest and most educated social backgrounds. Among wealthier family backgrounds it was easier to invest in the education of the daughters, particularly in the cohorts that experienced a wider educational gender gap. We can assume that this segment of more educated women were in a position to develop family agency further in the process of decision making on reproductive patterns.

We have also observed how literacy, at its very basic level, transformed the reproductive patterns and family life of working-class women of the first cohorts born at the beginning of the century, when the supply of schooling was not yet normalized and literacy was acquired in part at home. During the following decades and the early Franco years, the situation of poverty of the labouring classes and the reversal of welfare conditions in the years 1940–1955 shifted downwards the budgets of many low-income families.[35] Therefore working-class families were unable to afford many children, and when they were offered effective education for their children, that made them limit the size of their offspring. The basic education of working-class mothers willing to educate their children in the same standards as wealthier families did and the family budgetary restrictions to invest in human capital were the second set of endogenous variables fostering the observed low fertility model.

Although education in Francoist Spain was far from following the liberal model of social values based on individual freedom, from our analysis we can state that the impact of human capital investment on women had further consequences on family life. The education of mothers proves to be a powerful explanatory variable of the observed demographic behaviour.

35 See the evolution of living standards in the long run in Reher and Ballesteros (1993). The reversal of welfare conditions can also be observed by means of anthropometric analysis. Cohorts of births of the 1940s and 1950s were shorter. See Martínez Carrión (2002).

The Role of the Levels of Participation of Mothers in Paid Production

One problem with the analysis of female activity patterns in historical societies is that historical and demographic sources very rarely give information relating to the economic activity of women. Only widows, as heads of households and owners of the household economic assets, receive the same statistical treatment as men. In broad terms, although we are certain that married women and mothers performed paid activity in the open labour market, they are systematically omitted from statistical sources or simply under-registered, depending on their different economic situations, and also depending on the rules the local officers executing the census followed concerning the information they had to collect. This is the reason why the quality of the information we can find at the local level is very diverse depending on the locality, region or jurisdiction, and the historical period.[36]

In figure 1 we present the evolution of activity rates according to age of the cohorts under study. As a general remark we can stress that these results for female levels of participation in the workforce are significantly higher than those provided by the census returns.[37] The rates are exceptionally high between the ages of 18 and 25, corresponding approximately to the period before first marriage and before the conception of the first child. These activity patterns are consistent with the savings families needed to accumulate before the birth of their children and are also in line with the working hypothesis that regards women's paid work as a supplement to the family economy (including also the parental family in the period prior to marriage).

But apart from the aforementioned female pattern of activity we find a large proportion of women for whom participation in the labour force can be considered as central (and not a supplement) to the family economy. Activity rates among mothers after the age of 30 stand between 30 percent and 40 percent.

36 See on this topic Wrigley (1973). See for underregistration of female labour force in historical Spanish sources Gálvez and Sarasua (2004), Pérez-Fuentes (2004). This fact is obviously not particular to the Spanish case and continues to be a problem in most primary sources in historical demography.

37 See Nicolau Nos (1989).

Figure 1. Labour Force Participation (Proportions). Women, Spanish Birth Cohorts 1901–1950, ES

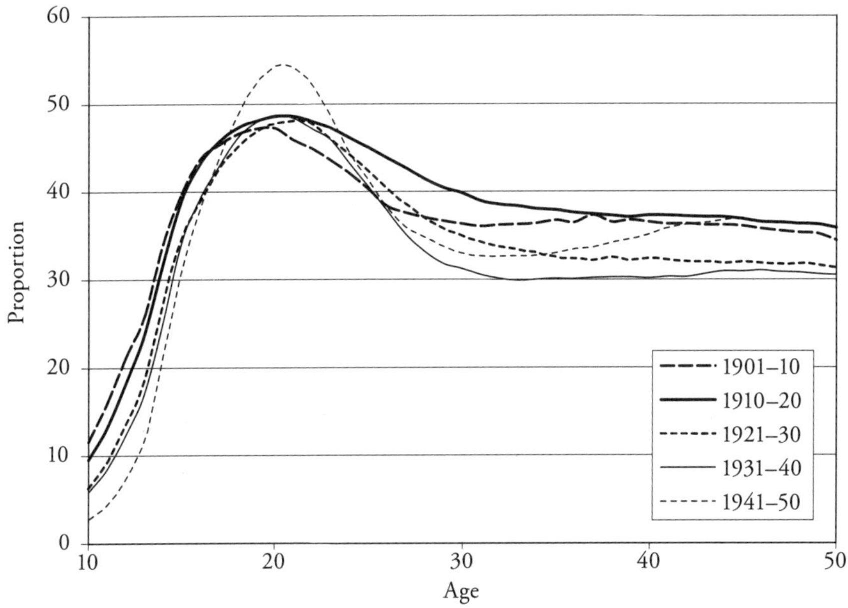

These rates are high for the period under consideration and present us with a female activity pattern similar to that obtained in the developed countries of Europe during the Golden Age.[38] Notice particularly the modern shape of the activity rate function of the 1941–1950 cohort, which is already similar to the stylized M model according to which fertility control allows women to leave the labour market when the first child is born and to return to it when the child conception time span has finished.

Among the first cohorts, women employed in industry also increased their share in employment particularly before the Civil War. During the first third of the twentieth century some regions of Spain were experiencing the second technological revolution, which in traditional sectors like the Catalan textile or the

38 See Janssens (2003). Nonetheless, our results may be overestimated according to other sources (Garrido, 1992).

Galician fish canning industries made intensive use of female work. Together with technological change and higher levels of women's human capital investment, during the 1920s and 1930s there was an increase in women's real wages having as an immediate outcome a decrease in fertility (see figure 2 for the Catalan case). As far as domestic chores are concerned, it must be stressed that contemporaneously with the second industrial revolution technologies for housework also improved with the appearance of new durable goods (household appliances, etc.).

Figure 2 compares the data on legitimate fertility constructed by Anna Cabré (1999) with the series of female real wages constructed by Montserrat Llonch (2005). In order to make the data comparable they have been converted to index numbers (1911–1915 = 100). The combined effect of the indices clearly shows that while women's real wages increased fertility levels declined. During the following decades, after the setback of the war and the years of reconstruction, the Spanish economy increasingly moved towards the services sector, during the 1950s and 1960s. In this new period the educational levels of women increased as well. In table 8 we can see that women in the higher social ranks employed in the services sector began to adopt fertility control measures as early as the cohorts of 1930–1940 and 1940–1950.

From the existing data provided by the literature it does not seem unreasonable to state that over the twentieth century the income gender gap continuously decreased. In the first third of the century, during the second industrial revolution, we have seen that the advances of women's labour productivity and the systems of specific human capital investment in trade schools had as a consequence a sharp increase in women's real wages relative to that of men. During the Second Republic a trend towards the levelling of wages and also towards a more egalitarian distribution of income had as an outcome the narrowing of the gender gap. During the Franco period, coupled with educational demands to work in the services sector, the minimum administrative real wages of women were relatively high compared to those of men. Or to put it in other words, a plausible assumption would be that the wage gender gap was eroded throughout the period under consideration[39] for most Spanish occupations. This outcome is in line with the results of our multivariate regression models,

39 And together with this the opportunity cost of women's work increased. See the data on women's real wages in Llonch (2004) and Vilar (2004).

Figure 2. Fertility and Women's Real Wage. The Catalan Model

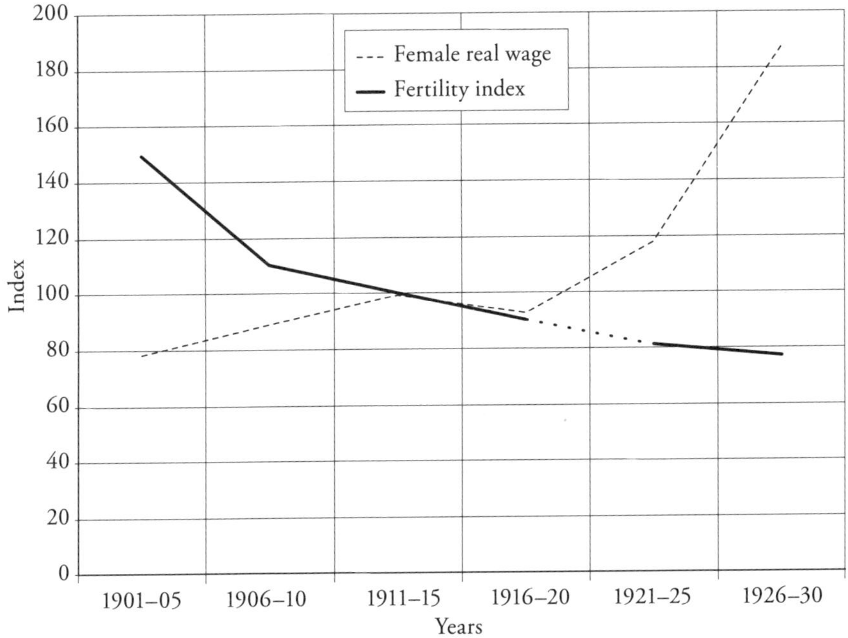

which show the strong incidence of women's work in terms of length of service and participation in high and middle rank and industrial jobs on the lower probability of having children (see tables 4, 7 and 8). These results can also be read as an indirect outcome of previous investment in women's education, which in turn made possible an increase in levels of participation of mothers in the workforce.

During the Franco period the shift towards budget constraint based on the real individual male wages for all salaried jobs should have impelled higher levels of participation of mothers. While individual incomes were artificially compressed expenditures on children's education constituted a major economic burden.[40] Together with the better educational backgrounds of women,

40 Even if children attended a public school this represented a financial cost for the parents because of the income derived from children's work they ceased to receive (Camps, 2003 and 2004).

higher levels of participation in the workforce by mothers enlarged the family income and were a means to adjust it to increasing expenditures to educate children. Moreover, among this segment of industrial wage earners, restricting fertility should have been another way to adjust expenditures to the family budget. But according to the model of parity progression ratios the incidence of this kind of employment on fertility control was lower than that of jobs with higher human capital investment requirements.

If we try to explain the trajectory of fertility patterns shown in table 2 (completed fertility according to women's birth cohort), we can conclude that the forces leading to the decrease in the number of children per mother were diverse and dynamic according to the historical period under consideration. In the cohorts of 1901–1910 and 1911–1920 fertility dropped from 3.1 to 2.7 despite the poor levels of education of mothers. We have nonetheless seen the adaptive family strategies to supply education at home at the literacy level. But the increase in the value of women's time in this period can also be explained by technological change in industry and the increasing use of female labour by the second industrial revolution. Notice for instance the steep increase in Catalan women's real wages during the first third of the century and the associated decrease in the size of the offspring in the region. Technological change during these decades actively fostered an increase in the levels of productivity of women's labour despite the modest achievements in education.[41]

The aforementioned trend of diffusion of the second industrial revolution and the improvement of the educational supply by the Second Republic were hindered by the Civil War. In educational terms we have seen that the Civil War affected cohorts from 1922 to 1939. These cohorts did not change their average completed fertility levels, which remained low at 2.7 children per mother. Uncompleted educational attainment and the influence of adverse vital, economic and professional circumstances caused by the war were all factors leading to low fertility rates.

The most notable transformations of women's educational and professional lives are those observed for women born during peacetime, from the 1940–1950 birth cohort. In figure 3 the Kaplan-Meier educational survival functions show that this is the cohort that put off leaving primary or secondary school

41 Most human capital formation at the time was specific, and training was acquired in *Escoles d'Arts i Oficis* (Llonch, 2004).

Figure 3. End of Educational Enrolment by Birth Cohort. Women, Spain. Source: ES.

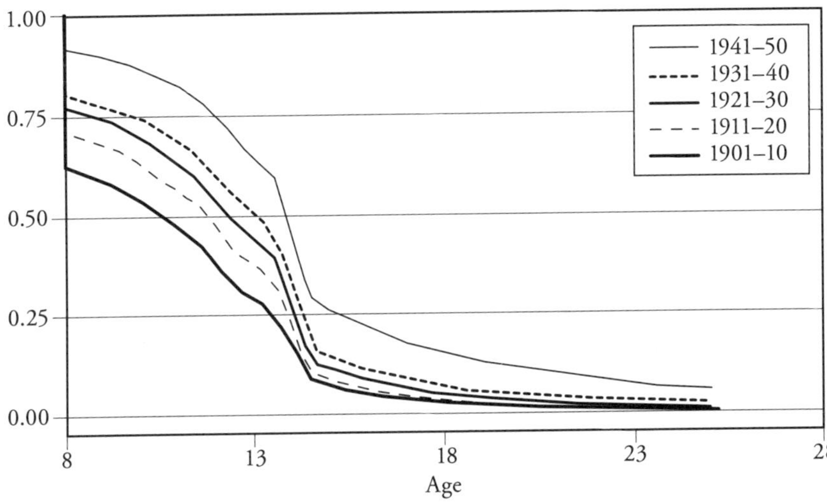

or tertiary educational institutions for longest. This is also the cohort that achieved the most modern activity rate function (see figure 1), and together with a higher investment in their education this cohort notably increased its share of participation in high (8.8 percent) and middle (21.3 percent) rank jobs. Because of all the human capital arguments we have inferred up to now, better educational backgrounds and greater professional achievement resulted in the completed fertility of this 1940–1950 birth cohort falling from 2.7 to 2.5. However, we must also make explicit the hypothesis that the sectors of society investing in the human capital formation of their daughters were on the side of the winners of the war, for whom the triumph implied a radical change in economic expectations.

Conclusions

In the above pages we have seen the role of women's education in the adoption of a model of low fertility rates in the context of the Spanish female cohorts of 1901–1950. Although the pattern of educational improvement was slow and modest it was the main driving force behind this model of low fertility levels. As a result of previous human capital investment, women's employment in the paid labour market also had an active role in fertility decline although its incidence was lower than that of education. The trend towards low fertility among the birth cohorts of the first half of the twentieth century can be explained in terms of the moderate but increasing supply of education, the narrowing of the wage gender gap it implied and the increasing costs of raising educated children by educated mothers. All the aforementioned factors actively encouraged a decrease in the quantity and an increase in the quality of children.

From our data this last statement, the role of educated mothers in raising educated children, can be proved for the most part indirectly. When exploring the family backgrounds of women we have seen that one of the most noticeable variables determining their education levels and their fertility patterns is the education level of their respective mothers (much more significant than that of their fathers). This last intergenerational result is clear in showing the centrality of women's education in all the associated human capital and demographic transformations. In order to foster economic growth it is important for women to be educated since this leads to lower fertility but also to higher levels of education of their children.

References

Auriat, N. (1996), *Les défaillances de la mémoire humaine. Aspects cognitifs des enquêtes rétrospectives,* Travaux et Documents de l'INED, no. 136, Paris, Presses Universitaires de France.

Baizán, P. (1998), «Transitions des jeunes vers l'âge adulte des générations espagnoles nées en 1940, 1950 et 1960», *Genus,* vol. 54, 233–263.

Baizán, P. (2001), 'Transitions to Adulthood in Spain', in Corijn M. and Klijzing E. (eds), *Transitions to Adulthood in Europe,* Series: European Studies of Population, no. 10, Dordrecht, Kluwer Academic Publishers, 279–312.

Baizán, P. (2002), *Formation des ménages et migrations: Une analyse biographique de trois générations espagnoles,* Louvain-la-Neuve, Academia-Bruylant/L'Harmattan.

Becker, G. S. (1981) (Revised and Enlarged 1991), *A Treatise on the Family,* Cambridge, MA, Harvard University Press.

Billari, F. C. and Rosina, A. (2004), 'Italian "Latest-late" Transition to Adulthood: An Exploration of Its Consequences', *Genus,* 60, 71–88.

Blossfeld, H. P. and Rohwer G. (1995), *Techniques of Event History Modeling, New Approaches to Causal Analysis,* Mahwah, New Jersey, Lawrence Erlbaum Associates.

Brown, J. C. and Guinnane, T. W. (2002), 'Fertility Transition in a Rural, Catholic Population: Bavaria, 1880–1910', *Population Studies,* 56, 35–50.

Cabré, A. (1999), *La reproducció de les generacions catalanes,* Barcelona, Proa.

Caldwell, J. C. (1982), *Theory of Fertility Decline,* New York, Academic Press.

Camps, E. (1995), *La formación del mercado de trabajo industrial en la Cataluña del siglo XIX,* Colección de Historia Social, Ministerio de Trabajo y Seguridad Social.

Camps, E. (2003), 'The Rise and Decline of Children's Labour Participation Levels during the Early Stages of Industrialisation. Catalonia (1850–1925)', CREA Working Papers, no. 51.

Camps, E. (2004), 'Wage Structures and Family Economies in the Catalan Textile Sector in an Age of Nascent Capitalism', *Continuity and Change,* 19:2.

Carreras, A. and Tafunell, X. (2004), *Historia económica de la España contemporánea,* Crítica, Barcelona.

Catalán, J. (1995), *La economía española y la segunda Guerra Mundial,* Ariel, Barcelona.

Coale, A. J. and Watkins, S. C. (eds) (1986), *The Decline of Fertility in Europe,* Princeton, Princeton University Press.

Cochrane, S. H. (1979), *Education and Fertility: What Do We Really Know?,* Baltimore, Johns Hopkins University Press.

Courgeau D. and Lelièvre E. (1992), *Event History Analysis in Demography,* Clarendon, Oxford.

Delgado, M. and Castro Martín, T. (1999), *Fertility and Family Surveys in Countries of the ECE region. Standard Country Report. Spain,* New York and Geneva, United Nations.

Dopico Gutiérrez del Arroyo, Fausto and Reher, David (1998), *El declive de la mortalidad en España, 1860–1930,* Madrid, Asociación de Demografía Histórica.

Erikson, R. and Goldthorpe, J. H. (1993), *The Constant Flux: A Study of Class Mobility in Industrial Societies,* Oxford, Clarendon Press.

Fernández Cordón, José Antonio (1992), 'Análisis longitudinal de la fecundidad en España', *Actas del simposio Internacional sobre Tendencias Demográficas y Planificación Económica*, Madrid, Ministerio de Economía y Hacienda, 49–75.

Galor, O. and Weil, D. N. (1996), 'The Gender Gap, Fertility and Growth', *The American Economic Review*, 86, 3–5.

Gálvez, L. and Sarasua, C. (2004), *Eficiencia o privilegios*, Instituto de Cultura Juan Gil-Albert, Alicante, Universidad de Alicante.

Garrido, L. J. (1992), *Las dos biografías de la mujer en España*, Instituto de la Mujer, Estudios no. 33. Madrid, Ministerio de Asuntos Sociales.

Goldin, C. and Katz, L. F. (2002), 'The Power of the Pill: Oral Contraceptives and Women's Career and Marriage Decisions', *Journal of Political Economy*, 110.

Gómez Redondo, R. (1989), La transición de la mortalidad infantil en España, Tesis doctoral, Facultad de Ciencias Políticas y Sociología, Universidad Complutense, Madrid.

Gómez Redondo, R. (1990), *Las causas de muerte en España, 1981–85. Análisis diferencial por sexo y edad*, Serie Documentos de Trabajo, no. 4, Madrid, Instituto de Demografía.

González, M. J. (2003), 'Who Marries Whom? Educational Homogamy in Spain', in Blossfeld, H. P. and Timm, A. (eds), *Who marries Whom? Educational Systems as Marriage Markets in Modern Societies*, European Studies of Population, Volume 12. Dordrecht, Kluwer Academic Publishers.

Hazan, M. and Berdugo, B. (2004), 'Child Labor, Fertility and Economic Growth', *The Economic Journal*, 112: 482.

Janssens, A. (2003): 'Economic Transformation, Women's Work and Family Life', in Kertzer, D.I. and Barbagli, M. (eds), *The History of European Family. Family Life in the Twentieth Century*, vol. 3, New Haven/London, Yale University Press, 55–110.

INE, Instituto Nacional de Estadística (1993a), *Encuesta Sociodemográfica 1991, Metodología*, Madrid, Instituto Nacional de Estadística.

INE, Instituto Nacional de Estadística (1993b), *Encuesta Sociodemográfica 1991. Hogar y Familia*, Madrid, Instituto Nacional de Estadística.

Inkeles, A. and Holsinger, D. B. (eds) (1974), *Education and Individual Modernity in Developing Countries*, Brill Academic Publishers, Leiden.

Le Vine, R. A., Le Vine, S. E., and others (1991), 'Women's Schooling and Child Care in the Demographic Transition: A Mexican Case Study', *Population and Development Review*, 17:3.

Llonch, M. (2004), 'Jornada, salarios y costes laborales en el sector textil catalán, (1891–1936)', *Historia Industrial*, 26.

Martínez Carrión, J. M. and Pérez Castejón, J. J. (2002), 'Crecimiento con desigualdad. Niveles de vida biológicos en la España rural mediterránea desde 1840', in *El nivel de vida en la España rural, siglos XVIII–XX*, Univeritat d'Alacant, Alicante.

Nicolau Nos, R. (1989), 'La población', in Carreras, A. and Tafunell, X., *Estadísticas Históricas de España*, Fundación BBVA, Madrid.

Nicolau Nos, R. (1991), *Modelos regionales de la transición demográfica en España y Portugal*, Instituto de Cultura Juan Gil-Albert, Alicante.

Núñez, C. E. (2005), 'Educación', in Carreras, A., Tafunell, X. (eds), *Estadísticas Históricas de España*, Fundación BBVA, Madrid.

Pérez-Fuentes, P. (2004), *"Ganadores del Pan" y "Amas de Casa". Otra mirada sobre la industrialización vasca*, Bilbao, Universidad del Pais Vasco.

Pujadas, I. and Solsona, M. (1988), 'Evolución reciente y modelos de nupcialidad en España (1975–1981)', in *La población española de 1970 a 1986*, Madrid, Editorial Síntesis.

Ramiro Fariñas, Diego and Sanz Gimeno, Alberto (2000), 'Childhood Mortality in Central Spain, 1790–1960. Changes in the Course of Demographic Modernisation', *Continuity and Change*, 15, 2, 235–267.

Regidor Poyatos, E. and González Enríquez, J. (1989), 'Social Inequality and Mortality in Spain', *Rev. Sanid. Hig. Pública*, Madrid, 63 (9–10): 107–16.

Reher, D. S. (1996), *La familia en España. Pasado y presente*, Madrid, Alianza.

Reher, D. S. and Ballesteros, E. (1993), 'Precios y salarios en Castilla la Nueva: la construcción de un índice de salarios reales, 1501–1991', *Revista de Historia Económica*, XI, 1.

Reher, D. S. and Iriso-Napal, P. L. (1989), 'Marital Fertility and its Determinants in Rural and in Urban Spain, 1887–1930', *Population Studies*, 43 (3), 405–427.

Reher, David S. and Sanz-Gimeno, Alberto (2000), 'Mortality and Economic Development over the Course of Modernization: An Analysis of Short-run Fluctuations in Spain, 1850–1990', *Population Studies*, 54 (2), 135–152.

Solsona, M. and Treviño, R. (1990), *Estructuras familiares en España*. Serie estudios, no. 25, Madrid, Ministerio de Asuntos Sociales, Instituto de la Mujer.

Trifiró, C. (1991), *La mortalité différentielle dans les provinces espagnoles. Causes de décès et facteurs de risque chez les adultes*, Working Paper no. 156, Louvain-la-Neuve, Institut de Démographie, Université Catholique de Louvain.

Vilar, M. (2004), 'El precio del trabajo industrial en las primeras fases del franquismo (1936–63)', Mimeo, Universidad de Santiago de Compostela.

Wrigley, E. A. (1973), *Identifying people in the past*, London, Edward Arnold.

Appendix

Table 4. Time to First Birth (Conception).
Piecewise Constant Exponential Model. Women. Spain

Variable category	Relative risk Model 1	Significance level	Relative risk Model 2	Significance level
Birth cohort				
1901–1910	1		1	
1911–1920	0.9828		0.9627	
1921–1930	1.0604	***	1.0216	
1931–1940	1.2280	***	1.1964	***
1941–1950	1.4384	***	1.5628	***
Region of birth				
South	1.0859	***	0.9969	
East	1		1	
Centre	1.0426	***	1.0053	
North	0.9982		0.9689	*
Place of birth				
Urban area	1		1	
Rural area	1.0268	**	0.9903	
Mother's educational level				
Illiterate	1		1	
Can read & write	0.9342	***	0.9375	***
Primary not compl.	0.8716	***	0.8849	***
Primary completed	0.8797	***	0.9273	***
Lower secondary compl.	0.8203	***	0.8856	***
Mother's labour force status at 15				
Out of labour force	1		1	
High or middle	0.8884	**	0.9422	
Self-employed	1.0792	***	1.1459	***
Agricultural worker	1.0186		1.0636	*
Other worker	1.0721	*	1.1902	***
Domestic service	1.0214		1.1266	***

Variable category	Relative risk Model 1	Significance level	Relative risk Model 2	Significance level
Father's educational level				
Illiterate	1		1	
Can read & write	0.9468	***	0.9536	***
Primary not completed	0.9930		1.0248	
Primary completed	0.8762	***	0.9230	***
Lower secondary completed	0.7871	***	0.8666	***
Father's labour force status at 15				
High	1		1	
Middle	1.0035		1.0123	
Self-employed	1.1356	***	1.0834	***
Agricultural worker	1.2298	***	1.2053	***
Other worker	1.1688	***	1.1676	***
Enrolled in education			0.4266	***
Educational level				
Illiterate			1.0237	
Can read & write			0.9554	**
Primary not completed			1	
Primary completed			0.9036	***
Lower secondary compl.			0.7950	***
Higher secondary compl.			0.8065	***
Labour force status				
Out of labour force			1	
High			0.4952	***
Middle			0.5029	***
Self-employed			0.7488	***
Agricultural worker			0.7726	***
Other worker			0.6140	***
Domestic service			0.6212	***
Historical period				
Before war			1	
War 1936–38			0.7315	**
After war			1.0850	***

Note: Baseline not shown (three-year time periods from age 13 to 45).
Significance: *** 0.99; ** 0.95; * 0.90.

Table 5. Time to End of Educational Enrolment. Piecewise Constant Exponential Model. Women. Spain

Variable category	Relative risk Model 3	Significance level
Birth cohort		
1901–1910	1	
1911–1920	0.8803	***
1921–1930	0.7901	***
1931–1940	0.7287	***
1941–1950	0.5456	***
Region of birth		
South	1.1670	***
East	1	
Centre	1.0037	
North	0.9131	***
Place of birth		
Urban area	1	
Rural area	1.1038	***
Mother's educational level		
Illiterate	1	
Can read & write	0.8294	***
Primary not compl.	0.7974	***
Primary completed	0.7082	***
Lower secondary compl.	0.6991	***
Mother's labour force status at 15		
Out of labour force	1	
High or middle	0.8009	***
Self-employed	0.7927	***
Agricultural worker	0.9656	
Other worker	1.0293	
Domestic service	1.1059	**
Father's educational level		
Illiterate	1	
Can read & write	0.9099	***
Primary not completed	0.8563	***
Primary completed	0.7188	***

Variable category	Relative risk Model 3	Significance level
Lower secondary completed	0.5295	***
Father's labour force status at 15		
High	1	
Middle	1.1975	***
Self-employed	1.3301	***
Agricultural worker	1.6210	***
Other worker	1.4265	***
Labour force status		
Out of labour force	1	
Participates	5.0820	***
Historical period		
Before war		
War 1936–1938	1.3228	***
After war	0.9606	*

Note: Baseline not shown (10 time periods between age 8 and 25).
Significance: *** 0.99; ** 0.95; * 0.90.

Table 6. Educational Attainment. Women. Spain

Variable category	Relative risk Model 4	Significance level
Birth cohort		
1901–1910	1	
1911–1920	1.371	***
1921–1930	1.802	***
1931–1940	2.325	***
1941–1950	5.140	***
Region of birth		
South	0.368	***
East	1	
Centre	0.818	***
North	0.897	***

Variable category	Relative risk Model 4	Significance level
Place of birth		
Urban area	1	
Rural area	0.773	***
Mother's educational level		
Illiterate	1	
Can read & write	2.232	***
Primary not compl.	3.453	***
Primary completed	6.851	***
Lower secondary compl.	8.141	***
Mother's labour force status at 15		
Out of labour force	1	
High or middle	2.181	***
Self-employed	0.881	***
Agricultural worker	0.614	***
Other worker	0.910	
Domestic service	0.770	***
Father's educational level		
Illiterate	1	
Can read & write	1.142	***
Primary not completed	1.276	***
Primary completed	1.369	***
Lower secondary completed	2.024	***
Father's labour force status at 15		
High	1	
Middle	0.496	***
Self-employed	0.282	***
Agricultural worker	0.149	***
Other worker	0.244	***

Note: Ordered logit with categories: 0 = illiterate (never went to school), 1 = can read & write (never went to school), 2 = primary school not completed, 3 = primary school completed, 4 = lower secondary, 5 = upper secondary, 6 = higher education.
Significance: *** 0.99; ** 0.95; * 0.90.

Table 7. Parity Progression Ratios: Impact of Family Background, Education, Labour Force Participation and Age at Marriage. Women. Spain

Variable category	Rel. risk Model 5	Signif. level	Rel. risk Model 6	Signif. level	Rel. risk Model 7	Signif. level
Birth cohort						
1901–1910	1		1		1	
1911–1920	0.719	***	0.742	***	0.717	***
1921–1930	0.663	***	0.689	***	0.628	***
1931–1940	0.681	***	0.705	***	0.548	***
1941–1950	0.612	***	0.677	***	0.421	***
Region of birth						
South	2.050	***	1.725	***	2.257	***
East	1		1		1	
Centre	1.580	***	1.437	***	1.799	***
North	1.153	***	1.108	***	1.372	***
Place of birth						
Urban area	1		1		1	
Rural area	1.085	***	1.039	**	1.060	***
Mother's educational level						
Illiterate	1		1		1	
Can read & write	0.909	***	0.950	**	1.032	
Primary not compl.	0.830	***	0.895	***	0.994	
Primary completed	0.825	***	0.946		1.094	**
Lower secondary	0.710	***	0.831	**	0.857	**
Mother's labour force status at 15						
Out of labour force	1		1		1	
High or middle	0.858	**	1.024		1.013	
Self-employed	1.039		1.175	***	1.020	
Agricultural worker	0.915		0.957		0.858	**
Other worker	1.005		1.189	***	1.012	
Domestic service	1.033		1.187	***	1.026	
Father's educational level						
Illiterate	1		1		1	
Can read & write	0.899	***	0.905	***	0.893	***
Primary not completed	0.925	***	0.947	*	0.905	***
Primary completed	0.857	***	0.877	***	0.856	***
Lower secondary	0.809	***	0.862	**	0.910	

Variable category	Rel. risk Model 5	Signif. level	Rel. risk Model 6	Signif. level	Rel. risk Model 7	Signif. level
Father's labour force status at 15						
High	1		1			
Middle	1.011		0.995		0.962	
Self-employed	1.262	***	1.111	***	1.010	
Agricultural worker	1.515	***	1.322	***	1.121	***
Other worker	1.220	***	1.125	***	0.953	
Educational level						
Illiterate			1.414	***	1.302	***
Can read & write			0.989		0.939	
Primary not completed			1		1	
Primary completed			0.842	***	0.917	***
Lower secondary			0.768	***	1.013	
Higher secondary			0.762	***	1.148	***
Years of labour force participation (up to 45)						
Never participated			2.282	***	1.542	***
Less than 8			2.487	***	1.317	***
8 to 20			1.818	***	1.273	***
More than 20			1		1	
Labour force status						
High			0.813	***	1.215	***
Middle			0.877	***	1.056	
Self-employed			1.430	***	1.243	***
Worker (agriculture)			1.684	***	1.426	***
Worker (other)			1		1	***
Domestic service			1.146	***	1.231	***
Age at union formation					0.869	***

Note: Ordered logit with categories: 0, 1, 2, 3, 4, 5 and over.
Significance: *** 0.99; ** 0.95; * 0.90.

Table 8. Parity Progression Ratios: Impact of Family Background, Education, Labour Force Participation and Age at Marriage. Birth-cohort Specific Models. Women. Spain

Birth cohort	1901–1910	1911–1920	1921–1930	1931–1940	1941–1950
Region of birth					
South	1.818***	1.803***	1.724***	1.687***	1.604***
East	1	1	1	1	1
Centre	1.819***	1.674***	1.424***	1.303***	1.116*
North	1.302***	1.264***	1.113**	1.059	0.881**
Place of birth					
Urban area	1	1	1	1	
Rural area	1.290***	1.162***	1.050	0.937*	0.890***
Mother's educational level					
Illiterate	1	1	1	1	1
Can read & write	1.073	1.041	0.852***	0.941	0.952
Primary not compl.	0.871	1.049	0.847***	0.840***	0.857**
Primary completed	1.083	1.006	0.956	0.959	0.796**
Lower secondary	0.767	0.940	0.746*	0.963	0.617***
Mother's labour force status at 15					
Out of labour force	1	1	1	1	1
High or middle	0.944	0.692**	1.324*	1.173	0.923
Self-employed	1.109	1.365***	1.166***	1.036	1.267***
Agricultural worker	0.903	1.096	0.989	0.802*	0.980
Other worker	1.238	1.174	1.236*	1.108	1.062
Domestic service	1.089	1.348**	1.112	1.010	1.428**
Father's educational level					
Illiterate	1	1	1	1	1
Can read & write	0.798**	0.901*	0.936	0.957	0.824**
Primary not completed	0.966	0.858**	0.984	1.049	0.897
Primary completed	0.676**	0.901	0.922	0.911	0.888
Lower secondary	0.634*	0.848	0.954	0.846	0.950
Father's labour force status at 15					
High	1	1	1	1	1
Middle	0.941	0.876	1.114	0.936	0.965
Self-employed	1.335**	1.128	1.218***	1.040	0.845**

Birth cohort	1901–1910	1911–1920	1921–1930	1931–1940	1941–1950
Agricultural worker	1.608***	1.360***	1.386***	1.319***	1.002
Other worker	1.166	1.039	1.255***	1.138	0.916
Educational level					
Illiterate	1.523***	1.381***	1.254***	1.492***	0.997
Can read & write	0.925	0.999	0.957	1.085	0.943
Primary not completed	1	1	1	1	1
Primary completed	0.833**	0.911**	0.776***	0.891***	0.768***
Lower secondary	0.530**	0.762*	0.765**	0.892	0.604***
Higher secondary	0.457***	0.576***	0.637***	0.817*	0.629***
Years of labour force participation (up to 45)					
Never participated	1.991***	2.019***	2.347***	2.305***	2.562***
Less than 8	2.446***	2.488***	2.441***	2.407***	3.241***
8 to 20	1.837***	1.766***	1.889***	1.728***	2.070***
More than 20	1	1	1	1	1
Labour force status					
High	0.770	0.702**	0.548***	0.807*	0.842*
Middle	0.861	0.674***	0.697***	0.732****	0.938
Self-employed	1.129	1.208***	1.382***	1.330***	1.291***
Worker (agriculture)	1.394**	1.514***	1.605***	1.514***	1.772***
Worker (other)	1	1	1	1	1
Domestic service	0.856	0.863**	1.084	1.242***	1.221***

Note: Ordered logit with categories: 0, 1, 2, 3, 4, 5 and over.
Significance: *** 0.99; ** 0.95; * 0.90.

'Master of Your Own Body and What Is In It' – Reducing Marital Fertility in Norway, 1890–1930

IDA BLOM

In 1915 the Norwegian feminist Katti Anker Møller in a speech entitled 'The emancipation of motherhood' made a vigorous attack on the Norwegian penal code that punished provoked abortion with years of emprisonment. She stated that 'the basis for all freedom is to be master of your own body and what is in it' (Mohr, 1976: 108). With this speech she intensified the long crusade she had started two years earlier to allow women to decide freely how many children they wanted. Her politics were important both in raising the question of marital fertility and in providing means to limit the number of births in a family. Nine years later, in 1924, she cooperated with women from the Labour Party in starting the Oslo Mothers' Clinic, patterned on Mary Stopes' work in London, and aiming at providing women with the possibility to control fertility irrespective of their husbands' will. A central theme in Norwegian discussions on the reduction of marital fertility was women's self-determination.

Reducing fertility was part of the demographic transition that between the late eighteenth and the middle of the twentieth century changed the Western world from a society with high mortality and fertility to a society where both mortality and fertility were low. The transition started with a reduction of mortality that led to a rising number of people. A reduction in fertility followed, especially from the late nineteenth century onwards, and by the late 1930s the transition was completed. This is of course a very simplistic description of a complicated process with numerous geographical, social and cultural variations, but it conveys the important demographic changes that have shaped modern societies. During the past decades, wide ranging historical research has supplemented demographic studies in attempts at understanding the many-faceted aspects of this development. The intention of this article is to present Norwegian women's involvement with the reduction of marital fertility and to examine whether some of the observations made concerning the fertility decline in Britain may also be valid for Norway.

The paper builds on my book, published in 1980, and a number of later Norwegian studies. My book went below the national level, concentrating on Oslo, the Norwegian capital. The main intention was to find expressions of Norwegian women's motives for reducing the number of births. Two groups of women's journals were analysed for this purpose. One group consisted of journals edited by and mainly read by middle-class women, another of journals mainly by and for women of the working class or women belonging to the Labour Party.[1] Arguments found in these journals cannot be related to specific geographical areas, but the contents of the journals show that they are especially valid for urban women. A collection of 4,361 letters addressed to the first Mothers' Clinic in Oslo between 1924 and 1929 further elucidates reasons for wanting to stop having babies. The letters came mainly from people of small economic means, and mainly from women.[2]

The other main intention of my book was to study the question of how to reduce fertility. For this purpose I analysed public discussions on contraception and abortion, raised by attempts to change legislation on these questions and by the work of the Oslo Mothers' Clinic. This part of the book builds on

1 The journals *Husmoderen* (The Housewife) 1989–1916, *Nylænde* 1887–1927 and *Urd* 1897–1920 were read and edited by urban middle-class women. While *Nylænde* represented the liberal Norwegian Women's Association, *Urd* and *Husmoderen* addressed a broader range of middle-class women. The journals *Social-Demokraten* 1885–1920, *Kvinden*, *Arbeiderkvinden* (The Women, from 1923 named The Working-Class Woman) 1909–1939 and *Klassekampen* (The Class War) 1919–1934 all mirror socialist perceptions.

2 This collection of letters was put at my disposal by the kind agreement of Tove Mohr, the daughter of the founder of the Clinic, Katti Anker Møller. In cooperation with the EDB-center at the Faculty of the Humanities at the University of Bergen the letters were coded and computerised to provide a numerical indication of their contents. In 79 percent of the letters the writer asked for information on contraception, in 6 percent the need for abortion was indicated. The main part of these letters came from the southern part of Norway. In 15 percent of the letters advice on child care was obtained. In 18 percent of all letters the writer was male, mainly husbands who wrote on behalf of their wives and some physicians requiring information on contraception in order to assist clients. Most of these letters were short and mainly asked to have contraception sent to the letter-writer. Since only 8 percent of the letters mention the occupation or social status of the letter-writer, the impression that most of the letters came from working-class mothers is derived from poor spelling, the use of expressions rarely found with middle-class people, etc. The letters are now deposited at the University Library, Oslo. For a full discussion of the use of this collection of letters, see Blom, 1980: 17–20, and tables 27, 29 and 35 on pages 288, 289 and 295.

parliamentary documents concerning legislation on contraception and abortion, on the archives of the Central Board of the Norwegian Association for Propriety *(Sentralstyret for de norske Sædelighetsforeninger)* as well as journals voicing the opinion of this association, of political parties and of religious groupings within the Lutheran church, the absolutely dominant religion in Norway. The archives of the Oslo Mothers' Clinic also constituted an important source material.[3] Together these sources reflect the culture surrounding women and men who strove to reduce fertility and within which important choices had to be made.

One or Several Fertility Declines?

In 1996 Simon Szreter published a major work on the reduction of marital fertility in Britain (Szreter, 1996). He revised earlier studies that had focussed on the macro level, on fertility as a national problem. These studies had posited a unilateral fall in fertility, starting in the urban middle class and spreading to working-class and rural areas. Szeter found that the fertility decline started within the non-manual occupations and their clerical and domestic assistants. But for the rest of the population, he drew the picture of a multitude of different fertility regimes, many geographically and chronologically disparate processes. In short, according to Szreter there was no such phenomenon as *the* fertility decline (Srzeter, 1996: 310–366).

Does this picture hold true also for Norway? Between 1880 and 1930 marital fertility in Norway fell from 302 to 148 births per 1,000 women aged 15–44 years. Census material indicates an early reduction in the upper social groups in urban areas spreading socially and geographically to workers and to agrarian and coastal districts (Myklebost, 1976). The problem was discussed by statisticians already in the 1920s, but only caught the attention of historians in the 1970s and 1980s (Jahn, 1920; Sogner et al., 1984; Sogner, 1986; Dyrvik and Alsvik, 1987; Dyrvik, 2004).

3 For a full account of source material see Blom (1980), 15–20 and 336–347.

The fertility decline was especially strong in Oslo[4], the Norwegian capital, and started out with distinct differences between the eastern and the western districts of the city (see figure 1). While marital fertility in the western parts of the city declined through the last decades of the nineteenth century, it was still rising in the eastern districts, reaching a peak in 1900. But thirty years later, the difference between the western and eastern districts had been seriously reduced and average marital fertility had fallen from 254 to 71 births per 1,000 women aged 15–44 years. The reduction was most marked during the 1920s.

Figure 1. Proportion of Children Born Alive per 1,000 Women Aged 15/20 until 44/49, 1890–1930

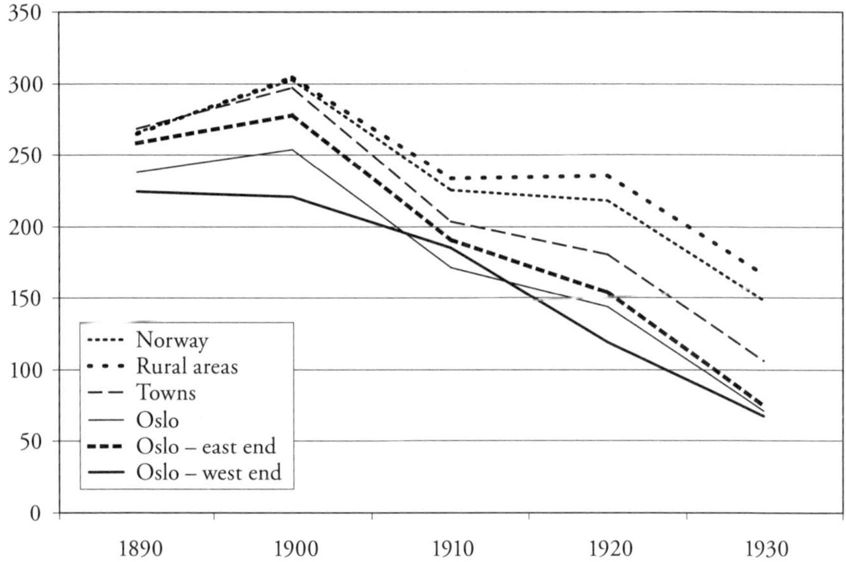

Sources: Blom 1980

4 Until 1924 the name of this city was Kristiania. To simplify understandings the modern name Oslo is used in this paper.

The city of Oslo was typically divided into the working-class areas of the eastern districts and the well off middle- and upper middle-class western districts. Housing statistics confirm marked differences between these two parts of the city. A preponderance of one-room-flats, almost all without bathroom facilities, characterised the east, whereas inhabitants of the western districts lived in spacious apartments, mostly including bathrooms. Servants were common in the west, but absolutely absent in the east. Around 1900 mortality from tuberculosis in the east was double that of the west (Blom, 1980: tables 6, 7, 8, 9 and 32). All this clearly indicated a city divided in a wealthy and healthy western part where marital fertility fell early and a poor and unhealthy eastern part where the reduction came a little later. No doubt, class was an important factor for neighbourhoods and also for the fall in marital fertility. But once the reduction started in the east, the difference in marital fertility between the two parts of the city quickly levelled out. Although there may have been two clearly distinct fertility transitions in the city, once they had started they followed parallel trajectories.

This result was later confirmed by a study of the city of Stavanger on the Norwegian west coast. Here neighbourhood and workplace had an important effect on the number of children families ultimately had. Regardless of individual characteristics such as profession or income people living in the same neighbourhood or working within the same trade tended to share reproductive behaviour (Dyrvik and Alsvik, 1987). This supports Szreter's point of the importance of what he terms 'communication communities', i.e. shared social practices and values of social groups (Szreter 1996: 546–558). It also indicates that local studies highlight variations in patterns of fertility that may not be discerned at the national level. A multitude of local fertility declines added up to the national reduction of births.

Why Reduce the Number of Births in a Family?

What exactly was it that made people start limiting the number of births in a family? This has been one of the big questions ever since historians started studying the demographic transition. Most attempts at answering this question have been made at the macro level.

A nation-wide Norwegian study published in 1984 confirmed that fertility fell in a modernising society (Sogner et al., 1984; Dyrvik, 2004: 12–15). Attitudes such as fear of the unfamiliar and unknown, a wish to preserve traditional society, to protect it against foreign influences and a negative attitude to women's emancipation made for condemnation of mechanical contraception and constituted a barrier to reduced fertility. It came as no surprise that reduction of marital fertility was marked in regions where women were breaking out of traditional perceptions of femininity, using their newly won suffrage rights and taking part in social and political activities.[5] Early reduction was also observed where a high proportion of the population was active within secondary and tertiary trades (Sogner et al., 1984: 99–105 and 139; Sogner, 1986).

Economists have focussed on the importance of the family economy. Before the demographic transition families with a high economic standard tended to have many children – since in these social groups women married young – while poorer families limited the number of births by late marriages. During the nineteenth century this picture changed. Upper-class families now began to reduce the number of births in attempts to uphold a high standard of living (Banks 1964; Dyrvik, 2004: 76–82). When poorer families at the end of the nineteenth century embarked on the same policies, this might be seen as attempts at attaining better living conditions (Easterlin, 1976; Caldwell, 1976; Leibenstein, 1976; Oppenheimer, 1976; Sanderson, 1976; Dyrvik, 2004). The question of children as potential contributors to the family economy also figures among economic reasons for limiting the number of births. When parents needed to spend money on the upbringing and education of children without the prospect of seeing them as future providers, limitation of the number of children became important. Consequently expenses involved in bringing up

5 Women's suffrage was introduced in Norway in 1913.

children grew with mandatory school attendance and the need for theoretical education to secure an acceptable future for the young generation. Further, the time involved in taking care of children may also be of importance in decisions on how many births would be accepted. In short, as Srzeter has pointed out, childhood was redefined as a period of training and financial dependence (Szreter 1996: 513–525).

Did Norwegian women share such considerations? Four main problems were discussed in the journals and the letters that served as sources for my study: the family economy, the future of the children, the health of mothers and infants and the question of women's emancipation. The last two problems both had to do with time and efforts involved in taking care of children. All four themes were important to middle-class women, while working-class women mainly focussed on the family economy and on health problems. When they touched on the future of their children they stressed very different aspects than those considered by middle-class women. This was also the case when working-class women discussed women's emancipation.

Economic Considerations

Arguments forwarded in the middle-class women's journals show that what was at stake was not the economic survival of the family, but the threat of being degraded by the quickly rising standard of living among workers and lower employees. Between 1900 and 1920 the difference between a working-class income and that of a higher employee in the Oslo municipality was more than halved (Økonomisk utsyn, 1900–1950, 1955: tables 91 and 92, 181; Blom, 1980: 70). Middle-class women complained:

> A middle-class woman certainly has a life not at all to be envied. She sees her husband work himself half to death 'in order to live' and she herself tries to make his income stretch as far as possible […] To attempt to make something out of little […] is her life. Servants are expensive, she herself has to be parlour maid, nanny, cook, repair clothes. Little time is left over for reading and music […] Two servants are usually needed for a family with two children if the housewife is not to be degraded to a slave (*Urd*, 1901: 233, 244–45 and 256–257).[6]

6 All quotations are translated by the author.

The overall theme was where economy would be the most efficient, whether cutting down on a husband's expensive habits of cigars and toddies, on woman's expensive clothes or on servants' wages. A discussion in the journal *Husmoderen* on whether it was at all possible to raise 6–7 children in a middle-class family suggested that this could only be done if the family led a frugal life. The budget did not allow an apartment in the most expensive part of town. The practical work involved in raising many children would have to be the responsibility of the mother. In order to avoid seeing the children as 'cinderellas in a school for rich people' mothers also ought to shoulder the education of the younger children in the home. Making friends in a school for all kinds of children was not a good idea. This was seen as especially important for young girls since it was believed that girls usually made friends for life at a much younger age than boys (*Husmoderen*, 1911: 107 and following and 134 and following; Blom, 1980: 78–79).

The discussions continuously stressed the need to cut down expenses on food, clothes, furniture, servants, parties and entertainment. Still, families were expected to have only two or three children, four was seen as exceptional.

> … having children today is no cheap pleasure since prices are rising all around. The wish for well-being and a little luxury has permeated all social groups. People want a spacious economy and consequently they cannot afford to have children; at least only as few as possible (*Husmoderen*, February 24th, 1917; similar ideas in *Husmoderen*, November 3rd, 1917).

A comfortable family economy was preferred to many children. The fall in marital fertility had already been accepted in these families. The question of income generated through children's work or through a wife's paid employment was never mentioned in the middle-class women's journals, nor was the possibility of children as providers for elderly parents. It may be assumed that such topics had no relevance for these families. The discussions confirm the widespread assumption that the family economy was important in determining the number of births. Women obviously shared their husbands' worries about loosing out to lower socio-economic groups. Levelling out economic differences in Norwegian society was not without effects for the reduction of marital fertility.

Turning to the working class we get a very different impression of the relationship between the family economy and fertility levels. The editor of the leading Labour Party paper, *Social-Demokraten,* wrote already in 1886 about the responsibility of raising a big family:

> The most important contribution to the misery is all the people that are not needed in today's society [...] There is no stronger warning for anyone to take seriously the responsibility of giving life to a big family and then send them out in the world devoid of everything in the fight for survival, they arrive without weapons and they have all possibilities of remaining breadless [...] (*Social-Demokraten*, February 27th, 1886).

Another short-lived socialist journal was even more explicit: 'It is frivolous and sinful to give birth to individuals whose lives in all probability will only be a continuous chain of suffering and deprivation' (*Mikkel* no. 2, 1987; similar remarks in *Mikkel* no. 6 and 8, 1888). Other sources picturing working-class lives leave the same impression (Karen Sundt in *Arbeideren*, March 18th, 1886; *Urd*, 1910: 559; *Kvinden* July 1st, 1915: 54).

There was no question of keeping up a relatively good standard of living. The problem was rather that of shear survival. A local economic crisis in the capital around 1900 helps explain why marital fertility started to decline in the east-end districts. Later, rising prices made it difficult to make wages suffice, and when prices fell in the 1920s unemployment set in again. Now the number of families on the dole rose abruptly (Blom, 1980: 127–129).

The annual reports from the Oslo Mothers' Clinic show that most of the women who consulted the clinic during the 1920s and 1930s were married to working-class men. Between 10 and 19 percent of the husbands were unemployed and a growing proportion of the women were registered as earning their own money.[7] About 60 percent of the clients lived in one-room-flats (Blom, 1980: 136). A few of the letters to the Oslo Mothers' Clinic between 1924 and 1929 mirror the situation of those who were better off. Typically, in these letters the motive for wanting to reduce the number of births was to retain a better standard of living (Blom, 1980: 137). Others fought for economic survival. The latter group argued very differently from the middle-class women:

> I am desperate [...] I have seven children and I cannot cope with any more, I am completely exhausted [...] My husband has been unemployed for a long time and everything is so dismal ... (Letter nr. 2481).

7 Between 1933 and 1939 the proportion of women contributing to the family economy among those who consulted the Oslo Mothers' Clinic rose from 10 to 29 percent (Blom, 1980: table 30, 290).

In another letter a woman pleaded:

> I hope you will answer my letter [...] I have had six children in eleven years, four are still alive [...] my husband has tuberculosis and has not worked for three years, I need to be healthy in order to work for him and my children ... (Letter nr. 410).

Unlike middle-class women, a working-class woman's income might be a last resort for the family. This woman wanted information on contraceptives, but some even asked for help with abortion – at the time a criminal act.

> As a last resort I hope you may help me [...] I might ask friends for assistance but I cannot use that kind of solution. Have mercy upon me. Maybe a physician could help but I cannot pay his fee. I hope you will keep this a secret and I fervently hope you do not forsake me [...] Try to imagine my situation if you can. Oh no, I am sure you cannot. Such things cannot be explained, they have to be experienced ... (Letter nr. 1610).

Also the journal *Kvinden*, (The Woman), from 1923 renamed *Arbeiderkvinnen*, (The Working-Class Woman), all through the interwar period stressed the importance of limiting the number of births. The right to decide how many children you wanted should not be a prerogative for middle- and upper-class women. Having large numbers of children should be outlawed also in a working-class family:

> Unemployment, poverty, suffering and the horribly unhealthy living quarters limit the number of children. Why should women suffer many births and become bodily and spiritually exhausted [...] when this can be avoided? This is a question that women should consider very seriously *(Arbeiderkvinden*, July 1910 and April – May 1925).

A contributor signing 'The Man' bluntly said: 'There will be no more children in my family until the labour exchange starts advertising for workers' (*Arbeiderkvinnen*, September 1931).

There is no sign of the argument that less frequent income from child labour contributed to a wish to limit the number of births. The explanation may be that the law of 1892 prohibiting gainful employment for children under the age of 12 and limiting the number of working hours also for those under 18, only applied to factory work. Between 1871 and 1912 about 30 percent of boys and 15 percent of girls in Oslo's primary schools continued to have waged work (Blom, 1980: 138–140). The reduction in marital fertility among the working class started before child labour had lost economic importance. Some resources still flowed from children to parents – when children could find work.

It is apparent that economic considerations were important motives for limiting the number of births, but also that these considerations differed widely between west-end and east-end families. One may almost speak of two groups of motives for a fertility decline.

Children's Education, Children's Future

The question of children's future worried west-end women, mainly because of the need for education. During the final decades of the nineteenth century, the Norwegian school system had been thoroughly reformed. Learning by doing was no longer the main way to education. Schooling in reading and writing became more important in an industrialising and urbanising society. As a parallel to political democratisation, the idea was to give all children access to the same schooling and let them attend the same schools. *Folkeskolen* (The People's School) introduced in 1889 was free and meant to teach all the younger children. Fees were only paid in private schools and in schools preparing for academic studies.

Nevertheless, until the 1930s middle-class parents generally preferred private schools, especially for girls. But the fees were high, and grew with the level of schooling required. After the third form paying for one year at a private girls' school was as expensive and sometime even more expensive than one year's wage for a maid servant (Blom, 1980: 97–100). The problem was that it was now seen as increasingly important not only to give sons the best possible education, but also to make daughters economically self-sufficient through a good education. Lack of suitable marriage partners had been caused by heavy immigration, especially among young men, and periods of unemployment, especially during the 1920s and early 1930s. A drastic fall in the marriage rate lasted until the late 1930s. The need for young girls to earn their own money was stressed again and again in the women's journals and some education was needed to fill jobs in offices, schools and hospitals that offered respectable possibilities for women who had to support themselves.

But in middle-class families marriage was still by far the preferred way for women to support themselves. The new possibilities on the labour market might be accepted only as a second rate solution. These problems were mirrored in the women's journal. Elderly women might voice a nostalgic view of

> the old cosy homes, filled with peace and harmony. An old housewife with white hair, surrounded by healthy and happy daughters. Nobody thought there were too many of them, they all had something important to do (*Urd*, 1904: 280–281).

But the worrying tone of a contributor to the emancipationist journal *Nylænde* seven years later painted another picture:

> The times have changed. It used to be only the sons who needed education because of their responsibility as providers. Now this also applies to daughters [...] It is not enough to offer an education for young women that might result in a temporary job, or, if she continues to work, in a miserable outcome. Also women must have an education that enables them to find inspiring work (så de kan vokse i og med sit arbeid) and have the prospect of a satisfactory future' (*Nylænde*, 1911: 49).

With east-end women the worry for the future of the children was very different. Nothing is said about education, not even for boys. This may seem strange in a society where schooling assumed an increasing importance for the possibilities offered young people. But children's earning capacities were still important for many families and there was often little understanding of the need for theoretical learning. School authorities had to organise the compulsory schooling according to parents' preferences. In rural areas that meant concentrating schooling to periods where there was less demand for child labour in the fields or in the fishing industries. In towns it meant taking care not to prevent children's work by demanding that they stay in school for long hours. Add to this that public authorities were not too eager to curtail child labour since that might mean more families to be supported by the poor law budget (Hagemann, 1992: 34–37). In any case it seems that more education than what was offered through the free and mandatory People's School was deemed to be out of reach. The dominating problem concerning children's future was the threat of unemployment. As a contributor to *Arbeiderkvinnen* wrote in 1929:

> It is irresponsible and suicidal of a working-class family that is already weighed down by destitution and misery to give life to even more children whom they cannot provide for or find work for. Many workers have now accepted that. Nobody knows better than working-class women what it means to the homes when unemployment flourishes as a consequence of over-population (*Arbeiderkvinnen*, February 1929).

Not lack of education, but lack of work to generate a minimum income was the worry for the future of working-class children.

Child Care and Health Problems

Srzeter points to changing relations between parents and children as one of many explanations for birth control. He underlines the change from the present patriarchal father to the absent and anxious breadwinning father, and sees mothering as differing widely by class, marking a distinction between the 'patrician' and the 'plebeian' worlds (Szreter, 1996: 460–465). My sources mainly stress the changing role of mothers and the growing expectations of child care. The father's role as breadwinner was also important, but mainly related to economic problems, not to fathering.

From the end of the nineteenth century rising expectations as to child care and increasing worries over the health of mothers might have been an important factor in decisions on whether or not to have another child. The journals *Husmoderen* and *Urd* repeatedly focussed on the importance of high quality child care, and saw this as the exclusive responsibility of mothers. Leaving the care of your children to a nanny was criticised as lack of responsibility. The increasing tendency for young women to concentrate on an education that had little to do with their work as married women and mothers was perceived as a threat to children's health. On the other hand, growing expectations as to what it took to care for a child were blamed for making women unwilling to have more than a few children (*Husmoderen*, 1899: 225, 1901, 78–80 and 289–290; *Urd*, 1900: 164–168, 179, 186, 237).

The conservative MP Ole Malm wrote ironically about child care:

> What hullabaloo about all that is needed [...] to have children: refined child care, bath-tub, thermometers, an overload of children's clothes, suitable artificial food if you cannot breast-feed, the assistance of midwives until the age of 15, nurses, attending courses and lectures and vocational training, all that costs money, time, work and servants ... (Malm 1916: 70).

Malm saw worries over the health of children as an important reason for the reduction of marital fertility. But also worries over the health of mothers had an impact.

Among the middle-class women's journals especially *Nylænde* was interested in the importance of women's health. It was recommended to reduce the use of corsets and to stop seeing pregnancy as a situation to be concealed by all means. Sports, skiing and skating was welcomed as a means for women to strengthen their health, and good health was seen as a help to reduce death in childbirth. But a reduction of the number of births was also suggested as a means to improve women's health (*Nylænde* March 15th, 1887; February 1st, 1888; June 1st, and October 15th, 1889; April 15th, 1891; December 1st, 1901).

The two other journals addressing middle-class women were less enthusiastic. *Urd* recommended seeing a physician before embarking on sports such as cycling, but soon published patterns of women's clothes to use for skiing and skating. *Husmoderen* was the most reluctant. Although skiing might be an encouragement for mothers and children, a contributor warned against 'the free tone' when sporting in the mountains together with young men. This might easily be misunderstood

> … We shall not dwell on the accidents so easily resulting from such free and easy behaviour with a broad-minded conscience, although there are phenomena that might tempt to do so … (Thea Christensen in *Husmoderen*, 1910: 94).

This journal defended the perception of women as first and foremost wives and mothers, while *Nylænde* was fighting for women's emancipation and *Urd* expressed a middle position in the question of how to understand femininity. But common for the middle-class women's journals was the idea that higher standards of child care, fewer births and, with some reservation, more sports for mothers were important means of improving the health of women and children.

Children's health did not seem to be the main preoccupation of working-class women. Worries over children's health left no traces in the journal of the *Kvindeforbundet* (the Labour Party's Women's Association). This may be surprising, not least since until the 1930s mortality from diseases such as tuberculosis and rachitis in the eastern districts of Oslo reached levels that were double of those for the western parts of the city. (Rachitis was a disease caused by lack of vitamin D (Blom, 1980: table 32, 292).) But these threats were understood as a problem to be solved by improving the family economy. When some of the letters to the Oslo Mothers' Clinic asked advice on child care, the reason was mainly that mothers' bad health made it difficult to care for the children.

The main focus of the letters was on mothers' health. This may in part have been a result of the fact that the Mothers' Clinic especially stressed the importance of family planning for 'worn-out mothers' and consequently made letter-writers concentrate on mothers' health, not on the health of children. In the letters women often described themselves as 'worn out, tired, wretched', indicating that clients may have seen bad health as an especially important justification for wanting to limit the number of births. But that was certainly not the only explanation. The annual reports from the clinic show that every fifth woman who consulted the clinic had health problems, and 12 percent of that group had tuberculosis. In their letters, women mainly ascribed their bad health to too many births.

> I have seven children [...] I spent three and a half weeks in hospital after the latest birth. The chief physician told me to have no more children. But I could not make myself ask him what he would recommend me to do about it ... (Letter nr. 3680).

> 'I have born eight children, two abortions, one has died. I have suffered once from puerperal fever, three times from swollen breasts [...] with the last birth I had kidney disease and infection of my bladder for two months, and lost blood twice before the child was born ... (Letter nr. 2396).

The great importance attached to the mother's health comes out clearly by the fact that while only 6 percent of all letters mentioned abortion; this question was raised by 24 percent of the mothers who suffered from health problems. There is no reason to doubt that worries over mothers' health were an important factor when attempting to limit the number of births in an east-end family.

It is worth noticing that worries over fathers' health were sometimes mentioned. Bad health made the role of provider precarious. Thus also a father's bad health would be seen as a reason for limiting the number of births (Letters nr. 2481 and 4101). This theme was completely absent with west-end women.

Class was obviously important when it came to arguments about the connection between the number of children and health. While east-end women seemed to have worried about their own extremely serious health problems and how to avoid the worst physical consequences of too many births, west-end women discussed child care, suitable clothes and sports. But to all of these women, reducing the number of births was seen as a means to overcome health problems.

Generational and Class Conflicts over the Role of Women

Around the turn of the century decades of efforts to open up new opportunities for women had given some results. Admittance to universities came in 1884, limited rights to vote at municipal elections were reached in 1901 and in 1913 general female suffrage was attained at national elections. New ideas of what a woman should be, where her priorities should be, caused conflicts, also among women, and these discussions had an important impact on women's attitudes to marital fertility. In a lecture in 1910, published in *Husmoderen,* it was said that

> if women need to be prepared for a career in the same way as men and to the same degree, I do not understand how she will find space for the education she as a woman must have [...] The home, the cornerstone of society, will be in danger. The woman too. Her deepest, purest instincts and thoughts [...] her full and whole womanly essence – will be hurt. The supporting forces, the complementing, the expiating element in women's nature, the mother love [...] the merciful will be endangered (*Husmoderen*, 1910: 219–222).

The lecturer, Marianne Nærup, was a widowed teacher with two children. She also took part in politics. Still she found women's responsibilities to be primarily with her children and her home. Other women expressing worries about these issues thought that the desire to not have children, or at least to postpone having them even after marriage, was due to a wish to enjoy life and avoid serious commitments. When finally such women had children, they were no longer prepared to give their children a proper education, since they themselves had never experienced deprivation. They might even find that they would no longer be able to have children. Children should be seen as a gift from God and a woman should prepare for this gift and be thankful for it (*Urd*, 1897: 237).

These misgivings about reduced fertility were characteristic of the elderly generation of women. In *Nylænde* a vivid discussion took place between what the editors called 'the elderly women' and 'the young women' (Blom, 1980: 116–122; Blom 1990: 131–147). Representatives of the elderly generation spitefully called the younger women 'the student-girls'. The elderly women defended the view of women as essentially wives and mothers, devoted to the welfare of the family, especially of the children, and submissive to the will of their husbands. In this respect it was important not to interfere with the number of children in a family. Again, the idea of children as a gift from God, to be gracefully accepted, was stressed.

But the younger generation already around 1900 protested against this way of understanding femininity and attempted to spread a different gospel. Intellect and restraint, not passive acceptance was of importance in the question of how many children to have.

> I think many women agree with me when I state that the intellect is important in these matters, intellect and self-control should be considered necessary especially in the question of the size of the family etc. It is equally important that women think of their own prosperous development and their own well-being, since the children, the husband and the home depend on this ... (*Nylænde*, October 15th, 1901).

This view was vividly supported by the founder of the first Mothers' Clinic, Katti Anker Møller. She found that it should not come as a surprise if women no longer felt content to concentrate on 'the bodily work in the house, the simple demands of the nursery or the second rate position as a spiritual mediator between the outer world and her flock of children' (*Nylænde*, 1902: 135–137).[8] Support for this position also came from the at that time famous Norwegian author, Bjørnstjerne Bjørnson. Already in 1899 he maintained that a woman should understand that her work in the home was not sufficient to support the future fate of her children. The future depended on society outside the home and it was important that women participated in shaping that society (*Nylænde*, 1899: 130–131). As mentioned earlier, in areas where women used their newly won right to vote at parliamentary elections to a higher degree than in other areas the fall in marital fertility was more outspoken than elsewhere (Sogner et al., 1984: 86; Dyrvik, 2004: 83–91). No doubt, middle-class women in a modernising society wanted fewer babies.

What were the ideas of working-class women on the connection between marital fertility and women's emancipation? None of the letters to the Mothers' Clinic mention the possibility that concern of marital fertility might be connected to women's desire to take part in politics or in other ways engage themselves in matters not directly of importance to home and family. Such ideas were, however, expressed in the journal of The Women's Section of the Labour Party *(Kvindeforbundet)*. In 1910, the year after the journal started appearing, the complaint was voiced that with many children women had no time to develop 'spiritual faculties' (*Kvinden*, July 1st, 1910). This problem was

8 For a full account of generational differences, also among men, in this discussion, see Blom, 1990. On the policies of Katti Anker Møller, see Blom, 1991.

later expanded. August Aasen, a prominent socialist woman, argued that a reduction of marital fertility was 'a precondition for women to heighten their own economic and cultural standard in order to be more fit for the ongoing class struggle.' But she disagreed that limiting the number of births on its own would be of help to women.

> ... I see only one solution to the emancipation of working-class women and that is the realisation of socialism. I see no solution in emancipating women as compared to men [...] there is no gender politics in the working class [...] In a socialist society all the little children will mean an absolute advantage and will be taken care of from the first moment and woman will have the position she deserves as a result of her competence (*Kvinden*, June, 1919).

During the 1930s the argumentation changed. In 1934 an article entitled 'Birth strike and social policies' used the reduction of marital fertility as an argument for social reforms. Only when a working-class family had economic safety would it be possible to expect the birth rate to rise again. Now the emancipation of women was also seen as one of the explanations for the falling fertility. 'The woman today rejects being seen as the man's plaything or to be considered a childbearing machine' (*Arbeiderkvinnen*, January, 1934).

As in a number of other questions, during the 1930s socialist and bourgeois women and men, and socialist and non-socialist political parties, gradually build up cooperation that had until then been unthinkable. This may explain that arguments that had so far been exclusively used when addressing middle-class families were now also found in a journal aimed at working-class women.[9]

There is no doubt, then, that many women considered a limitation of the size of their family on the grounds of economic and health problems, and that the question of women's role in the family and in society also played a part in their discussions. The generational differences observed by Szreter between the attitudes of the elderly generation of feminists and 'the new women' is perceivable also in Norwegian sources. While the themes are similar in Norway also class differences coloured the argumentation of both west- and east-end women.

9 For a further introduction into this theme, see Ida Blom (1998A and 1998B).

How to Reduce Marital Fertility?

Szreter maintains that a variety of means were applied to achieve a lower fertility, but within what he terms a general culture of abstinence he finds sexual abstinence and coitus interruptus to be the most widespread contraceptives. He reasons that the low estimated figures of provoked abortions proved that the risks and fears involved in this way of avoiding a pregnancy were too great to make abortion important for the fertility decline (Szreter, 1996: 367–440). Since men controlled the most frequently used means of birth control, according to Szreter, women were dependent on their husbands' good will (Szreter, 1996: 566). Kate Fisher has lately confirmed this point of view. She has interviewed working-class people in Wales and Oxford and maintains that they did not plan their families, that husbands were responsible for birth control and that wives passively accepted their husbands' decisions (Fisher, 2000).

Who controlled fertility in Norway, husbands or wives? This would be an important question in case of disagreement between spouses. Is there reason to believe that men disagreed with women over the problem of birth control? Sources tell very little of husbands' attitudes. A few contributions from men may be found in the women's journals, but men mostly voiced their opinions in other journals. When men discussed the reduction of marital fertility, their arguments were mainly part of discussions on population developments, general economic theories, the function of marriage as an institution or the importance of religion. They sometimes referred to the importance of sexuality for personal development, but they rarely voiced concern for personal problems or wishes expressed by women (Blom, 1980: 122–124). In left wing political journals men already in the 1880s expressed worries over the family economy and suggested that an important means to control expenses would be to use 'the so-called contraceptives to reduce the members of the family to a restricted number' (*Mikkel*, 1888, nr. 3). Most of the letters to the Oslo Mothers' Clinic written by men quite simply asked for contraceptives to be forwarded to the letter-writer, without indicating what kind of contraceptive was wanted. None of this signals any disagreement between wives and husbands. It may also be asked why husbands should oppose birth control as long as this helped preserve the family economy, strengthened the health of mothers and children and made the future look more promising for both sons and daughters.[10] The only

10 This conclusion is also reached by Seccombe (1992: 66–84).

reason to oppose a wife's wish to avoid a pregnancy would be the inconvenience this might cause for sexual pleasures. If a husband insisted on intercourse and refused to use 'self-control', a wife's final solution might be abortion. This may have been what happened in a number of cases, since the estimated numbers of illegal abortions among married women rose three fold between 1920 and 1933 (Blom, 1980: table 12, 274).

Discussions on how to achieve a lower number of births in a family suffered from the tabooing of sexual questions. There are no indications in the journals used for this study of birth control means other than 'common sense and self-control', 'self-denial' or 'to outwit the evil powers of nature' (Discussions in *Nylænde*, October to December, 1901; Knut Wicksell in *Samtiden*, 1890; Blom, 1980: 119 and 123). The collection of letters to the Oslo Mothers' Clinic during the last part of the 1920s shows that the wish to apply prophylactics was considerable: in 71 percent of all letters advice on contraception was asked for. Most of these letters came from women in poor socio-economic groups and so did the majority of women who consulted the clinic in person. This testifies to women's will to regulate fertility without depending on husbands. The letters also bear witness to the interests in mechanical prophylactics, in this case in the cervical cap that was the favoured contraceptive recommended at the Mothers' Clinic. Further, ethnological studies based on interviews with women in two local communities confirm an outspoken intention of not having too many children (Kvåle, 1981; Danielsen, 2000). Women who had grown up in big families did not wish to repeat their mothers' experiences. Despite the firm intention of avoiding too many pregnancies, these women maintained that they did not 'do anything special' to avoid pregnancies. Thus, it seems to be sheer chance that they ended up with only two or three children. But conversations among these women showed that they agreed that husbands' sexual urges made it necessary for wives to take over responsibility for avoiding another pregnancy. They laughingly exchanged views on the best means to reach this goal, varying from leaping out of bed to 'telling the old man that if he did not provide himself with some kind of prophylactics, he would have to sleep in the pigsty' (Danielsen, 2000: 89). In this way they supported the concept of men's irrepressible and irresponsible sexuality, but also of women as strong and responsible individuals. Fisher's impression that working-class women passively accepted their husband's decisions and that working-class families left the problem of the number of children to pure luck definitely cannot be applied to these women. On the contrary, they behaved according to Coale's thesis of conscious choice (Coale, 1973: 65). But on the other hand this also shows that there was not always sufficient communication between spouses on the matter of marital fertility, and that this was not necessarily a precondition for limiting the number of births. One may speculate, as Fisher also does, whether problems of oral history – possible worries over decorum and embarrassment during interviews – may have coloured the interviews with British working-class women (Fisher, 2000: 312). Or was it quite simply that coitus interruptus and sexual abstinence did not count as 'something special', when spouses decided on sexual activities?

As Szreter argues these means were well-known and what is more, they did not contravene the culture of abstinence that was very pronounced also in Norwegian society before the Second World War. Writing about or lecturing about contraception could, according to the penal code, be stamped as grossly indecent behaviour warranting forced labour or imprisonment. The use of condoms was seen as an expression of immorality since this had been introduced in brothels to hinder the spread of venereal diseases. Employing condoms in a marital relationship could be interpreted as introducing innocent women to indecent behaviour. Opposition to contraception continued to be strong throughout the inter-war period (Blom, 1980: 171–222). The Association for Propriety *(Sædelighetsforeningen)* found support within medical and clerical circles and among members of the Housewives Association *(Hjemmenes Vel)* for continued attacks on contraception, at least until they lost a law suit against the Oslo Mothers' Clinic in 1927 (Blom, 1980: 181–189).

But although contraception was condemned as *'a sin against nature and consequently against God'* this did not mean that the Lutheran church advised against birth control as long as acceptable means were applied. The journal of the Association for Propriety explained: *'In principle, from a Christian point of view, marital abstinence is the only advisable solution when child birth has to be avoided because of sickness or when mothers are worn out.'* (*Værn*, 1926: 86).[11] There was no correlation between religiosity and a late reduction of fertility. The Lutheran church absolutely dominated the Norwegian religious landscape and had a much weaker tradition than the Catholic Church for interfering with marital behaviour. It should also be noted that the Norwegian clergy was among the earliest social groups to experience a reduction of marital fertility,

11 See also Blom 1980: 219–222.

although at a slightly later moment than other academics. It seems more than likely that this was achieved by sexual abstinence (Blom, 1980: 219–222; Sogner, 1984: 99–102).

Not only religious quarters but also most physicians condemned the use of mechanical prophylaxis at least until the early 1930s (Bull, 1977; Blom, 1980: 214–222). The Labour Party was divided on the issue and the attitude of leading men within this party remained conservative as to women's emancipation (Blom, 1998B). It was not until the 1930s that the Labour Party gradually began to accept contraceptives, now as part of 'the socialist planned society' (Evang, 1930: 89; Tranmæl in *Arbeiderbladet*, February 17th and July 19th, 1935; Nilsen, 1978). But women within the Labour Party cooperated with Katti Anker Møller to start the Oslo Mothers' Clinic in 1924. This clinic was patterned on the clinics established by Mary Stopes in Britain, but without the negative attitude to abortion. The lawsuit against the clinic in 1927 resulted in acquittal and this helped spread mothers' clinics to other cities during the late 1920s and 1930s. Most of these clinics offered advice on contraception, prioritising the cervical cap that would allow women to take over control of fertility. But the clinics only reached a minority of the population and support for these institutions remained weak until the 1950s. It should also be remembered that it was mainly middle-class urban families who had the hygienic preconditions for employing the cervical cap (Blom, 1980: 209–210).

All this activity witnessed to the initiatives taken by women within the Labour Party and supports the impression that working-class women eagerly attempted to control fertility. There is little sign of passive attitudes such as those charted by Kate Fisher in Wales and Oxford. On the other hand it also seems convincing that the prime contraceptives were coitus interruptus and sexual abstinence. The culture of abstinence prevailing in Norwegian society during the fall in marital fertility certainly did not promote other means of reducing the number of births.

Abortion was an even less possible solution. Only 5 percent of the letters to the Oslo Mothers' Clinic mention abortion, not surprisingly since according to the penal code having an abortion was a criminal offence. If convicted, a woman would risk up to three years imprisonment while the abortionist risked six years imprisonment. When in 1915 Katti Anker Møller raised the question of decriminalising abortion she argued that: 'The basis for all freedom is the right to decide over your own body and what is in it' (Mohr, 1976: 102–130). She postulated that husbands had free disposal of their wives and that if a wife denied her husband sexual gratification he could divorce her. In Katti Anker Møller's opinion abortion was the revolutionary expression of women's despair and suppression (Mohr, 1976: 102–130). Public discussions over the question of decriminalising abortion raged on and off until 1919 and were resumed in the 1930s. No revisions of the penal code were made until 1960. Further changes were made in 1975, but it was only in 1978 that the decision of abortion was left to the mother (Blom, 1980: 223–251; Blom and Elvbakken, 2001). Only then had women become 'masters of their own body and what is in it'. It may safely be said that the fertility decline took place in a climate of strong opposition to both mechanical contraception and abortion.

Conclusion

A variety of individual choices and individual experiences have accompanied the reduction of marital fertility. Norwegian studies support some of the findings concerning the fertility decline in Britain. Szreter's picture of multiple fertility declines may well be applied also to what happened in Norway between roughly 1890 and 1930. Discussions in middle-class as well as in working-class women's journals, the contents of the letters to the Mothers' Clinic and the activities of that clinic leave no doubt that women were preoccupied with the question of birth control. Considerations of the family economy, worries over the children's future and over the health of mothers and children were forwarded as important motives for limiting the number of births. But these motives meant widely different things to middle-class and to working-class women. Finally, a new understanding of womanhood, as comprising more than motherhood and devoted child care, had started among middle-class women, while working-class women saw the possibility of taking better care of children as an important future goal that, to some, might only be reached in a socialist society.

It is hard to say to what extent women's motivation for birth control differed from men's, but it is striking that while women took their arguments from private family life, men mainly considered the importance of the number of births for society as such, for the public world. However, given that the family economy as well as the health of mothers and children was certainly of great importance also to husbands there is little reason to believe that a fundamental disagreement on limiting the number of births existed between spouses. Public discussions abundantly demonstrate a culture of abstention, where the use of contraception, not to speak of abortion, was deemed highly unacceptable. It is sensible to accept that Szreter's picture of British families, falling back on the well-known means of sexual abstinence and coitus interruptus is valid also for Norway. This does of course mean that some wives had to suffer unwanted pregnancies when husbands were not careful. But Kate Fisher's assumption that working-class women knew nothing about family planning and left all such questions for husbands to decide does not apply to Norwegian working class women. Writing in their own journals or to the Mothers' Clinic, they had no reason to pretend ignorance or lack of interest in matters so important to their own lives and to that of their families. Although some women upheld the understanding of male sexuality as an undisciplined urge, they at the same time assumed responsibility for handling that problem without letting it result in unwanted pregnancies. Both middle-class and working class women presented themselves as individuals with a clear goal of avoiding further pregnancies.

Still, despite these many signs of women's determination the rise in estimated numbers of illegal abortions for married women also shows that some wives found themselves with an unwanted pregnancy. In such cases unknown sufferings have accompanied efforts to reach lower fertility.

References

Banks, J. A. and Olive (1964), *Feminism and Family Planning in Victorian England*, Liverpool, Liverpool University Press.

Blom, Ida (1980), *Barnebegrensning – synd eller sunn fornuft?*, Bergen, Universitetsforlaget.

Blom, Ida (1990), 'Changing Gender Identities in an Industrialising Society', *Gender and History*, 2, 131–147.

Blom, Ida (1991), 'Voluntary Motherhood 1900–1930 : Theories and Policies of a Norwegian Feminist in an International Perspective', in Bock, Gisela and Thane, Pat (eds), *Maternity, Visions of Gender and the Rise of the European Welfare States, 1890–1950*, London, Routledge, 21–39.

Blom, Ida (1998A), 'Prelude to Welfare States: Introduction', in Gruber, Helmuth, Greeves, Pamela (eds), *Women and Socialism/Socialism and Women: Europe Between the World Wars*, Providence and Oxford, Berghahn Books, 415–424.

Blom, Ida (1998B), '"A Double Responsibility": Women, Men and Socialism in Norway c. 1918–c. 1940', in Helmuth Gruber and Pamela Greeves (eds), *Women and Socialism/ Socialism and Women: Europe Between the World Wars*, Providence and Oxford, Berghahn Books, 425–449.
Blom, Ida and Elvbakken, Karitove (2001), 'Linjer i norsk abortlovgivning og abortpolitikk', *Tidskrift for velferdsforskning*, 4, 30–48.
Bull, Ida (1977), 'Norske legers holdning til spørsmålet om barnebgresning', *Historisk tidskrift*, 4, 398–432.
Caldwell, John C. (1976), 'Towards a Restatement of Demographic Transition Theory', *Population and Development Review*, 2, 321–366.
Coale, Ansley (1973), 'The Demographic Transition', *International Population Conference, Liege 1973*, vol. 1, Liege.
Danielsen, Hilde (2000), *Dei moderne kvinnene i Odda. Ein studie imødrehygiene og barneavgrensing i mellomrigstida*, Norsk Vasskraft- og Industristadmuseum, Tyssedal.
Dyrvik, Ståle (2004), *Den demografiske overgangen*, Oslo, Det Norske Samlaget.
Dyrvik, Ståle and Alsvik, Marit Karin (1987), *Gjennombrotet for fødselsreguelering i Stavanger 1900–1935*, Bergen, Bergen University.
Easterlin, Richard A. (1976), 'The Conflict between Aspirations and Resources', *Population and Development Review*, 2, 417–425.
Evang, Karl (1930), *Fødselsregulering. Dens berettigelse og dens praktiske gjennemførelse*, Oslo, Fram.
Evang, Karl (1934), *Rasepolitikk og Reaksjon*, Oslo.
Fisher, K. (2000), 'Negotiating the Fertility Transition: Birth Control Practices and Family Planning Strategies in Britain, 1925–50', *Population and Development Review*, 26, 295–317.
Freedman, Deborah (1976), 'Fertility, Aspirations and Resources: A Symposium on the Easterlin Hypothesis', *Population and Development Review*, 2, 411–415.
Hagemann, Gro (1997), *Skolefolk. Lærernes historie i Norge*, Ad Notam Gyldendal, Oslo.
Jahn, Gunnar (1920), *Barnetallet i norske ekteskap*, NOS VII, 97, Folketellingen i Norge 1920, Sjette hefte.
Kvåle, Ingrid (1981), *Alt hva mødrene har kjempet ... Bernebegrensning i et lokalsamfunn 1910–1940, – utbredelse, metoder og motiv*, Unprinted master thesis, University of Oslo.
Leibenstein, Harvey (1976), 'The Problem of Characterizing Aspirations', *Population and Development Review*, 2, 427–431.
Malm, Ole (1916), *Barneformindskelsen i Norge og dens aarsaker*, Kristiania.
McLaren, Angus (1978), *Birth Control in Nineteenth Century England*, London, Croom.
Mohr, Tove (1968), *Katti Anker Møller – en banebryter*, Oslo, Helm.
Myklebost, Hallstein (1976), 'The Decrease of Fertility in Norway: The Spread of an Innovation', *Norsk geografisk Tidskrift*, vol. 30, 179–186.
Nilsen, Kåre H. (1978), *Det norske arbeiderparti og befolkningsspørsmålet i mellomkrigstiden*, Unpublished master thesis, University of Bergen.
Økonomisk utsyn 1900–1950 (1955), Samfunnsøkonomiske studier nr. 3, Central Bureau of Statistics, Oslo.
Oppenheimer, Valerie Kincade (1976), 'The Easterlin Hypotheses: Another Aspect of the Echo to Consider', *Population and Development Review*, 2, 433–457.

Rainwater, Lee (1960), *And the Poor Get Children. Sex, Contraception and Family Planning in the Working Class*, Chicago, Quadrangle Books.
Sanderson, Warren C. (1976), 'On Two Schools of the Economics of Fertility', *Population and Development Review*, 1, 469–477.
Seccombe, Wally (1992), 'Men's "Marital Rights" and Women's "Wifely Duties": Changing Conjugal Relations in the Fertility Decline', in Gillis, John R., Tilly, Louise A. and Levine, David (eds), *The European Experience of Declining Fertility. A Quiet Revolution 1850–1970*, Cambridge Mass. and Oxford, Blackwell, 66–84.
Sogner, Sølvi, Randborg, HegeBrit and Fuire, Eli. (1984), *Fra stua full til tobarnskull. Om fruktbarhetsnedgangen i Norge ca. 1890–1930*, Oslo.
Sogner, Sølvi et al. (1986), 'Le déclin de la fécondité en Norvège', *Annales de démographie historique*, 361–375.
Szreter, Simon (1996), *Fertility, Class, and Gender in Britain 1860–1940*, Cambridge, Cambridge University Press.

Women Who Controlled Their Fertility and Women Who Did Not

An Analysis of Women's Fertility Behaviour in Late 19th and Early 20th Century Spain*

Fernando Gil Alonso**

1. Introduction

The demographic transition, and more specifically the transition of marital fertility, is a multifaceted process that has generated a large amount of research. The role of women in this process however has been blurred by research traditions based on the use of macro-data taken from aggregated sources. This situation is even worse in countries such as Spain where the application of gender perspectives in the social sciences, and specifically in demography, is still in its first stages. Nevertheless, there can be little doubt that Spanish women played a key role in the adoption of low fertility patterns and in the choice of specific fertility control methods. This article, which summarizes some of the findings of my PhD thesis (Gil Alonso, 2005), intends to throw some light on the complex relationships between gender and the marital fertility transition in Spain. It will be done, firstly, by setting up a theoretical

* This research has been elaborated in the framework of the R+D project SEJ2004-00846 / SOCI, funded by the Spanish Ministry for Education and Sciences, through the *Plan Nacional de Investigación Científica, Desarrollo e Innovación Tecnológica*.

** Fernando Gil Alonso is a researcher at the Centre d'Estudis Demogràfics (CED) of Barcelona, and holder of a *Juan de la Cierva Program* grant for doctors, funded by the Spanish Ministry for Education and Sciences. He is also coordinator of the consolidated research group *Grup d'Estudis de Demografia i Migracions* within the CED, funded by the Autonomous Government of Catalonia (ref: 2005SGR00930).

framework which takes into account women's contribution in this process, and secondly, by using retrospective fertility data for the calculation of indicators on parity and on the use of fertility control methods. Thus, some knowledge of women's participation in the marital fertility transition process can indirectly be obtained from aggregated census data. This may enable us to establish an association between the evolution of these indicators and the evolving role of women in the process of reproduction control in a changing historical context marked by social and economic modernisation.

The main objectives of this paper are threefold: firstly, it aims to investigate patterns in the marital fertility decline in Spain, and more specifically the spatial differences at the provincial level in the final decades of the nineteenth century and the beginning of the twentieth century. Secondly, it intends to throw some light on the type of birth control methods – spacing or stopping – used by ever-married women in those provinces where marital fertility was decreasing. And thirdly, it tries to link the first two points to the role that women played in the demographic transition. These three issues are very relevant, as they are closely linked to the debate within demography on the validity of the demographic transition as the dominant paradigm explaining the changes experienced by the European (and world) population in the last two centuries.

This research uses information on children ever-born by married and widowed women recorded in the 1920, 1930 and 1940 Spanish censuses. Most research previously done on the fertility transition in Spain is based on two different methodologies: one using data from the *Registro Civil* (Civil Register) which allows for the estimation of age-specific fertility rates at the national level from 1922 up to the present day (Fernández Cordón, 1977; Sàez, 1979); and another approach using indirect demographic techniques applied to the age and sex structure of the population in order to calculate fertility indicators like the Princeton indicators or the child-woman ratios (Leasure, 1963; Livi Bacci, 1968; Coale and Watkins, 1986; Nicolau, 1989). This is the first time that retrospective data on fertility from the 1920, 1930 and the 1940 censuses are used extensively. This fact, and the well-known biases inherent in retrospective data – such as memory errors in elderly people, not-at-home errors, zero errors, possible biases due to differential mortality and migration, etcetera (El-Badry, 1961; Brass, 1975; Auriat, 1996) – made it necessary to exercise a rigorous data critique based on an assessment of the internal consistency of the recorded data and a comparison with other sources, and the application of data correction when required. More specifically, the data on 13 provinces contained in the 1920 census as well as on the 50 provinces in the 1930 census, were corrected using the so-called El-Badry technique (Gil Alonso, 2005). This technique tries to correct the data for women without children who have mistakenly been classified under the category 'without response' (El-Badry, 1961). Once data were corrected, the critical evaluation of the obtained data produced positive results for all three censuses, with the exception of half a dozen provinces in the 1920 census. Therefore, retrospective fertility census data may be considered of good quality and a reliable source of information to analyse the process of the marital fertility transition in Spain. The following pages summarise the main results obtained from the analysis of this type of data.

2. What Retrospective Data on Marital Fertility Show

2.1. Marital Fertility Decline in Spain

The mean parity of ever-married female cohorts born before 1905 can be reconstructed from the number of births reported in each of the censuses by married and widowed women who at the time of the census had finished their reproductive cycle, either entirely or for the greater part of it.[1] Table 1 presents these data. Ever-married women born before 1865 (55 years old and over in 1920) reported an average parity of 4.71 children, which figure increases to 4.94 for those born between 1865 and 1869. It is assumed that this upward trend is caused by memory failures concerning the exact number of births women had ever had, a bias which increases with age, resulting in an underestimation of real fertility for these groups[2] (Brass, 1975; Auriat, 1996). For the

1 Women who were 55 years or older at the time of the 1920 census (and 45 years or older for the 1930 and 1940 censuses) were collected into one big group so that it is impossible to distinguish between those aged 55–60, 60–65, 65–70 et cetera. This means that the number of female birth cohorts whose mean parity can be calculated is limited: it is not possible to go back further than the 1865–1869 birth cohort.

2 Memory failures increase with the age of the individuals and with the passing of time. This is a problem well-known by UN experts working in the implementation of censuses in developing countries (Brass, 1981). In general it affects all retrospective questions but

following five-year cohort it goes down to 4.92 and from then on it continues to diminish steadily. Women born between 1885 and 1889 (41 to 45 years old in 1930) declared a mean parity of 4.69 children, while those born ten years later (41 to 45 years old in 1940) had given birth to 4.17 children, that is to say, half a child less.

Together with average parity calculated from census data, table 1 also presents an estimated series of final fertility – calculated through a fertility model[3] – in order to correct for the underregistration of births. Underregistration of births was caused by two different reasons. Firstly, the already mentioned memory failures affecting female respondents in the oldest age groups, resulting in an underestimation of real parity for the corresponding age cohorts. And secondly, other female cohorts are truncated – e.g. women born in 1880–1884 were 36–40 years old in 1920, which means that they had not yet finished their reproductive cycle at the time of the census. Both series of data however present very similar trends in marital fertility decrease.

The data on retrospective fertility from the 1920, 1930 and 1940 censuses show that over a period of 30 years (from 1910 to 1940) marital fertility fell by more than one child. By overlapping the three censuses we can also observe that this process accelerated in the 1930s, due to the economic, social and political crisis that affected this decade and that led to the outbreak of the Spanish Civil War. The fall of marital fertility was more important for women whose reproductive cycle partly coincided with this decade. Parity declared by married women and widows who were between 26 and 35 years old and those who were between 36 and 45 years old diminished by 4 percent and 3.1 percent respectively between 1920 and 1930. However, between 1930 and 1940

in particular the number of children ever-born. Indeed, memory failures produce an underestimation of the parity declared by (older) women in censuses, compared with the real fertility that they actually had (Auriat, 1996). This type of underregistration does not affect women under 40 years of age. Omission of children ever-born starts to appear among women aged 40–44 years, and it has a significant importance from age 45 onwards (Brass, 1981). If data on parity is classified by marriage duration, this problem may appear beginning with the group of 15–19 years of marriage duration (UN, 1983).

3 The fertility model applied here to complete the series of retrospective fertility for incomplete (truncated) birth cohorts is the standard pattern for cumulated age-specific fertility rates designed by Zaba (1981) in order to represent a typical fertility pattern for high parity countries (Gil Alonso, 2005).

Table 1. Average Parity of Ever-married Women Calculated from the Number of Children Ever-born in the 1920, 1930 and 1940 Spanish censuses. Cohorts born before 1865 (> 55 Years Old in 1920) to 1900–1904 (36–40 Years Old in 1940)

Cohorts	Calculated average parity	Estimated average parity
born before 1865	4.71	+5
1865–1869	4.94	+5
1870–1874	4.92	+5
1875–1879	4.84	around 4.9
1880–1884	4.22	between 4.6–4.7
1885–1889	4.69	around 4.75
1890–1894	4.10	around 4.5
1895–1899	4.17	around 4.25
1900–1904	3.59	around 3.9

marital fertility fell by 9.4 percent and 11.9 percent respectively for the two age groups; that is to say, by a pace which was on average three times higher when compared to the previous decade.

Obviously, this process did not have the same speed in all Spanish provinces. On the contrary, figures on marital fertility as recorded by the censuses show that the phenomenon evolved along very different spatial patterns.

2.2. Spatial Patterns in Marital Fertility

Charts 1 to 6 show average parity levels for the different provinces in Spain for a selection of cohorts. Charting the number of children ever-born in the 1920, 1930 and 1940 censuses by ever-married women belonging to cohorts which had concluded the greater part or more of their reproductive cycle reveals the existence of five big regional areas with different patterns of marital fertility behaviour and with an unequal pace in their transitional trajectory during the period under investigation.

1) *Central Spain* (Old and New Castile – except for Madrid – part of León and Extremadura) is characterised by a 'traditional' type of reproduc-

tive behaviour, with high marital fertility during the entire period.[4] In 1920 the provinces of this large central region did not show any transitional signs towards more controlled fertility. The process only started in the following two decades and it was initially very slow. The *Canary Islands* also share these characteristics, and during practically the whole period under study this archipelago showed the highest parity levels in Spain, followed by those of the central-northern region of Old Castile.

2) The *Northern coast* (Cantabrian Sea) had marital fertility levels in the 1920 census which were very similar to those of central Spain at that time. However, this started to change from 1930 onwards, when a process of quick decrease began, especially in the two Basque coastal provinces. In consequence, by 1940 the whole Cantabrian fringe already had an intermediate level of fertility – or even a low-intermediate one in the case of the Basque provinces of Biscay and Guipúzcoa – which was, in any case, much lower than the one found for central Spain.

3) The *Eastern territories* pertaining to the old Crown of Aragon (Catalonia, Balearic Islands, Valencia and Aragon) may be seen as the pioneers in the Spanish demographic transition with fertility levels which were the lowest in Spain for the entire period analysed here. In the first two regions – Catalonia and the Balearic Islands – fertility levels were initially much lower than in the two other provinces, Valencia and Aragon. Especially in Catalonia fertility patterns in 1920 were practically post-transitional – with evidence of an increasingly wider use of birth control methods. From there, the pattern of low fertility was diffused towards the south (Valencia) and the west (Aragon). The provinces of Madrid[5] (in central Spain) and Huelva (in Andalusia), although not geographically belonging to this region, were also characterised by low fertility in 1940.

4) The *north-western quarter*, with intermediate-low fertility in 1920, includes Galicia and the surrounding provinces: Asturias, León and Zamora. High emigration and late marriage seem to have affected fertility levels in this

4 There are authors – Leasure (1962), for example – who explain this 'traditional' reproductive behaviour by claiming that these regions more strictly adhered to the moral guidelines of the Catholic Church and, were therefore, less influenced by the secularisation process.

5 Results on the province of Madrid are heavily influenced by the city of Madrid where fertility levels were well below those existing in the rest of the province.

Chart 1. Average Parity of Ever-married Women Born before 1865 (>55 Years Old in 1920)

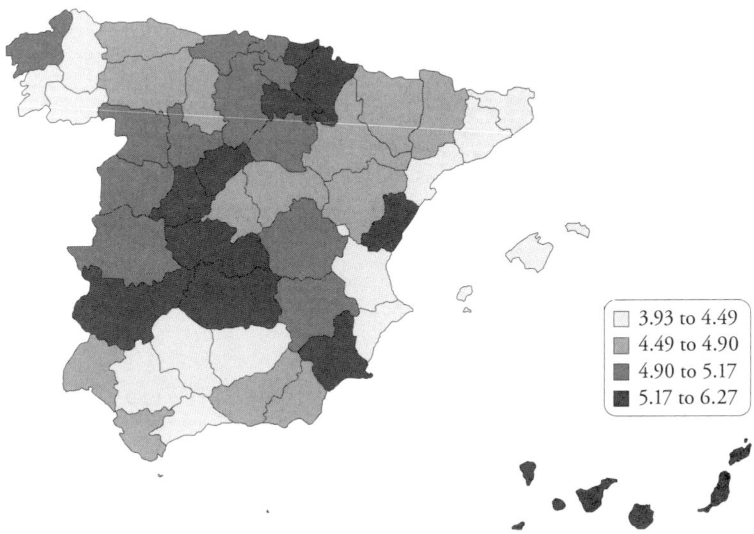

Chart 2. Average Parity of Ever-married Women Born between 1865 and 1869 (51–55 Years Old in 1920)

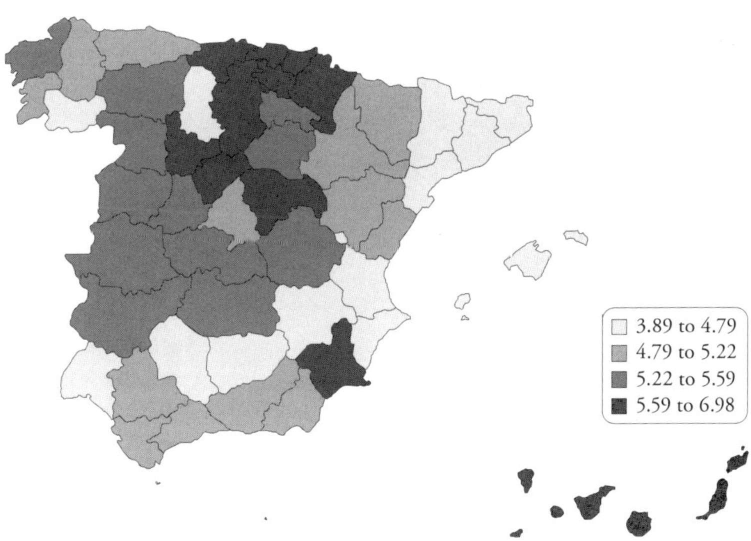

Chart 3. Average Parity of Ever-married Women Born between 1870 and 1874 (46–50 Years Old in 1920)

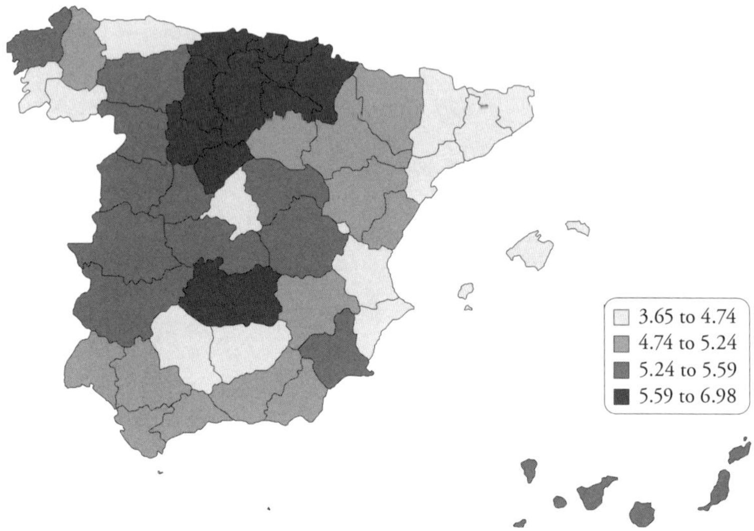

Chart 4. Average Parity of Ever-married Women Born between 1875 and 1879 (41–45 Years Old in 1920)

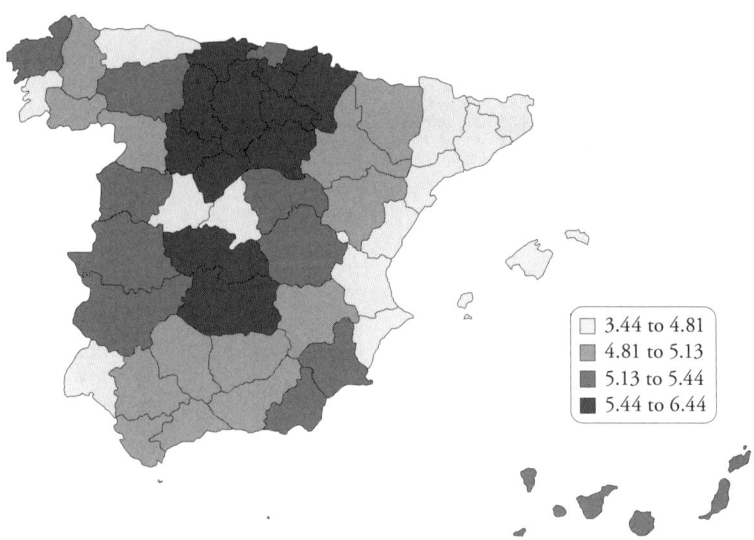

Chart 5. Average Parity of Ever-married Women Born between 1885 and 1889 (41–45 Years Old in 1930)

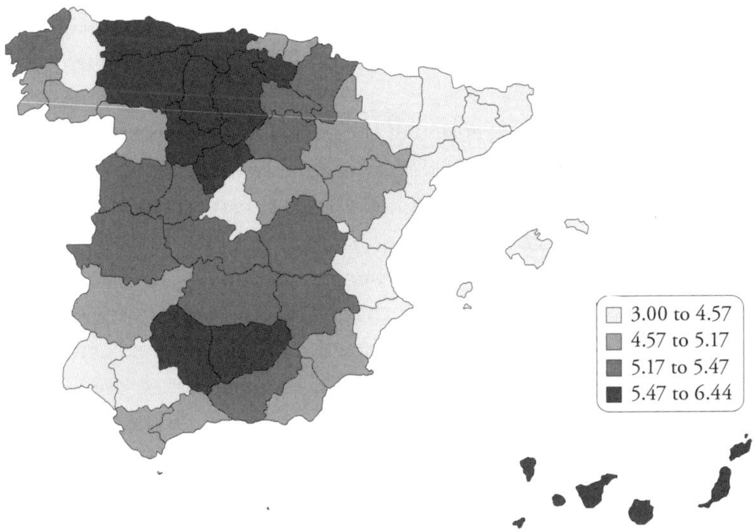

Chart 6. Average Parity of Ever-married Women Born between 1895 and 1899 (41–45 Years Old in 1940)

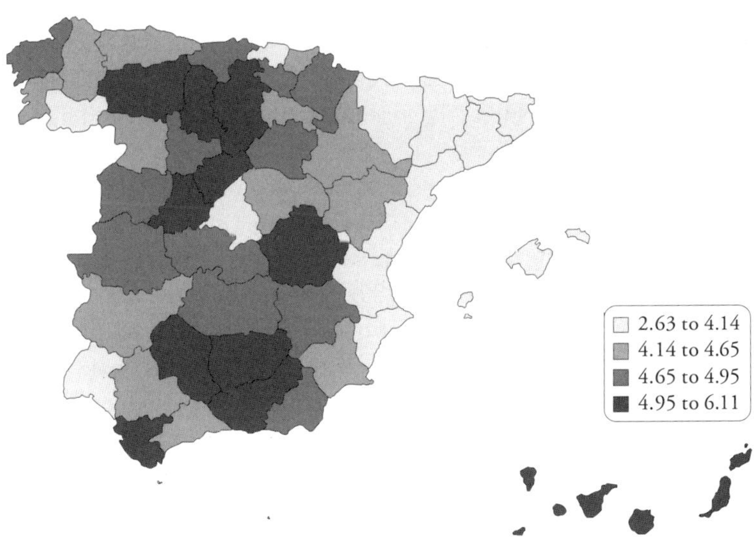

region, which were lower than those existing in central Spain. The pace of the decline in marital fertility between 1920 and 1940 was quite slow. Therefore, by the end of the period under study (1940) it appeared like an area of intermediate fertility which, due to the decrease experienced by the neighbouring Cantabrian provinces, ran all the way from Navarra and Guipúzcoa to the Portuguese border.

5) *Andalusia*, with the exception of the province of Huelva, is characterised by a fertility pattern which deviates considerably from developments found in the other areas of Spain. Although the 1920 census data corresponding to the provinces of Granada, Córdoba and Jaén appear rather doubtful – as they seem to underestimate fertility – on the whole, Andalusian data show intermediate levels of marital fertility for that particular year. However, between 1920 and 1940 Andalusian female cohorts do not show the expected decrease in marital fertility; in fact, in several provinces, parity levels are even higher in 1940 than in 1920. Therefore, this region (together with the Canary Islands and the central-northern part of Spain) came to be one of the areas with the highest fertility levels in the 1940 census.

These five geographical areas may be classified in two big groups depending on the speed with which fertility declined. On the one hand we have the eastern part of Spain and the northern coast, together with some specific provinces such as Madrid or Huelva, which show a quick decrease in parity levels. On the other hand, there are the provinces in central Spain, the north-western provinces, Andalusia and the Canary Islands, for which we found a very slow pace in fertility decrease. Here, the marital fertility transition still had a long way to go in 1940.

Both the geographical patterns and the pace of the decline in marital fertility inferred from retrospective census data are similar to those produced by previous authors using different data sets (Leasure, 1963; Livi Bacci, 1968; Coale and Watkins, 1986; Nicolau, 1989). Spatial results are also very close to those obtained by Pau Baizán and Enriqueta Camps using the 1991 Spanish Socio-Demographic Survey, which are also presented in this book. This similarity reinforces the reliability of the data used in this research and thus confirms the geographical patterns of the marital fertility transition in Spain, which process started first in Catalonia, with the Centre (Castile, except for Madrid), the South (except Huelva) and the Canary Islands being amongst the laggards.

3. Introducing Gender: Women Who Control Their Fertility, Women Who Do Not

3.1. The Marital Fertility Transition as a Transition of Birth Control Methods

Following on from Louis Henry's definition of 'natural' fertility (Henry, 1959, 1961a, 1961b), the process of fertility transition has been defined by a school of demographic thought, as reflected by the Princeton European Fertility Project, as the process of transition from a stage of 'natural' or un-controlled fertility to one of controlled fertility (Coale, 1973; Coale and Watkins, 1986; Knodel, 1979; Knodel and Van de Walle, 1979). As opposed to 'natural' fertility – when fertility control is not dependent upon the number of children ever-born – 'controlled' fertility is defined as a behaviour where parents decide the maximum number of children they wish to have, and act to avoid new births once that desired size has been reached. This type of control, called 'parity-specific limitation' by Coale or 'stopping' methods by other authors, would be the result of an 'innovation' within a pioneer group whose behaviour would later be 'diffused' to other social groups and other regions. The innovation by the pioneer group is seen as the end of the old demographic regime and the beginning of the fertility transition.

Other authors, however, argue that there is no clear distinction between a pre-transitional fertility pattern and a transitional one with parity-specific control (Carlsson, 1966; Blake, 1985). These authors claim that there have always been various methods of birth control, and that couples decided if they used them or not. These 'traditional' methods to control fertility were basically aimed to space births through breastfeeding, abstinence of sexual intercourse for longer periods after childbirth, sexual taboos, etc. (not to speak of voluntary abortion or even infanticide). In this sense, the fertility transition involves an increase in the proportion of the population beginning to use some previously well-known birth control strategy when the existing social, economic or demographic circumstances changed. Among the reasons for this 'adjustment' we might find, for example, higher survival rates for descending children due to a decrease in infant mortality.

Some studies have tried to combine both views, defining the marital fertility transition as a process of transition in the methods of birth control. More specifically, Hionidou (1998) created a theoretical model of transition with three successive phases: a first phase of adjustment to a new demographic and socio-economic context through spacing methods; a second phase of innovation of methods implying the introduction of stopping methods; and a third phase of innovation of ideas when couples start to fix the desired family size from the outset. Starting from this model, but adapting it to the findings from the Spanish censuses, I have elaborated a theoretical framework which seeks to explain both provincial differences within the marital fertility transition process and the different type of methods (spacing or stopping) used to obtain these fertility levels (figure 1). At the same time, this model highlights the role of women as an actor of increasing importance in the process of reproduction control.

Figure 1. Proposal for a Model of the Marital Fertility Transition in Spain

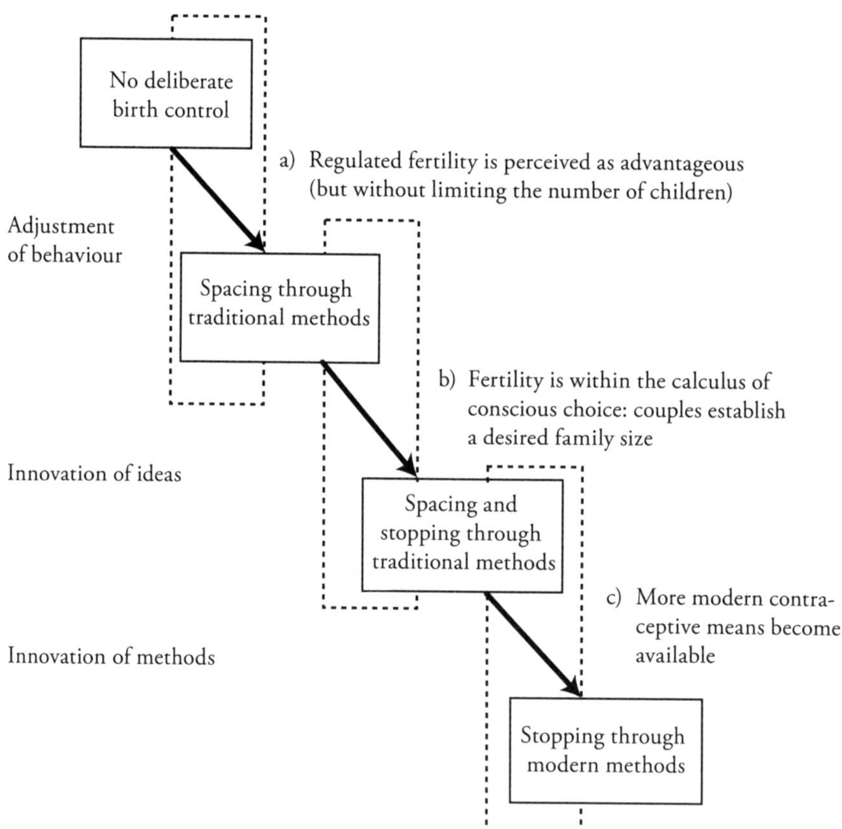

According to this model, the marital fertility transition consisted in the gradual adoption of birth control by couples through a series of successive stages in which not only the proportion of women who controlled fertility varied, but also the predominant methods used and, therefore, the role that women and men played in this process. This model describes this transition from high to low marital fertility as a complex process that consisted of: a) an initial adjustment of reproductive behaviour using traditional birth control methods followed by b) an innovation of ideas, and finally by c) a process of method innovation, that is to say, a transition in the types of control methods. Therefore, there are three transitions in one.

- In the first transition, couples who previously did not control their fertility perceive that it is advantageous to do so and begin to space births ('adjustment of behaviour') with traditional methods already known to them. Therefore, the proportion of couples using these traditional methods increases – but they do so without fixing a limit to the number of children they ultimately want to have.
- This only takes place in a second transition, when the idea is introduced that family size is one of the conscious choices a couple can make ('innovation of ideas'). In this second stage the reduction in marital fertility is probably more significant than in the first one: if spacing was the only procedure used in the previous stage, now stopping is added to the former, but still by traditional and low performance methods.
- The last transition, with the highest decrease in marital fertility, takes place with the spread of new and more effective contraceptive methods, which allow to completely stop fertility ('innovation of methods').

The successive transitions described by the model can be interpreted as a gradual shift from a social control of reproduction to different forms of individual control, in a context of modernisation, secularisation, industrialisation and the diffusion of bourgeois values. As Jutta Schwarzkopf, Anne-Françoise Praz and Sofia Kling explain in their chapters in this volume, the values associated with the ideas of 'femininity' and 'masculinity' – prescribing different behaviour regarding sexuality and contraception – changed along with this process. As a consequence, during this prolonged transition, the progressive empowerment of women (through increasing education and participation in the labour market) and the changing relation between husbands and wives, as well as the improvements in contraceptive technologies, conditioned the replacement of some birth control methods by others. As figure 1 shows, the three steps in the control method transition define four stages in the historical process of marital fertility decrease. In each of these phases, the types of control methods that were predominantly used are different. During the first (pretransitional) phase social control of reproduction through delayed marriage was probably the most important form of limiting the number of children. The second stage, characterised by the introduction of spacing techniques, was probably implemented through prolonged breastfeeding, periods of sexual abstinence and withdrawal. *Coitus interruptus* also played a protagonist role in the third phase, when stopping was implemented through traditional methods. Finally, the popularisation of condoms and the later introduction of other more sophisticated contraceptive methods (but still combined with the use of traditional ones such as withdrawal) are the main characteristics of the final phase of the transition.[6]

The model represented in figure 1 illustrates that, in the debate between adjustment or innovation/diffusion in the marital fertility transition, both positions are right, but for different stages of the process. The adjustment theory may explain the beginning of the transition: the number of children born inside marriage is adjusted by a wider use by couples, or by more social groups, of control techniques – mostly spacing – previously known and used, although to a smaller extent. The innovation/diffusion theory shows up more clearly in a later phase, when the more effective control methods applied to limit family size are known and accepted by an increasingly higher proportion of the population through a diffusion process which is not only helped by geographical vicinity, but also by shared linguistic or cultural links. This would explain the diffusion of fertility control patterns from the initial Catalan nucleus to the surrounding regions which were not only part of Barcelona's migratory hinterland but also shared a number of cultural and linguistic ties (Valencia, Balearic islands). The following section of this chapter is aimed at verifying the way in which the model that has just been defined fits in with Spanish data on retrospective fertility from the aforementioned censuses.

6 This process is what some authors call the 'first contraceptive revolution' or 'birth limitation', in opposition to the 'second contraceptive revolution' or 'birth planning', in which the number of children and the timing of their birth is already decided at the moment of couple consolidation. This phase is much later; it starts during the 1960s with the diffusion of the pill and other modern contraceptive methods (Ryder and Westoff, 1977; Leridon et al., 1987).

3.2. A Typology of Spanish Provinces by Stage in the Fertility Transition Process

Making the model I have just described operative has not been easy. First of all, the census data do not inform us on the intentions of parents regarding their fertility, that is to say, whether they were planning any specific limit to the size of their family and, if so, which techniques, of either spacing or stopping, they applied. Secondly, the theoretical framework does not explain which are the parity thresholds that separate one phase from the following one.

These inconveniences have been overcome by calculating two types of indicators from data on retrospective fertility to fix the different transitional phases. First, mean parity levels calculated from census data allowed the classification of Spanish provinces by fertility level and, therefore, by their progress in the fertility transition process.

Second, parity progression ratios were calculated from census data (figure 2) after which a mathematical transformation (logit) was applied to the parity progression ratios. When the result is a straight line, it means that stopping techniques are not significantly spread throughout the population. When by contrast, the line linking parity logits adopts a concave shape, it means that stopping techniques were applied by substantial numbers of women. Therefore, the correlation of the logits' curve to an adjusted straight line linking parity progression 1 to parity progression 7 allows us to know if the decrease in marital fertility was caused by the use of stopping methods (resulting in low correlation), or if (high correlation), other procedures such as spacing were used.

Figures 3 and 4 illustrate this mathematical procedure with two extreme examples: the Catalan province of Lérida (figure 3), placed in the pioneer region with early marital fertility decrease, shows parity progression ratios with concave shape; following logit transformation the concavity of the curve is even more pronounced and, therefore, the correlation coefficient is relatively low: $r^2 = 0.879$. This low correlation supports the existence of a wide diffusion of stopping techniques among the women living in this province.

Figure 2. Parity Progression Ratios. Ever-married Women Born in 1890–1894 (36–40 Years Old in 1930)

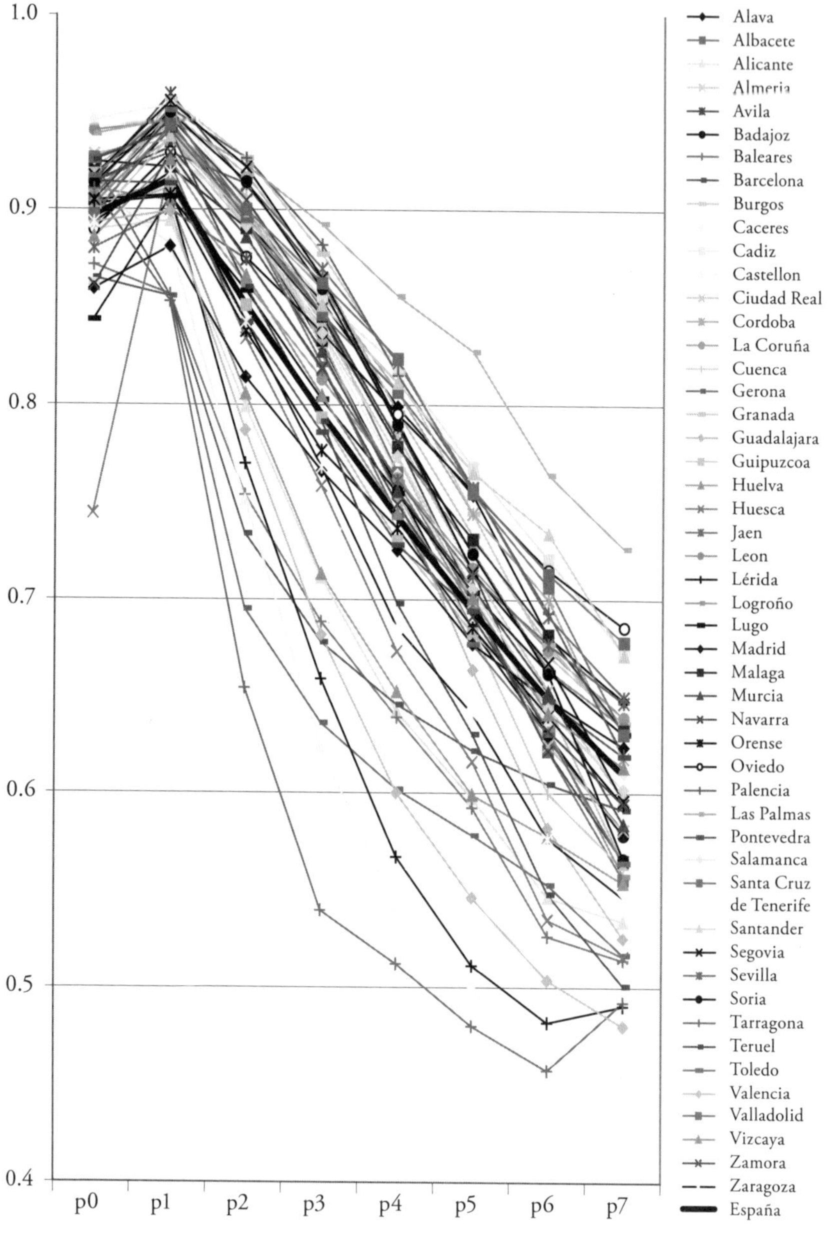

Figure 3. Parity Progression Ratios and Their Logits. Province of Lérida (Catalonia), Ever-married Women Aged 41–45 Years Old in 1930

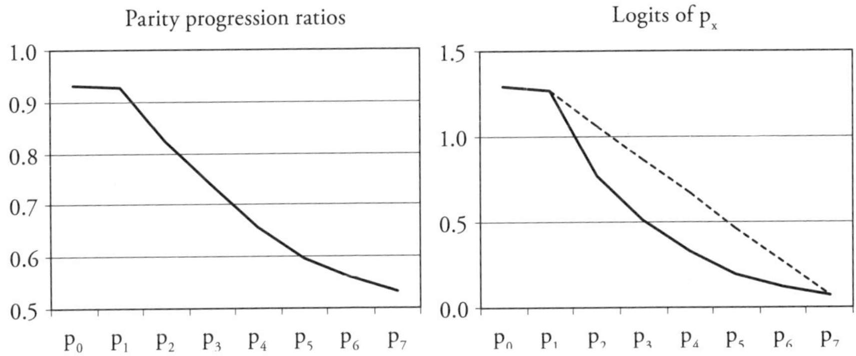

Figure 4. Parity Progression Ratios and their Logits. Province of Las Palmas (Canary Islands), Ever-married Women Aged 41–45 Years Old in 1930

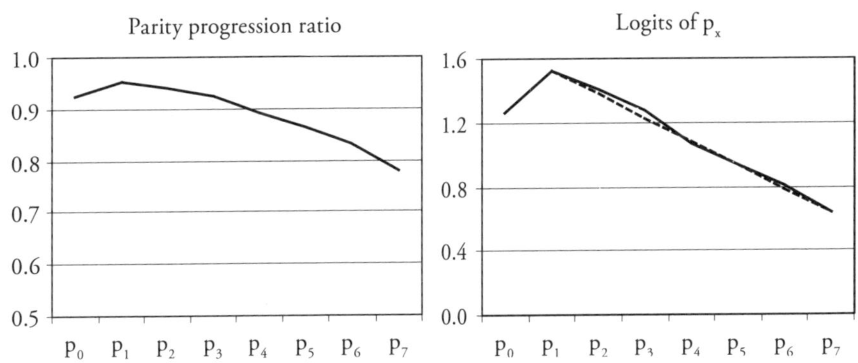

Source for figures 3 and 4: indicators calculated from 1930 Spanish Census data.

At the other end of the scale, there is the province of Las Palmas, in the Canary Islands (figure 4), showing a very different profile for the same female cohorts. The parity progression ratios' curve draws a convex curve and, after logit transformation, the resulting curve is nearly straight. Its high correlation with the adjustment line ($r^2 = 0.996$) indicates that stopping methods were practically absent in this province.

By consequence, the theoretical model with three transitions defining four stages has become a typology with four types of provinces depending on the progress made in the transition of marital fertility, as defined by two criteria: 1) the change in parity level between 1920 and 1930 for female cohorts born between 1885 and 1894; and 2) the correlation coefficient (r^2) showing the relationship between the parity progression ratio's logits curve and the adjustment line, that is to say, the concavity of the curve calculated for the same female cohorts.

Using a clustering technique depending on the above criteria, the 50 Spanish provinces have been classified into four groups (figure 5):

- Most provinces in the centre of Spain and some provinces in Andalusia are still in the first phase of the transition, characterised by 'natural' fertility: a high level of marital fertility, with an important increase in mean parity between 1920 and 1930, combined with the absence of any type of stopping behaviour (the logits' curve is straight).
- Other provinces in Andalusia, in Galicia, some Basque provinces, the two provinces of Extremadura and other specific provinces like Logroño, Santander or Santa Cruz de Tenerife are in the second stage: they do not show any significant use of stopping, but their marital fertility levels have started to decrease. This means that couples (or at least some of them) are using spacing methods in order to regulate their fertility. Therefore, these provinces are now in the phase of adjustment to the changing socio-economic and demographic circumstances.
- The three provinces of the Valencian region, the Balearic islands, the Catalan province of Lérida and provinces such as Madrid, Huelva, Huesca (in Aragon), and Lugo, Orense and Zamora (in the north-western part of Spain) are in the third stage of the transition (innovation of ideas): the significant decrease in fertility levels has been accompanied by an increase in the degree of concavity of the logits' curve that announces a wider use of stopping methods once the desired family size has been reached.
- Finally, three Catalan provinces (Barcelona, Tarragona and Gerona) are in the last phase of the transition (innovation of methods), characterised by very low parity levels combined with very concave curves of parity progression ratios' logits, which demonstrate a widespread use of modern stopping techniques.[7]

7 Some evidence exists that big numbers of latex condoms, industrially manufactured since the second decade of the twentieth century, were imported through Barcelona harbour.

Figure 5. Clusters of Provinces Depending on Parity Growth between 1920 and 1930, and Logits Correlation in 1930. Ever-married Women Born between 1885 and 1894 (36–45 Years Old in 1930)

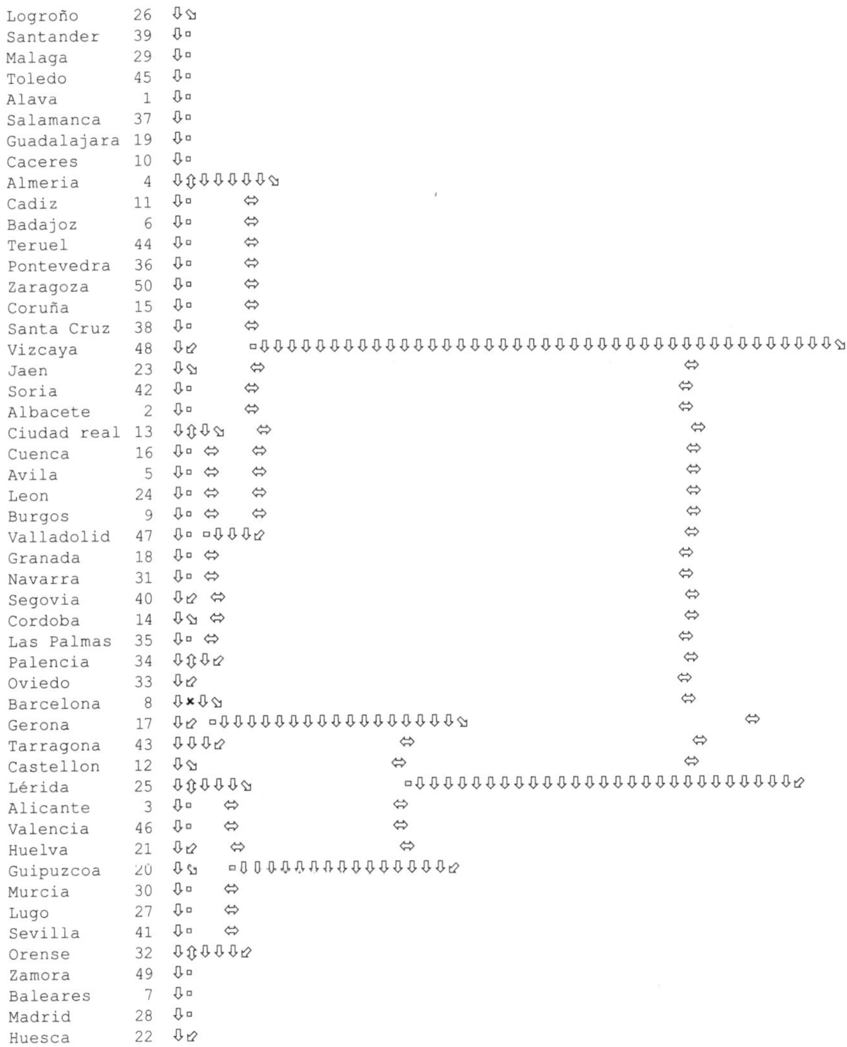

This typology of the Spanish provinces by parity levels and the use of birth control methods give us important information about the transition in marital fertility in this country. What the data show is not that different provinces were choosing different strategies of birth control, but that the marital fertility transition was a common phenomenon that affected all areas, but with very important timing differences. Indeed, the typology of Spanish provinces for the 1885–1894 female cohort, presented above, is the result of a snapshot, one specific image taken from a continuous film which was developed along several decades. What results show is that, for the period and generations picked up by those censuses, some provinces were in the initial stage of the transition, whilst other provinces were in the intermediate or final stages of this process.

Why did these large differences between regions exist in the marital fertility transition in Spain? It is difficult to answer this question with the type of data used here. However, Pau Baizán and Enriqueta Camps' research presented in this book highlights the important role of women's education[8] in decreasing fertility levels in Spain during the first half of the twentieth century. The increasing participation of women in the non-agrarian labour market

The widespread prostitution in this city may have had the effect of a better familiarity, at least amongst men, with the use of this contraceptive method. Other authors however think that a widespread use of *coitus interruptus* within marriage in all social groups is the most plausible explanation of Catalonia's very low marital fertility levels (Cabré, 1999).

8 The importance of education and its link with decreasing fertility is also mentioned in other contributions in this volume, notably by Alison Mackinnon and her co-authors. These latter authors think that, rather than literacy *per se*, one of the main contributors towards reducing the number of years spent in reproduction was the level of female schooling, i.e. the spread of mass education. However, this does not seem to be the case in the Netherlands, following the work presented by Angélique Janssens: The effect of women's education in the adoption of low fertility behaviour is not clear, at least not in the two towns analysed in that paper. Concerning Spain, the link between education and fertility decrease has been the subject of debate as evidence points in opposite directions. On the one hand, the regions with the highest level of literacy during the period under study (Old Castile and the Basque Country) are characterised by high fertility levels (Reher and Iriso Napal, 1989: 410), therefore 'the relation between illiteracy and fertility has remained significantly different from what would be expected on the basis of traditional demographic theory' (Reher and Iriso Napal, 1989: 418). On the other hand, Catalonia, the leading region in the process of fertility decrease, showed, following the same authors, a parallel increase in literacy: 'Despite low original levels, the increase in literacy was far greater than the national average' (Reher and Iriso Napal, 1989: 426).

(Camps-Cura, 1998), in a context of technological change in industry, and the role of big cities as pioneers in social modernisation (Reher and Iriso Napal, 1989), probably also had an impact on fertility levels in Spain. Urban women pertaining to the wealthier social classes (bourgeoisie) and some sectors of the industrial working class[9] were among the early female groups in adopting a low fertility pattern, groups which were better represented in Catalonia (Reher and Iriso Napal, 1989; Nash, 1984). This could explain the leading role of this geographical area in the process of marital fertility transition in Spain (Cabré, 1999). At the other end of the scale, those regions – such as central and southern Spain – where women employed in agriculture seem to be over-represented, were the laggards in the adoption of fertility control methods. This means that the position of each province within the different transition stages would be determined by the internal socio-economic composition of different groups of women, with each group showing different behavioural patterns regarding fertility. On this latter issue the retrospective census data may provide some information.

3.3. Parity Differences within Each of the Provinces

The aforementioned typology, set out in figure 5, is based on average parity data for each of the provinces, hiding an enormous amount of individual variety. Indeed, in each of the analysed regions, women with very different degrees of birth control may be found, as well as those who did not practice any control at all. Indeed, women living in the same place and at the same time probably adopted, in a conscious or unconscious way, different reproductive strategies due to different combinations of influences such as family pressure, regional culture and traditions, local social and economic conditions, church's moral influence, etcetera. All these influences were mutually modified and conditioned by individual knowledge, perceptions and desires. This individual variety is reflected in the provincial histograms based on the frequency distribution of ever-married women according to the number of children ever-born. Figures 6 and 7 show the histograms for Spain and for a selection of 7 provinces representing different Spanish regions for two female

9 Mary Nash studied the influence of the anarchist movement on the diffusion of birth control methods within the Catalan working class, especially during the II Republic period (Nash, 1984).

cohorts: those born before 1875, aged more than 45 years in 1920; and those born between 1890 and 1894, aged 36–40 years in 1930.[10]

These histograms reflect different stages in the marital fertility transition process. Therefore, by overlapping the histograms we obtain a movie – much in the way that Festy (1979: 77) did with the data corresponding to different European countries – of how the distribution of ever-married women by number of children evolved along the transitional process.

In the first phase, before starting the transition, the distribution is very flat, with a scarcely marked modal value around 6 children and high percentages of women with very high numbers of children. When the transition begins a modal value starts to build up, due to the decrease of the biggest family sizes (7 children and more), concentrating around parity 5 or 6. When the transitional process continues, the modal value grows and it progressively moves to the left, towards the lower parity orders. At the end of the transition, the modal value is two children and the proportion of women that have this parity is around or over 20 percent, while the proportion of women with a large number of off-spring begins to be insignificant. While Barcelona, with a modal value of two children, was well into this last phase in the five-year cohort born between 1890 and 1894, Burgos, with a modal value of 5 children, had only just entered the second stage, that is to say, it had only just begun the transitional process. The remaining provinces were in an intermediate situation on the road from one stage to the other.

At the same time, these histograms show that in all the populations studied here there were women with high numbers of off-spring next to others without any children at all or those with only very few. What varies is their proportion, that is to say, the share of women who, one way or another, controlled their fertility – in a more or less efficient way –, and those who did not. It may be interpreted in the sense that the theoretical model with three transitions of birth control methods, such as was defined before, not only successfully explains differences between provinces but also differences within provinces. In other words, the model is able to explain the differences between women belonging to different social groups with different values and behaviours regarding fertility control at one particular moment in time (Szreter and Garrett, 2000, give a similar explanation for Britain).

10 These data do not exist in the 1940 Spanish census, where only mean parity at the provincial level may be calculated.

Figure 6. Distribution (%) of Ever-married Women* of Cohorts Born before 1875 Depending on the Number of Children (1920 Spanish census)

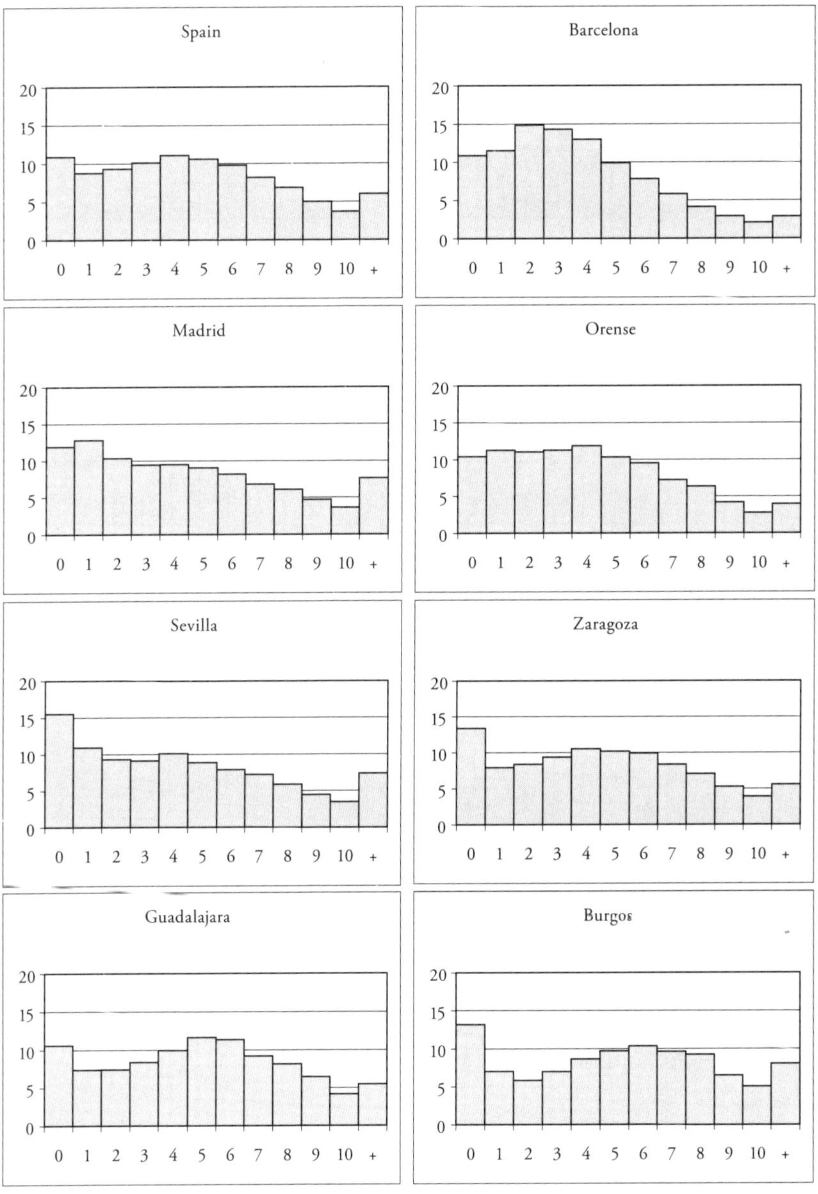

* Women without declaration not included.

Figure 7. Distribution (%) of Ever-married Women* of Cohorts Born between 1890–1894 Depending on the Number of Children (1930 Spanish census)

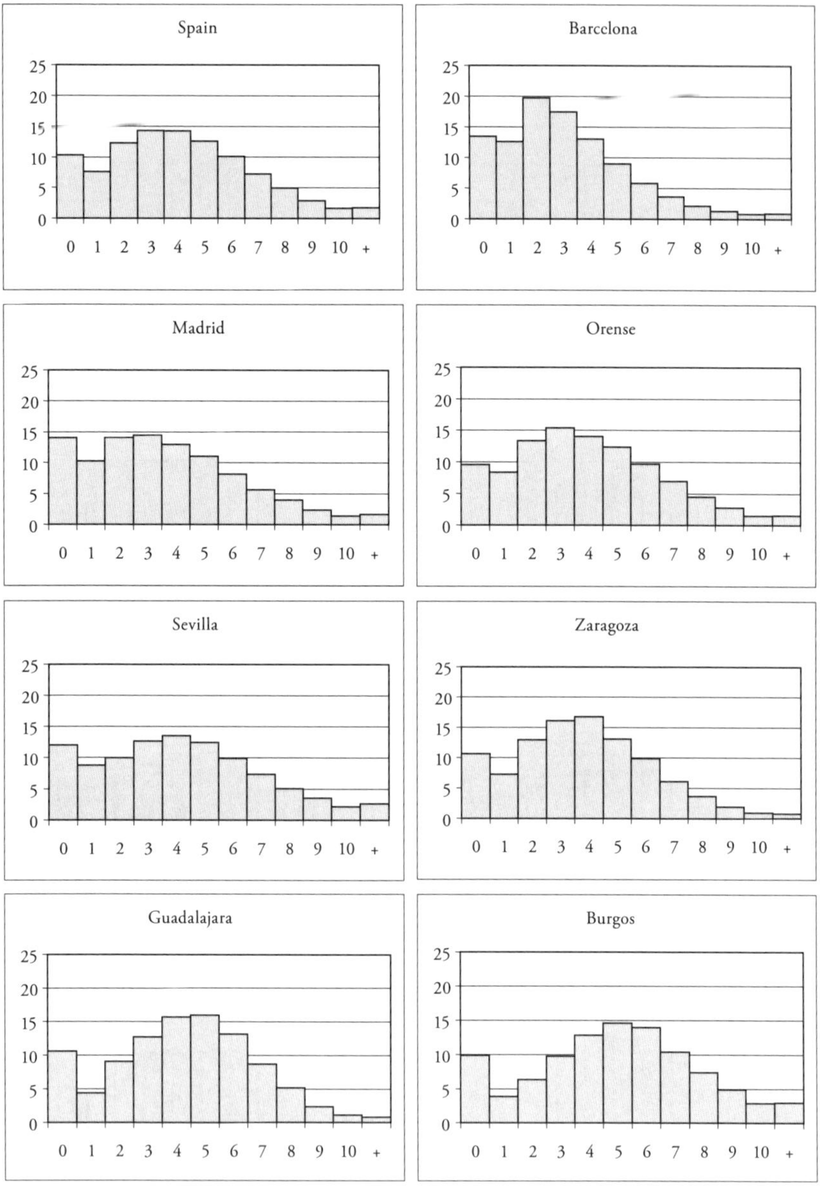

* Women without declaration not included.

4. Final Considerations on the Marital Fertility Transition in Spain and the Role of Women

The results of this research have shown the diversity of marital fertility transition situations existing across Spain in the late nineteenth and the early twentieth century. Differences in reproductive behaviour are important between provinces but also within provinces, that is to say, between groups of women. Although the census data used in this research cannot give us information on the socio-economic characteristics of women by parity level, there can be little doubt that differences in women's educational levels, in their participation in the labour market, as well as differences in the degree to which they accepted religious moral norms or traditional ideals of femininity, or differences in their bargaining powers with their husbands are probably behind the diverging patterns that census data on retrospective fertility show for Spain in that period.

The gradual empowerment of women, which lies behind this shift from a socially controlled pattern of reproduction to one based on individual control, was a process which was neither quick nor easy. It was a process moving through a number of generations and with an uneven pace across Spain, depending on local conditions. I have tried to illustrate this long and uneven process of change through a marital fertility transition model which interprets it as a succession of phases defined by the main type of birth control method used by couples. Following the three conditions defined by Coale (1973) for the adoption of fertility control – it has to be acceptable, advantageous and available – this model is based on the argument that couples first have to assume the necessity of regulating their fertility somehow before a specific contraceptive method is chosen by both members of the couple. Once this pre-condition has been met, couples will adopt the technique (spacing or stopping) most suited to their interests through an interaction process between spouses. This marital interaction process itself evolved as well, with the role of women becoming progressively more important and their power in reproductive decisions increasing as a result of rising levels in female education and labour market participation. More efficient birth control methods replaced the previous ones, and spacing techniques were gradually substituted by stopping methods as values, norms, and the demographic and socio-economic context changed.

Undoubtedly, fertility decisions were influenced by the historical contexts in which couples and individuals found themselves. For this reason, the use of stopping methods to control the number of children diffused diversely through space and time and social groups depending on the local and regional demographic and socio-economic conditions but also depending on moral (secularisation) and cultural (common cultural and linguistic trends) factors. The combination of individual characteristics and contextual factors would explain why the transition in Spain varied so much between social groups and between regions. The regional differences in the transitional trajectories have led some authors to defend the idea of the existence of several regional demographic systems in Spain, with different combinations of fertility, mortality and migration levels (Livi Bacci, 1968; Delgado, 1988; Cabré 1999; Nicolau, 1989; Reher and Iriso Napal, 1989). However, retrospective census data seem to demonstrate that the existence of only one transitional model distinguishing different phases is the most plausible explanatory framework regarding marital fertility in Spain.

In conclusion, retrospective analysis, cohort by cohort, of the differences in marital fertility in the 1920, 1930 and 1940 Spanish censuses has given some answers to certain questions, such as which territories maintained traditional reproductive patterns longer or which provinces were pioneers in birth control adoption, and which techniques were adopted by couples in different areas of Spain. We have also established where the transitional process was slower or quicker in relation to the birth control methods used. Finally, this research has tried to introduce a gender perspective by interpreting the differences between women who controlled their fertility (using spacing or stopping methods) and those who did not, as successive stages in the process of women's empowerment. However, these results are incomplete answers that deserve more in-depth research using qualitative data.

References

Auriat, N. (1996), *Les défaillances de la mémoire humaine. Aspects orientatifs des enquêtes rétrospectives*, Paris, INED / PUF.

Blake, J. (1985), 'The Fertility Transition: Continuity or Discontinuity with the Past?', *International Population Conference*, Florence.

Brass, W. (1975), *Methods for Estimating Fertility and Mortality from Limited and Defective Data,* Chapel Hill, Poplab, University of North Carolina.

Cabré, A. (1999), *El sistema català de reproducció,* Barcelona, Proa.

Camps-Cura, Enriqueta (1998), 'Transitions in Women's and Children's Work Patterns and Implications for the Study of Family Income and Household Structure: A Case Study from the Catalan Textile Sector (1850–1925)', *The History of the Family. An International Quarterly,* 3, 137–153.

Carlsson, G. (1966), 'Decline of Fertility: Innovation or Adjustment Process?', *Population Studies,* 20 (2), 149–174.

Coale, A. J. (1973), 'The Demographic Transition Reconsidered', *Proceedings of the International Population Conference,* Lieja, vol. I, 53–73.

Coale, A. J. and Watkins, S. C. (eds) (1986), *The Decline of Fertility in Europe*, Princeton, Princeton University Press / Office of Population Research.

Delgado, M. (1988), *El descenso de la fecundidad en España*, Tesis Doctoral, Universidad Complutense de Madrid.

El-Badry, M. A. (1961), 'Failure of Enumerators to Make Entries of Zero: Errors in Recording Childless Cases in Population Censuses', *Journal of the American Statistical Association,* 56 (296), 909–924.

Fernández Cordón, J. A. (1977), *Etude démographique de la fécondité en Espagne (1922–1974).* Thèse pour le Doctorat de 3e cycle en Travail et Ressources Humaines, Université de Paris I.

Festy, P. (1979), *La fécondité des Pays occidentaux de 1870 à 1970*, Paris, INED / PUF.

Gil Alonso, F. (2005), 'El descenso histórico de la fecundidad matrimonial en España. Análisis territorial retrospectivo a partir de los Censos de 1920, 1930 y 1940', PhD Thesis, Autonomous University of Barcelona, Department of Geography.

Henry, L. (1953), 'Fondements théoriques des mesures de la fécondité naturelle', *Revue de l'Institut International de la Statistique*, (3), 135–151.

Henry, L. (1961a), 'La fécondité naturelle: observation-théorie-résultats', *Congrès UIESP*, New York, UIESP, 47–55.

Henry, L. (1961b), 'Some Data on Natural Fertility', *Eugenics Quarterly*, vol. VIII (2), 81–91.

Hionidou, V. (1998), 'The Adoption of Fertility Control on Mykonos, 1879–1959: Stopping, Spacing or Both?', *Population Studies*, 52 (1), 67–83.

Knodel, J. (1979), 'From Natural Fertility to Family Limitations: The Onset of Fertility Transition in a Sample of German Villages', *Demography*, 16 (4), 493–521.

Knodel, J. and Van de Walle, E. (1979), 'Lessons from the Past: Policy Implications of Historical Fertility Studies', *Population and Development Review,* 5 (2), 217–245.

Leasure, J. W. (1963), 'Factors Involved in the Decline of Fertility in Spain, 1900–1950', *Population Studies,* XVI (3), 271–285.

Leridon, H., Charbit, Y., Collomb, P., Sardon, J.-P. and Toulemon, L. (1987), *La seconde révolution contraceptive: la régulation des naissances en France de 1950 à 1985*, París, INED / PUF, Travaux et Documents, nº 117.

Livi Bacci, M. (1968), 'Fertility and Nuptiality Changes in Spain from the Late 18th to the Early 20th Century', *Population Studies,* 22 (1 (part I), 2 (part II)), 83–102 (part I), 211–234 (part II).

Nash, M. (1984) 'El neomaltusianismo anarquista y los conocimientos populares sobre el control de la natalidad en España', in Nash, M. (ed.), *Presencia y protagonismo. Aspectos de la historia de la mujer*, Barcelona, Serba, 307–340.

Nicolau, R. (1989), *Trajectoires regionales dans la transition demographique espagnole.* Thèse pour le Doctorat. Institut d'Etudes Politiques de Paris.

Reher, D. S. and Iriso Napal, P. L. (1989), 'Marital Fertility and its Determinants in Rural and Urban Spain, 1887–1930', *Population Studies,* 43 (3), 405–427.

Ryder, N. B. and Westoff, C. F. (1977), *The Contraceptive Revolution*, Princeton, Princeton University Press.

Sàez, A. (1979), 'La fécondité en Espagne depuis le début du siècle', *Population*, 34 (6), 1007–1022.

Szreter, S. and Garrett, E. (2000), 'Reproduction, Compositional Demography, and Economic Growth: Family Planning in England Long before the Fertility Decline', *Population and Development Review*, 26 (1), 45–80.

United Nations (1983), *Manual X. Indirect Techniques for Demographic Estimation*, New York, United Nations.

'Because They Are too Menny ...' Children, Mothers and Fertility Decline

The Evidence from Working-class Autobiographies of the Eighteenth and Nineteenth Centuries

Jane Humphries

Introduction

This paper brings new evidence to bear on the forces that shaped the demographic transition. The source is British working-class autobiography.[1] In a larger project based on over 600 published and unpublished working-class memoirs, material about the autobiographers' families of origin is used to investigate aspects of childhood and specifically to construct an account of children's experience of work during the Industrial Revolution (Humphries, forthcoming). Although all male, these working-class autobiographers saw women, particularly mothers, as the beating heart of family life and their experiences and perception of that life bears on the origins of the demographic transition.[2]

Mothers were almost invariably the central caring figures in family life. Theirs was the burden of making ends meet, of stretching their families' resources to cover needs. As has often been demonstrated, mothers sacrificed their own consumption standards in the interests of their children, scrimping on their own food and clothing, and working long hours though often only in their own homes. But what the autobiographical evidence makes clear is that they also presided over transfers of time and resources from one child to another, primarily from older working children to younger dependent brothers and sisters.

1 For the classic introduction to the genre see Vincent (1981).

2 Rather than attempt to include the few working-class autobiographies written by women in this survey a separate project focused on female experience is planned.

Widespread evidence from modern populations documents that children's social, educational and economic outcomes vary inversely with the size of their families of orientation (see the voluminous literature cited in Preston, 1976). The same appears true for the autobiographers, with various measures of wellbeing such as age at starting work and years of schooling inversely correlated with size of sibling group. At the hubs of their households, responsible for sharing out scarce material and emotional resources, mothers must have recognized the costs new babies meant to existing children. Evidence from the autobiographies shows mothers painfully aware of the Sophie's choices they made among their children, and uncovers a powerful motive for seeking to limit family size.

But another key finding from the autobiographical evidence is that children were the most important secondary earners in working-class families through the period of the Industrial Revolution and on until the middle of the nineteenth century. They shared the burden of breadwinning with fathers, provided resources for hard-pressed mothers, and helped to support dependent siblings. Indeed the support that children provided to mothers in their efforts to stretch fathers' earnings may have blunted women's preferences for smaller families. But even when those preferences were dominant they waited on men's agreement before they could influence practice. Understanding and dating this agreement has always been difficult for demographic historians, who have tried, with only partial success, to link it to the increasing isolation of men as responsible for their families' economic survival. As women and children retreated from the labour market and became dependent, men, saddled with the task of their support, became convinced of the desirability of smaller families.

While the chronology of the conventional wisdom was never totally clear, the autobiographical evidence makes it even less convincing. The accounts of family life in the Industrial Revolution suggest precocious development of some aspects of the male breadwinner family form. Fathers were already the economic mainstays of their families. But men's specialized economic role rather than persuading them of the desirability of fewer children detached them from family life and insulated them from the problem of making ends meet. During the late eighteenth and early nineteenth centuries, fathers became aloof and distant, separated from their families by the cares of breadwinning, which involved long hours, and sometimes long periods, away from home. Male leisure, such as it was, did not commonly involve childcare or playing with children but was spent with other men. Ironically, while the male breadwinner family form assigned economic responsibilities increasingly to men, at the same time its demands detached men from the very families that they were required to support, and blunted their perception of the costs of additional children. What then eventually convinced men and women of the desirability of smaller families?

Here the autobiographies provide an important insight, and one which helps synchronize the explanation of fertility decline with the empirical trends. Recognition of the costs that additional children imposed on their older brothers and sisters came perhaps too late to influence mothers' fertility, but it had a lasting effect on the boys and girls who grew up in the large families of the era. Hitherto accounts of fertility decline have turned on the changes in the perceived relative costs of children to mothers and fathers and neglected the costs of family size to children themselves. The generation of children who grew up in early industrial Britain lived at the sharp end of the high fertility regimen. As child workers and household consumers their living standards suffered when additional babies appeared. The legacy was a preference for smaller families, carried forward when these boys and girls grew up and became parents at the end of the nineteenth century.[3] The new preference was then consolidated by the gradual disappearance of child labour and the dawning recognition of the importance of schooling, which not merely raised the perceived costs of additional children but deposited them squarely on the shoulders of parents. This latter part of the story may be familiar, but its taproot in children's experience has been ignored. In Thomas Hardy's masterpiece *Jude the Obscure*, Sue, Jude's wife becomes convinced that her several children 'would be better out o' the world than in it', but it is Old Father Time, Jude's eldest son who is moved by this Malthusian perception to act, hanging himself and his little brothers and sisters neatly in the family's cupboard 'because they are too menny (sic)' (Hardy, 1985: 406 and 410).

3 Demographic historians frequently make use of models where experience in childhood influences adult reproductive behaviour. For example, Wrigley and Schofield (1981) argued that the distinctive decline in marriage age in the eighteenth century represented a lagged response to the robust real wages of the previous generation.

The Fertility Decline and the Male Breadwinner Family

Historians are generally agreed on the overarching framework within which to study fertility decline. The chosen framework, borrowed from mainstream economics, emphasizes rational behaviour with smaller families promoted by changes in the perceived relative costs of child-rearing (PRCC model). But the need to link individual decisions not to the costs and benefits of children in narrow economic terms but rather to the perception of these costs and benefits complicates the otherwise 'beguilingly straightforward' model (Szreter, 1996). A key factor explaining both occupational/industrial differences in fertility levels and changes over time was the extent to which women and children contributed to family subsistence. Other family members' economic participation rates were in turn conditioned on the ability of the male wage to support a whole family and on attitudes to deviations from the male breadwinner standard. Trends in the relative costs of child rearing cannot be separated from the economic, social and cultural consequences of both the gendering and adulting of labour markets. Thus explanations of fertility decline rested on changes in the family economy.

Smaller families were causally linked to the emergence of the male breadwinner family and its corollary the demise of the domestically-based and involved father, as men were required to spend longer hours and more days away from home and in centralized and formalized workplaces. Burdened with total responsibility for their families' survival and status, husbands and fathers came to prefer fewer 'higher quality' children.

For the middle class, dependence on husbands and fathers was established early in the nineteenth century and its implication for family dynamics and affective relations have been carefully explored (Tosh, 1999; Mintz, 1983). For the working class, these changes were slow to materialize. In the first half of the nineteenth century, few working men could earn breadwinner wages. The majority of families were supported also by economic contributions from women and children who often competed in local labour markets with husbands and fathers. Historians went on to explain variation in fertility levels as responses to the perceived costs of child-rearing in different economic, social and cultural settings, with high fertility coal-mining communities and low fertility textile towns providing graphic illustrations. Changes over time were then explained by the increasing dominance of the male-breadwinner family form which made it possible for children to retreat from the labour market and by associating other family members' work with parental inadequacy branded as unrespectable those families in which women and children continued to contribute. By the last quarter of the nineteenth century the state's insistence on an expanded dependent childhood raised child-rearing costs and by providing official support for the male breadwinner norm leant weight to the stigma against parents who failed to conform. Thus as the male breadwinner standard trickled down from the middle and upper classes, working-class men were converted to a preference for fewer children.

But the timing of secular trends proved problematical. The changing role of fathers was dated from the 1830s and 40s while working-class conversion to small family size was not widespread until the twentieth century. There was little empirical work on shifts in household economics among the working class and the evidence that demographers assembled was circumstantial. Fertility levels were geographically or occupationally or (less successfully) temporarily correlated with economic conditions assumed to be embedded in community norms and values and rational response inferred. Motivation was inferred from the relationships identified in the data and assumed in the (economic) theory of ideal family size.

In a series of important contributions (Seccombe, 1993; Seccombe, 1990; Seccombe, 1992), Wally Seccombe focussed directly on motivation and thus challenged 'The standard models of fertility regulation […] framed at the level of the reproductive *couple*, as if spouses have symmetrical interests and make harmonious joint decisions in all matters of sex and procreation' (Seccombe, 1990: 173). Seccombe argued that since women bore the direct burdens of repeated pregnancy, childbearing, and childcare, they likely wanted small families, compared with their husbands whose primary concern was with their conjugal rights.[4] But the contraceptive methods of the day required men's

4 Seccombe cited qualitative sources, the Lewis Faning survey and Stopes correspondence, to illustrate women's aversion to additional children and the reasons for their anxieties. The latter included both economic reasons, the claim that the family could not afford more children, and concern about their own health and the perils that future pregnancies brought. An increase in the relative net costs of raising children is a central feature of most models of fertility decline. But as Seccombe says demographers have perhaps underestimated the fear of complications in childbirth as a motive force in women's desire to stop.

co-operation hence there was a disjuncture between female motivation and male capacity to act. The result was a 'simmering tension, if not open conflict, between spouses over the terms and conditions of intercourse' that would only be resolved when men came to fear the prospect of another child strongly enough to exercise sexual self-discipline (Seccombe, 1990: 187).[5] But Seccombe returned to the standard story in his explanation of men's conversion to the small family ideal, which he dated from the 1870s, associated with the spread of the male-breadwinner family among the working class. The costs of supporting additional children fell on working-class men and they responded by preferring smaller families.

While Seccombe should be applauded for recognizing potential conflicts of interest between husbands and wives over ideal family size, his development of the PRCC model has been criticized. If women's preferences for fewer children were of long-standing it becomes difficult to explain their late eighteenth and early nineteenth century collaboration in early marriage and almost universal nuptiality. Moreover demographer Robert Woods (1992) found Seccombe's explanation of changes in men's attitudes unconvincing. The 1870s, while a turning point in demographic behaviour, seemed too late a date for children to be seen as 'burdensome' when outside 'peasant society' children were always dependent. He saw no reasons to search for changes in the family economy in order to account for changes in men's attitudes. The explanation for women's burgeoning influence over their husbands lay instead in the spread of mass education, which drew men and women's views closer together.

Clearly changes in the sources of income and patterns of dependency are crucial in understanding fertility decline. This paper suggests that historians' account of the rise of the male breadwinner family within the working class is empirically under-developed, and out of touch with economic historians' understanding of changes in the labour market in the eighteenth and nineteenth centuries. It uses a source, working-class memoirs, that could be dismissed as anecdotal although it attempts to treat autobiographies systematically, where possible to extract quantitative evidence about family structure and functioning, and to relate this evidence to the economic history of the

5 This tension too was suggested by the qualitative sources consulted. Fertility decline thus waited on the convergence of men and women's interests and the former's collaboration in sexual restraint within marriage.

period. Working-class autobiographies, as historians of the genre note, almost never describe intimate relationships or discuss sexual practices. They do not document the simmering tensions between husbands and wives that historians have thought accompanied the clash between men's 'conjugal rights' and women's fears of childbirth. But they can be used to cast new light on the sourcing of family incomes and the related emotional and affective structure of the working-class family. In this way they uncover the perceived costs of children to mothers and fathers and how these differed. But they also highlight another victim of large families, namely the children who grew up in them and particularly the older children who were expected to work and contribute to their siblings' upkeep.

Working-class Household Economics

Much work in the larger project has gone into establishing that the autobiographers' sample is (or can by suitable re-weighting be made) representative in demographic, occupational and economic terms. It can then be used to explore aspects of working-class family life. While the book (Humphries, forthcoming) concentrates on children's experience of work during the Industrial Revolution, here attention is on the economic roles of husbands, wives and children, the implications for family dynamics and the different motivation of mothers and fathers to limit family size.

Fathers' Economic Roles

The autobiographers gave priority and status to the father's economic role in the family. Fathers were introduced in terms of their occupations and ability at those occupations, *defined* as miners, weavers, agricultural labourers and so on. The cardinal importance of the father's economic status is reflected in the almost universal provision of information on fathers' occupational group. In only 57 cases (9.4 percent) of the sample of 606 autobiographies used in this analysis, was there insufficient information to assign the father to an occupational group and in only 87 (14.4 percent) insufficient information to indicate a more detailed occupational title. A father's occupation was usually noted very early on in a memoir consistent with its centrality in the story that followed. Over two hundred separate occupations are mentioned, more often than not accompanied by a detailed description of skills, work and employment history. This depth of description stands in sharp contrast to the paucity of information provided about mothers' economic activity (see below) and clearly points to the father as the family's economic mainstay.

The priority accorded to the father's economic activity suggests that the primary responsibility for household support even in early industrial Britain already rested on the male head, the breadwinner, whose 'job' linked the family to the economy. Roger Langdon (born 1825) praised his father's breadwinning prowess: 'He rose very early and took rest late that he might maintain his children in what he termed "poor independence"' (Langdon, 1894: 13). The vital importance of a male breadwinner is reflected in the many cases of desperate women seeking to retain links to unstable men. Edward Rymer (born 1835) described the attempts of his mother to re-connect with his absconding father and obtain support and Francis Place (born 1771) his mother's struggle to reunite her family under the infuriating headship of Place senior (Rymer, 1976; Place, 1972). Neither Mrs. Rymer nor Mrs. Place was a timid, incapable woman. But both judged it better to cling to an inadequate man than to struggle without assistance (see Wall, 1994).

Of course it is possible that the autobiographers depictions of their families as already crucially dependent on men and male earnings as early as the end of the eighteenth century reflects a stereotype that took increasing hold as the nineteenth century wore on rather than economic reality. Undoubtedly the mid-Victorian fusion of respectability with a dependent wife and children and an adult male breadwinner became a frame through which the working-class authors looked back upon their early life and provided a standard according to which they measured their mothers and fathers. But how congruent was this vision with working-class reality? Even if men were economically dominant how dependent were other family members?

Mothers' Economic Roles

Fathers possessed in their child's imagination the status and standing of their specific occupations. In contrast, the role of mother crowded out any occupational identity. Mothers were infrequently described by an occupational designation and even where one was provided it was not assigned the centrality afforded fathers' jobs. Yet mothers without occupational titles were sometimes revealed as economically active. For one thing although fathers sometimes practiced dual occupations, mothers regularly did many jobs, patching together seasonally and cyclically available work. Henry Price (born 1824) lived with his grandmother whom he described as taking outwork from a local silk factory and frequently involved in agricultural work including gleaning: 'All these little jobs help'd to keep the pot a boiling' (Price, 1904, not paginated). Moreover mothers' activities were fitted around domestic tasks and childcare and so conflated with and submerged into housewifery. David Barr (born 1831) recalled 'Excursions [...] for the purpose of gathering mushrooms, hazelnuts, cowslips, and anything else that might be lawfully appropriated. These were sent to market and converted into cash ...' (Barr, 1910: 20; see also, Humphries, 1990). Several children remembered their mothers' taking on work put out by local merchant capitalists. Joseph Ricketts (born 1777), was early on integrated into his mother's economy of makeshift fitting his schooling around agricultural opportunities and in the spring assisting his mother and sisters at spinning and carding wool (Ricketts, 1965: 121).

One response to the limited job opportunities for married women and convenience of working from home, as other historians have noted (see Parkinson, 2002), was to operate a small business rather than work for wages. Several mothers, for example, ran dame schools. Others processed foodstuffs for sale or operated small retail shops. More commonly, wives helped in their husbands' enterprises, underlining the historical reality that marriage often provided the means whereby women could be productive, means that were lost if husbands died or absconded.

Some mothers did contribute by actively participating in the labour market. But these women were in the minority. There is a contrast here with the French and German working-class autobiographies studied by Mary Jo Maynes (1995). The European autobiographers reported mothers' as well as fathers' occupations and the great majority described their mothers as having done paid work throughout their childhood. In the British cases, work by mothers was often associated with a family crisis. When Joseph Arch's (born 1826) blacklisted father could get no work, his mother kept the family going by doing laundry work. Although Mrs. Arch was an excellent nurse and laundress 'and [...] did not hide these talents in a napkin' (Arch, 1898: 9), her labour was something to be resorted to when times were desperate. Continuous work especially if it took mothers out of their homes appears to have been a last resort.

Computations of married women's participation rates are extremely sensitive to both how economic activity is conceptualized and how characteristically shadowy information on mothers is treated. Here two conceptualizations of work are combined with two treatments of missing information to provide four estimates as shown in table 1. Participation is generously defined with any reference to productive activity, including self provisioning, counted. Where nothing like this is mentioned women were assumed inactive. The problem is how to treat cases where the autobiographer provides very little or no information about his mother. Even her presence during his childhood may be uncertain.[6] Column 1 of table 1 provides lower and upper bound estimates of mothers' economic activity according to the treatment of these uncertain cases though both involve the same broad definition of participation. The lower bound estimate includes all doubtful cases as inactive. It is possible that some mothers' efforts were simply not mentioned but more likely these cases contain a relatively high proportion of mothers who were limited to caring and domestic roles. Alternatively an upper bound estimate involves dropping all cases that lack information about mothers. Column 2 provides further estimates that broaden the already inclusive definition of participation. Here the strategy of the census takers of 1851 and 1861 to include the wives of farmers, inn, beer and lodging house keepers, shop keepers, shoemakers and butchers as active by dint of their husbands' work is adopted (see McKay, 1998). This definition yields two further estimates of participation according to whether mothers about whom there is little information are included as in active or excluded from the analysis.[7] Requiring reference to specific economic activity and assuming inactivity as the default gives rise to the lowest estimate in column 1, while the inclusion in addition of wives as active through their husband's occupation and the exclusion of uncertain cases from the analysis provide the highest estimates in column 2 (see table 1 below).

Between 30.5 and 46.1 percent of the autobiographers' mothers were economically active according to the definition of activity and the strategy with respect to shadowy information. These estimates lie above computations from the earliest reliable censuses of 1851 and 1861, which of course not only relate

6 Mothers who died in childhood are retained.

7 Mothers with no individual occupational designation and about whom the autobiographers said little may be counted as active in the extended definition by dint of their husbands' occupations.

Table 1. Participation of Married Women by Husbands' Broad Occupational Group (Sample Sizes in Parentheses)

	Participation percent (sample size)	Participation including by dint of husbands' occupation percent (sample size)
All mothers	30.5–36.6 (606–505)	41.6–46.1 (606–505)
All mothers with husbands' occupation known	32.6–38.4 (549–466)	44.8–48.7 (549–466)
Husbands' occupations		
Agriculture	30.8–36.9 (133–111)	58.7–59.5 (133–111)
Mining	21.6–25.6 (51–43)	21.6–25.6 (51–43)
Factory	41.7–45.5 (36–33)	41.7–45.5 (36–33)
Domestic manufacturing	45.8–52.4 (72–63)	56.9–61.9 (72–63)
Trades	26.5–33.8 (98–77)	30.6–37.7 (98–77)
Casual	47.5–52.8 (40–36)	47.5–52.8 (40–36)
Clerical	12.5–15.4 (16–13)	12.5–15.4 (16–13)
Soldiering	41.7–45.5 (12–11)	41.7–45.5 (12–11)
Sea	26.7–28.6 (30–28)	26.7–28.6 (30–28)
Services	31.1–37.3 (61–51)	60.7–64.7 (61–51)
Widows	31.9–32.6 (97–95)	n.a.
Deserted wives	52.3–56.1 (44–41)	n.a.

Notes: For the definition of participation and treatment of missing values see text. Differences by husbands' occupational group are statistically significant for both definitions of participation and both samples. Differences according to whether or not husbands were living are not significant in either sample. Differences according to husbands' presence are statistically significant in both samples.

to a snapshot in time and likely undercount women's spasmodic engagement but also are based on the population as a whole and not just the working class (for comparable evidence extracted from the nineteenth-century censuses, see Humphries, 1996; McKay, 1998; Anderson, 1999). For reference, the 1861 census returned 24 percent of married women under other occupations including the wives of 402473 farmers, inn, beer and lodging house keepers, shop keepers, shoemakers and butchers (Parliamentary Papers, 1863).

However the estimates based on the autobiographies are consistent with, though perhaps a little below, other estimates of working-class married women's participation rates from pre-census sources (see Horrell and Humphries, 1994; Earle, 1983). What might seem surprising is that mothers in these working-class families participated so sparingly in the burgeoning economy (but see Richards, 1974 for an early conclusion along similar lines).

According to the estimates from the autobiographies, participation of married women changed little over the course of the Industrial Revolution.[8] However participation does appear to vary with fathers' broad occupational group in ways consistent with the conventional wisdom as can be seen from table 1, which reports both upper and lower bound estimates by occupational group, along with the relevant sample sizes.[9] The wives of soldiers and casual workers, some of the lowest-paid and least reliable male workers were forced more upon their own resources. The wives of factory workers and domestic manufacturers had relatively high participation rates too. They enjoyed a robust market for their labour, the latter being able to contribute within a domestic setting. In contrast, miners' wives, likely resident in areas with few opportunities for married women, had low participation rates. The participation rates of women married to agricultural workers, domestic manufacturers and men in service occupations are boosted by including as active the wives of farmers, inn, beer and lodging house keepers, shop keepers, shoemakers and butchers whether or not their sons acknowledged their productive activity. The ranking of wives' participation rates by husbands' occupational group is consistent with the ranking of wives' participation by husbands' occupation

8 Time trends were statistically insignificant even when controlling for other possible explanatory variables.

9 The variation in participation by husbands' occupational group does not distort the aggregate picture as the sample occupational structure is broadly consistent with overall trends in the male labour force (see Humphries, forthcoming).

on the basis of household accounts (see Horrell and Humphries, 1995) and detailed exploration of census enumerators' books (see Anderson, 1999).

Sample sizes are too small to support an analysis by cohort and fathers' broad occupational group. But for relatively large occupational groups, variation in mothers' participation rates reflects patterns seen in data from other sources. For example, women in factory districts showed steadily increasing participation while domestic workers' wives' participation remained high throughout the period (for comparison see Horrell and Humphries, 1997).

Significantly too married women's participation rates varied according to the presence or absence of husbands. One surprising result is that widows' participation rates were not significantly different from married women with husbands present, in contrast to the much higher participation rates of mothers whose husbands were not present though probably still living. It may be that widows were older than were other lone mothers or that the Poor Law treated these women differently thus affecting their labour supply. Direct observation of poor relief supports the latter conjecture (see Humphries, 1998).

How were the majority of economically inactive wives and mothers regarded? Occasionally such women were thought dependent even burdensome, 'very helpless' as one anonymous chimney boy (born 1834) put it (Anon, 1901: 19). Much more commonly they were seen through their domestic efforts as doing the best they could for their families. Husbands and fathers almost without exception remained detached from these efforts as Emmanuel Lovekin's (born 1820) eloquently if ungrammatically makes clear. His mother was 'a big strong woman and not cast down with a little thing but strugled (sic) through with a family of seven sons and tow daughters [...] with a man that did not seem to take very little interest in home matters' (Lovekin, no date, p. 1).

When mothers were economically active, their returns were often pitifully small. The convenience of working at home or from home crowded their labour into a few badly paid occupations. George Acorn's (born 18?) mother made matchboxes at home, the archetype sweated labour, for 'a paltry two pence-farthing a gross complete!' (Acorn, 1911: 36). Daniel Chater's (born 1870) mother took work home from a local shirt factory, being paid 2½d per dozen and she had to find her own cotton (Chater, n.d.: 6). In agricultural districts, the seasons gave mothers' money-making activities a natural rhythm; times of demand for labour left them with aching backs, but spread over the whole year, earnings were small. Only in the textile districts was relatively well-paid and regular work available and then only to those mothers who could combine factory hours with childcare and domestic work (see McKay, 1998; Anderson, 1999).

Children's Economic Roles

But if the autobiographies reveal perhaps surprisingly low married women's participation, they also point up perhaps surprisingly high children's participation. The majority of autobiographers pinpointed the age at which they started work. In a number of additional cases, it was possible to identify age at starting work from contextual information. In only 97 cases (16 percent) was age when work began indeterminate. To illustrate trends over time, the autobiographical data was sub-divided into four cohorts according to the birth date of the memoirist.[10] Looking only by birth cohort, age at starting work first fell then rose as shown in table 2 below. Formal testing suggests that this degree of variation is unlikely to have occurred as a result of sample fluctuation.[11]

Table 2. Age at Starting Work by Cohort

Cohort	Median	Mean	Sample size	Standard deviation
≤1790	12.00	11.47	85	2.84
1791–1820	10.00	10.32	122	2.59
1821–1850	10.00	9.99	141	2.58
1851–1874	12.00	11.38	156	2.34
Total	11.00	10.75	504	2.63

10 The first open-ended cohort includes all boys born before and during 1790 (19% of the sample), the second those born between 1791 and 1820 (24% of the sample), the third those born between 1821 and 1850 (28% of the sample) and the fourth those born between 1851 and 1875 when the sample ends (27% of the sample). There are 9 boys whose date of birth is unknown (1% of the sample) but context allows two of these to be placed in a birth cohort. Dropping those cases where age at starting work is unknown leaves these proportions practically unchanged (17%, 24%, 28%, 31% and 1%).

11 The inverse U shape is not the product of the particular chronological subdivision adopted. A number of curve-fitting exercises confirm that a quadratic equation provides the best fit with age at starting work falling until around 1800 when it slowly began to increase.

The second and third cohorts of children that lived through the Industrial Revolution were more likely to be at work than were the same age children in the previous generation.[12] Only for the cohort born after 1851 was there a clear increase in the age at starting work as the clustered bar chart below shows. But even for this generation, child labour was not some dinosaur that rapidly became extinct. The nature of children's jobs may have changed, very young working ceased, and limitations on hours was more successfully enforced, but almost half of the children were at work by the age of eleven even after 1850. Industrializing Britain was not a peasant society and working children may not always have covered their own subsistence but neither were they 'burdensome' as Woods (1992) contended.

Figure 1. Participation by Age

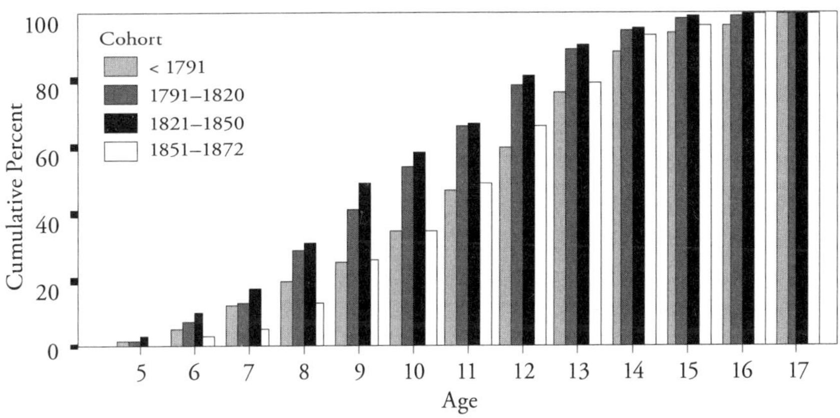

12 Does this increasing likelihood of early working during the middle periods of the Industrial Revolution capture a real trend or simply reflect other differences across the cohorts? Humphries (forthcoming) argues that the sample of autobiographies represents the population of boys in each phase of the Industrial Revolution. Their family circumstances and fathers' occupational affiliation for example are shown to vary but more or less in line with the changes known to have affected the population overall. Moreover on the basis of a very different type of information Horrell and Humphries (1995) concluded that the 1820s and 30s saw an increase in child participation rates and younger children at work.

By the time boys in the sample were ten years old their activity rates exceeded those of their mothers.

The scene in which boys brought their first wages home to contribute to the family purse constitutes a set-piece in working-class memoir. Boys surrendered their wages not to their fathers but almost always to their mothers whose loving and proud observance crowned the act of giving. William Rawstron (born 1874) 'well remembered' his mother when he proudly put his first week's wage of 3/- in her hand 'reckoning to spit on it' (Rawstron, 1954: 14). Moreover children's earnings almost without deduction found their way into the family exchequer. There was no regular top-slicing or even occasional withholding as with men's pay packets and the income was for mothers to dispose of. There were no strings attached.

Not only did mothers command children's earnings, they also frequently found children their first job and ensured their punctuality and performance. Jack Goring's (born 1861) mother, for example, had been employed in the service of a celebrated bread and biscuit maker, and when Jack left school she persuaded them to take him on (Goring, n.d.). When the job proved uncongenial, Mrs. Goring helped him to persist until something better came up. Protective labour legislation did not stop these mothers if their children's employment seemed the optimal family strategy. As George Cooper (born 1824) put it: 'The crux in those days was for us young people to pass the doctor. Our mothers used to pad our feet in order to add an inch to our stature' (Cooper, n.d. no pagination).

Children's work was regular in comparison with the work patterns of their mothers. The reliability of their earnings must have been attractive. Frank Forrest's (born 1816) father was transported and the family forced to migrate to Dundee in search of work for his mother and the children. Mrs. Forrest wound pirns for handloom weavers at home, working long hours but on her own schedule, while Frank worked from six in the morning until 9 or 10 at night in the spinning mills (Forrest, 1850). Nor was agricultural work necessarily intermittent. William Arnold's (born 1860) first job was scaring crows, a seasonal task. But for William and probably many of his peers it dovetailed with other agricultural work (Arnold, 1915).

Thus children were important secondary earners within working-class families, supplementing the resources provided by fathers in most families and taking the place of fathers in female-headed households. This finding corroborates earlier independent evidence on the sources of working-class family incomes (Horrell and Humphries, 1993). How did child labour impact upon the economic participation of mothers? Did children substitute for mothers in the labour market or could mothers' efforts to earn allow children to be withheld from the labour market?

In fact, mothers' economic participation was a complement and not a substitute for boys' early working. For the sample for which there is information on age at starting work and mothers' participation, boys whose mothers were economically active on average started work at a younger age (10.45 years) than did boys whose mothers remained at home (10.90 years), a difference that was statistically significant (t-statistic = 1.86, significance level = .063). Clearly mothers' economic efforts signaled the need of households while their earnings were insufficient to protect sons from the pressures of poverty. Even restricting attention to households where husbands were present, the age at starting work was lower for boys with active mothers. Moreover although schooling and work were not always alternatives in the period under review, a similar relationship holds between mothers' economic activity and years of schooling. Active mothers had sons with lower schooling attainments, 2.30 years on average, than mothers who worked only in the home, whose sons went to school for 2.58 years on average (t-statistic = 2.27, significance level = .023). Nor apparently could sons relieve economic pressures on mothers by starting work. In households where sons started work younger than average 36.2 percent of mothers were at work while in households where sons started work older than average 28.8 percent of their mothers were at work.[13]

Thus relatively precocious child labour and working mothers were concentrated in the same sub-set of presumably poorer families. This complementarity extended to mothers combining with their own children to engage in self-provisioning and home-working activities (see above, p. 121). But by the time boys were 10 years old their participation rates exceeded those of their mothers suggesting that children were a more common source of earning power than mothers. Even where mothers were not economically active, 55 percent of families at some stage contained a working child aged eleven or younger.

The evidence from the autobiographies supports the hypothesis that the dominant family strategy involved sending children rather than their mothers out to work (for census evidence corroborating this point, see Anderson,

13 T-stat. = 1.76; sig. level = .079.

1999). It was rare for mothers to seek employment if they had sons over ten at home not employed. Thomas Cooper's (born 1805) mother worked explicitly so that he might continue with his education. But this response, made possible by Thomas's status as an only child and Mrs. Cooper's enterprise, was clearly unconventional and frowned upon by their community (Cooper, 1872). Frank Galton's (born 1967) family labour supply was more conventional, Mrs. Galton only entered the labour market in a severe family crisis and then after her two older boys aged 11 and 13 were already working (Galton, n.d.).

Families' apparent preferences for sending children rather than mothers out to work must have reflected a rational response to earnings opportunities relative to the value of family members' time in the home, with comparisons refracted of course through perceptions of respectable behaviour. How did boys' wages compare with those of adult women? Age-earnings profiles for males and females in farm and factory work suggest that teenage boys could earn as much as 40-year-old women in farm work in the nineteenth century (Burnette, 2005). In textile factory work they lagged further behind, but could still earn between 60 and 70 percent of an adult female daily wage (Boot, forthcoming). Such differentials could be easily offset by children's ability to work more regularly than their mothers.

The comparative advantages of children in the labour market are well illustrated by cases introduced above. Frank Forrest's mother, who lacked the skills and confidence to get factory work, could earn only 3s 3d per week from winding pirns though she worked from 5 o'clock in the morning until 9 or 10 at night. Frank's first job in the mill paid 1s 6d but before he was 12 it had risen to 3s 6d. William Arnold earned 1s 6d a week crow scaring (plus all he could eat for Sunday dinner), enjoyed a 6d a week rise on the acorn harvest, and was up to 2s 6d by the end of the agricultural year, the regular mid-century wage for plough boys. But he really moved up the pay ladder as a sprigging boy when he regularly earned between 3s and 4s a week. Before he was eleven William's wages were 12 shillings a week, almost as much as his father could earn 'with his big family to keep' and completely beyond the earnings capacity of Mrs. Arnold for all her strength and industry both in the fields and beside her husband's bench.[14] And even in textile communities where substitutability

14 At this time William lived as economically as possible to be able to give his mother money as 'at that time there were five or six little ones to be kept. My money was a wonderful help to mother, I knew' (Arnold, 1915: 31).

between mothers for sons in the labour market appears to have been a more economic proposition, it was not always seen as an optimal strategy. In 1859 when his father was unemployed, Joseph Burgess's mother 'had to turn out at half-past five in the morning to a weaving job' (Burgess, 1927: 26). Several circumstances made this option possible: his mother had been a weaver before her marriage and had skills and connections; a local child-minder was available to nurse the youngest child; and the family was surrounded by supportive kin including a maiden aunt who was 'a second mother' to Joseph and the other children (Burgess, 1927: 29). But when the next crisis hit the Burgess family, circumstances were different. Another Burgess had been born delicate which 'mother attributed to the diet of bread and treacle and the "Ten Hours a Day" work on which she had had to bear him' (Burgess, 1927: 29). Mrs. Burgess stayed home. Three months short of his seventh birthday Joseph started punching cards for Jacquard looms. Thus a combination of factors from employment opportunities to potential relative earnings and including the problems of substituting for mothers in the home meant that boys were preferred to mothers as secondary workers in family strategies.

Affective Relations

The economic structure of working-class households imprinted affective bonds between children and their parents. Most writers testified to their parents' care and affection. 'The first certainty in my mind is that my mother and my stepfather were parents as good as any boy could have desired', stated the future Baron Snell (born 1865) (1936: 5). A small minority told of neglect, even abuse. More common, however, was the view that parents did their best but poverty, unemployment, and hard times generally, blighted childhood. Although both fathers and mothers were generally held to have cared for their children, the relationships revealed in the autobiographies were powerfully gendered with important implications for understanding family life.

Fathers

Breadwinning took fathers out of and away from the home even in the eighteenth century, but increasingly so as the Industrial Revolution gathered momentum. This modern family form took a toll on the relationship between boys and their fathers, who were often distant and unfamiliar. George Healey (born 1823) reported: 'I cannot say much about my father, for he was a man who had to do much with those in high life. I was little under his care' (Healey, 1823: 1). Emanuel Lovekin (born 1820) ungrammatically but vividly conveyed the alienation of his father, describing him as '… a man that did not seem to take very little interest in home Matters' (Lovekin, n.d.: 1).

In the second half of the eighteenth century both the working day and working week became longer, separating early-industrial breadwinners from their families for longer and longer periods of time (Voth, 2000). Moreover in the nineteenth century, work was increasingly undertaken away from home in centralized and specialized workplaces or in distant locations where railways were being built, ports constructed or harvests brought in. The extent to which economic change demanded an increasingly mobile workforce and the effect this had in creating quasi-fatherless families has perhaps been overlooked. Construction workers for example spent long periods away from home. Even men in more settled jobs were forced by low wages in the agricultural sector or competition from factory production to work longer hours. George Hardy's (born 1886) father was an agricultural labourer in East Yorkshire. He worked 'twelve hours a day on the farm and then worked in the big gardens round our cottage until it was dark' (Hardy, 1956: 1).[15]

Soldiers, sailors and other men were forced by their jobs, the law, or financial embarrassments into long periods of absolute absence. Frank Forrest's (born 1816) benign childhood was shattered when his father was transported for killing a man in a drunken brawl. His mother tried to keep her family together but faced an unequal struggle. She and Frank's brother eventually perished in a cholera epidemic leaving him alone. His relationship with his father was destroyed forever. Forrest senior, after remarrying (bigamously?) and fathering additional children, never reconnected with his surviving child even when he returned to Scotland having served his sentence (Forrest, 1850).

15 Healy is not included in the data analysis given his post-1875 birth date.

Politics too could draw fathers away. Walter Freer's (born 1846) father was a chartist, imprisoned for his radical beliefs, and preoccupied by politics. As a result his son barely knew him. 'To me my father remains a misty and somewhat mysterious being …' (Freer, 1929: 19).

There were boys who were close to their fathers but strong emotional ties often rested on some quirk of circumstance that threw them together in opposition to respectable society. The fierce affection exhibited by John Wilson (born 1835/6?) for his father was founded on the latter's determination following the death of his wife to keep his son close by and deepened by the hardships they shared while on the road together (Wilson, 1910).

Beyond the benign neglect born of their breadwinner role, some fathers descended into unkindness and even cruelty. Significantly, as in modern times (Gelles, 1979), intolerable physical violence was almost always accompanied by a simultaneous falling short of the breadwinner standard. The anonymous King of the Norfolk Poachers (born c. 1860) despised his father, who struggling to meet the standard of sole provider, substituted petty domestic tyranny for the legitimate authority that would have flowed automatically from economic provision (Anon, 1982). Abusive fathers were often drunkards, and alcoholism and misuse were often a prelude to the worst betrayal of all, the complete abrogation of the breadwinner role: desertion. John Edward Reilly (born 1860?) who grew up in the workhouse began bitterly: 'I have no recollection of a mother, but many recollections of a father and drink, and at an early age I was handed over to the care of the Guardians of an institution where we were under law and not under Grace' (Reilly, 1931: 9).

The testimonies to a handful of abusive fathers should not be taken out of proportion. Their incidence in what may well be a representative British sample lies between 2–4 percent, a much lower frequency than in autobiographies by European workers (Maynes, 1995). Physical force did not constitute a stable self-reinforcing system of familial control especially if it had to be applied by men who were neither continuously nor regularly on the scene. Abuse signaled the last gasp of a bankrupt patriarch and was bound to breed rebellion in sons who had time on their side. From the father's point of view violence was dominated by an alternative strategy, which was to abrogate responsibility and leave.

Unlike mothers, not only death removed fathers from their children's lives. They went to serve in the army, were press-ganged, were transported, worked away from home or simply deserted their responsibilities either before or after marriage.[16] Fathers who left their children to be supported by women alone or to the tender mercies of the overseers or guardians were hated. James Burn's (born c. 1802) moving comparison of his feelings for his stepfather and father illustrate the depth of the animosity. McNamee when drunk was abusive to little James but this was nothing compared with the pain inflicted by his biological father's initial desertion and subsequent indifference (Burn, 1978). Men who betrayed either families or pregnant women occur with more frequency than do fathers who abused their children. Given the physical and emotional toll breadwinning took, this low manifestation of irresponsibility must be the ultimate proof of fatherly devotion.

The majority of fathers were neither cruel nor particularly affectionate. They were decent men who as a result of economic exigencies spent much of their time away from home. When not about their work they were often exhausted or needed relaxation away at the pub. As the Industrial Revolution gathered momentum, work and home became increasingly separated and hours of work increasingly long (Voth, 2000). Working men, who had long found little time to spend in joint leisure or learning with their sons, saw their last opportunities for shared activities disappear, and they became increasingly remote figures.

Mothers

In contrast to the fathers, distanced from their sons by the exigencies of breadwinning, mothers were close and involved. Fathers fulfilled their role by 'providing' but mothers had to love, and according to their sons they almost to a woman did so. Sons rewarded fathers by respect, but mothers by devotion. Andrew Carnegie (born 1835) was almost choked with emotion when he wrote of his mother '… about whom I cannot trust myself to speak at length. […] Perhaps some day I may be able to tell the world something of this heroine, but I doubt it. I feel her to be sacred to myself and not for others to know' (Carnegie, 1920: 6).

It is possible that such effusive outpourings of filial devotion are merely stylized adoptions of Victorian artistic conventions. But their very excess seems

16 Not counting the 54 fathers about whom nothing is known, a further 51 were reported never present or hopelessly delinquent during their sons' minority, (8.4 percent).

to signal authenticity. Sometimes an autobiographer with a less hackneyed style broke through the conventions. But his point was the same: a deep and abiding love for his mother. The King of the Norfolk Poachers (born c. 1860) painted a grim picture of a childhood regimented by authority and religion relieved only by a mother who was 'quite the reverse of that' and concluded simply 'God Bless her' (Anon, 1982: 4).

What prompted such devotion? Mothers, though their economic efforts could be crucial in crises, were not the economic mainstays of their families. When forced, their efforts were cited as testimony of motherly love. George Acorn (born 18?) was one of the few writers to criticize his mother. He nonetheless records her efforts to support the family by making matchboxes when an accident to his father rendered him unable to work.

> My mother had never appeared to be particularly tender, and it was a revelation to me, this unfolding of the great, loving, maternal instinct. She would work like one possessed, her dexterous fingers moulding box after box almost too quickly for the eye to follow – and all for a paltry two-pence farthing a gross complete! (Acorn, 1911: 36)

Mothers were particularly commended for their attempts to earn because it was acknowledged that these went above and beyond the call of duty and women by and large were ill-prepared for the challenge.

Lone mothers in particular were extolled for their efforts in holding their families together. Their unmistakable greater frequency in comparison with lone fathers testifies to women's more dogged resistance to family breakup and in particular to alienation from their children. Attempts to cling on to an even unsatisfactory breadwinner might have been economically rational for many women, since their allowance from his wage might well have topped their own ability to earn (see Wall, 1994). But single-handedly raising a family even with help from other kin and poor relief was surely harder than renouncing children and going it alone even in the female-unfriendly labour market of early industrial Britain. After all a woman alone could hope to remarry a prospect that was much less likely if she had children to support.

While celebrated mothers' economic support was neither the primary manifestation of maternal love nor the taproot of boys' devotion. In the eyes of the autobiographers, just as important was the creation of domestic comfort. As shown above the majority of mothers devoted themselves to home-making even when their families were very poor and were thought no less of for so doing. Housework was an enormous task in the eighteenth and nineteenth centuries when families were large, housing poor and domestic equipment rudimentary. Women's struggles against dirt were celebrated with almost as much frequency as their struggles against want, suggesting the error that is made in overlooking the contribution of cleanliness to comfort. In the autobiographers' times, a family's wellbeing was closely associated with a mother's ability to transform earnings into food, clothing and shelter; a good manager could work wonders, a bad one could wreak havoc. Harry Snell's (born 1865) mother does not appear to have worked outside the home but she was celebrated alongside his provident stepfather. Snell gave his reasons.

> I have never known or heard of anyone who excelled her in forethought and matronly concern for those dependent upon her. My stepfather used teasingly to insist that her frugal hands could spread a pound of butter over the whole of the neighbouring churchyard and then have sufficient left to cover the gravestones on both sides (Snell, 1936: 4).

The wellbeing of children hung on the ability to stretch the wage, to conjure tasty and nourishing meals out of nothing much, to squirrel away resources for a pair of winter boots. The breadwinner's needs could not be gainsaid; they were a fixed charge on earnings. The mother's 'scratting and scraping' (Hardy, 1956: 10) was done for the children. Food for example was something that mothers provided and many of the grown up writers remembered its vital importance in their childhood vistas. Running through the autobiographies like a golden thread, cheering up all but the most-bitter experiences, were memories of good meals conjured up by caring mothers. Similarly when children were ill or infirm, it was mothers who nursed them and were their immediate source of relief sometimes at great cost to themselves. Mrs. Arch's nursing skill reputedly saved her children's lives twice over (Arch, 1898). Children's illnesses cast new light on mothers hardened by deprivation. George Acorn (born 18?) described his generally bitter mother nursing her younger child, 'trying to still its fitful cries by strange, sweet, soothing invocations' while George and his father could only look on (Acorn, 1911: 35).

Mothers loomed large not only for their provision of food and care when ill. They were for almost all boys the abiding presence of childhood. An unintended consequence of the nascent division of labour between husbands and wives was that children were not only alienated from their fathers; they were thrown together and identified with their mothers. Mothers had the flexibility in their household role to nurture, read to, teach and even play with their children. 'Mothers often have more to do with the training of children than fathers, for they are more under the mother's eye …' (Smith, 1870: 176). A great deal rested on mothers' performance.

Despite the tone of many autobiographies, mothers were not all saints and some resorted to physical chastisement. Theirs was the responsibility of order in the home and where corporal punishment was applied it was more likely to be administered by the parent on hand and in charge. But while a father's violence was a serious experience, a mother's lashing was often represented as justly-deserved by a boisterous boy who had exhausted the patience of an overworked but nonetheless loving parent. Mothers were, of course, not as large or strong as fathers and so less able to hurt. Significantly, for mothers violence was a last resort. They controlled their sons in other ways, often ostentatiously vouchsafing corporal punishment. Roger Langdon (born 1825) had a father 'who […] acting upon King Solomon's advice, never spared the rod' (Langdon, 1909: 12). In contrast, his 'kind and loving mother […] did not smack me […] but she would call me and speak to me […] and somehow, whenever she spoke she was obeyed' (Langdon, 1909: 12).

Mothers tried to soften the hardships of their children's lives. Elizabeth Ashby, first an unmarried mother, then in quick succession a wife and widow, worked hard all her life in the fields and houses of her community to support herself and her children. Amazingly she still found time to read them the bible and helped model and play with little clay figures (Ashby, 1974). Elizabeth's action in this story introduces the final link in the unassailable bond between many mothers and sons: the sacrifices that the former made on behalf of the latter. Fathers sacrificed too in their daily struggle to earn enough to keep the family. But these sacrifices were at one remove from the child's experience. Only later might some autobiographers appreciate the toll that breadwinning took, understand the deadliness of the lead industry or the rigors of arctic whaling. On the other hand, mothers' sacrifices were part of everyday life, immediately visible, and indeed often ritualized. They ranged from abstention from all luxury to ostentatiously going without food or eating only after the rest of the family. Patrick Barclay's (born 1852) beloved mother showed 'untiring energy, unfailing health and hope and faith, and never a new dress, never a holiday, never any leisure or amusement, never I fear even a generous meal of victuals' (Barclay, 1934: 9).

The nature of the mother-son relationship as glimpsed through the autobiographies has important implications. Mothers, not fathers, were able to extract the support that their families needed from working children. Fathers lacked the emotional closeness that leavened duty while their very need to call upon their children manifested failure in their own paternal role. They could exact a levy by physical force but it was a fragile mechanism, certainly in comparison with the ties that bound boys to mothers. These latter bonds often held working-class families together both economically and emotionally. Edward Davis (born 1828) suffered a childhood of unremitting toil while ill-fed and clothed owing mainly to the 'intemperance and irregular habits' of his father. He describes the reception afforded him by his mother after very long working days in the Birmingham toy trades:

> … on reaching home my dear mother would meet me with a kiss, wipe my face, and say how it troubled her that my brother and I were compelled to go to work so young; but we have the deep satisfaction of knowing that it was not through any fault of her's that we were forced to go through so much privation for she was our "good angel" in the home, and the one on whom we all had to lean (Davis, 1898: 9).

After several years in the labour force, aged about ten, Edward had a chance of a coveted post in a confectioners' bakeshop. His father's opposition on the grounds that it paid less than Edward's current job would maybe not have held him back but the master wanted him to live in. In view of conditions at home, Edward felt that this 'would have been the best thing for me'. But he could not only think about himself 'My mother depended a great deal upon me at that time, and I would not leave her' (Davis, 1898: 8). 'Trying to make the best of this disappointment' Edward, like so many boys of his time, soldiered on.

Mothers, Children and Family Size

The economic and emotive ties that secured the survival of working-class families emerge clearly from the autobiographies. Sustained contributions by fathers were essential if the families were to avoid poverty and obtain a modicum of security. But support from this quarter was not always reliable. It is useful to put this insecurity into historical context.

Many of the autobiographers' fathers died while they were still young although the boys in the sample were not any more unlucky in this respect than the population as a whole in these high-mortality times (Humphries, forthcoming). In the eighteenth century Britain fought several major wars with a number of countries, and such bellicose times had unsettling effects on family stability. Men who had served in the forces did not always come home when they were de-mobilized. Many of course were dead. Greenwood estimated that loss of life among servicemen was proportionally as high between 1794 and 1815 as between 1914 and 1918 and acknowledged that behind this frightening calculation was the unknown human sorrow and human suffering of families swept up in the war (Greenwood, 1942; see also Wrigley and Schofield, 1981: 221). If many men could not return to their breadwinning duties, others chose to default. As the autobiographies again show, a significant minority of men could not be kept in line by either ties of affection or duty, and de-camped. Deserted wives and families were a commonplace feature of pre- and early industrial England (Outhwaite, 1981; Stone, 1977; Snell, 1985). The temptation to shirk responsibility was perhaps exacerbated by new forms of work and structural changes that weakened family ties by taking men away from home and distancing them from their families, and by the new opportunities to simply disappear in an increasingly mobile and even global population (see also Kent 1990).

Even if fathers did not abscond, as the autobiographers have shown, their wages were not always devoted to supporting their families. Setting drunkards aside, many other men regarded it as acceptable for them to top-slice their earnings to smoke and drink. Others even if they worked hard and long and gave up their earnings in their entirety, could not as their sons often said 'keep the wolf from the door'. Of course when fathers were ill or unemployed, these problems multiplied.

Families responded to these pressures in a variety of ways. As we have seen mothers could be energetic and enterprising, but their main strategy was to stretch the resources coming into the household by more careful management or by increasingly desperate self-provisioning activities. Where possible they resorted to wage labour themselves but such a response was conditional on both local employment opportunities for married women and the availability of a substitute in the home. The more common response to either endemic economic pressure or a family crisis was to send a child out to work or engineer a higher paying (and harder?) job for an existing child worker. Children were the flexible resource in these households and not surprisingly they were mobilized according to need, and one primary source of need was a large sibling group.

A big family was a millstone around the necks of working men and women. Alan Davenport (born 1775) described his father as 'occupied in one continued struggle, having nothing but the products of his daily labour to provide for himself and his numerous family, six boys and four girls' (Davenport, 1986: 10). Infant and child mortality reduced the burden for some albeit in the cruelest way. 'There was a wonderful large family of us – eleven was born, but we died down to six' reported Bill H___ (born circa 1820) with grim humour (H____, 1862, p. 3). The death of George Acorn's brother allegedly 'really lightened our burdens for a while' (Acorn, 1911: 40).

But not only mothers and fathers suffered. Where children were numerous resources had to be shared around, and this could become hard if they were limited. At its simplest level more brothers and sisters meant smaller shares of food. Edward Davis (born 1828) with an intemperate father and many siblings, early noted that 'everything in our home seemed to be more sparingly served out than in our neighbours' (Davis, n.d.: 1). Boys were not backward in recognizing the negative effect that new babies had on their own diet. Benjamin Brierley (born 1825?) gave such sibling rivalry a humorous turn. 'Before I was of sufficient age to be sent to school I had a brother born. I did not give him the heartiest welcome, as I had fears that he might claim joint possession of my spoon. I hated the sight of "Owd Jacky Wife" for bringing him into the world …' (Brierley, 1886: 3). But Francis Crittall (born 1860) found no room for comedy. His father's business was quite successful and

> with a moderately-sized family he might have been comfortably off. But with ten children his means were sadly inadequate to provide anything but the plainest living […] In all my boyhood I cannot recall ever having eaten more than one good meal a day […] For breakfast and for tea there was an unvarying diet of bread, with butter spread on it as lightly as a butterfly's kiss (Crittall, 1934: 9–10).

Schooling was another item likely to fall by the wayside in large families. The only schooling Abraham Holroyd (born 1815) obtained was at the expense of his grandfather as his parents were 'too poor to do anything, as they had four little ones all younger than myself' (Holroyd, 1892: 10). And if large numbers of siblings crowded out schooling they crowded in early and onerous employment. Davis (born 1828) again was only six years and eight month old when 'compelled to join the ranks of the breadwinners of the family' (Davis, 1898: 6). Moreover the pressure on any one child of large numbers of siblings needing support meant that opportunities for advancement could not be seized if they involved a short-run cut in earnings. Thus Davis was not able to take up a coveted opportunity to work in a confectioner's bakeshop because it involved a cut in wages that his large family could ill-afford. The pressures on him finally abated when 'each member of the family grew old enough to work, they had to go, and this enabled us to fill our cupboard better than it had ever been before' (Davis, 1898: 10).

The inverse relationship between family size and both educational and economic outcomes is clear in the data (see table 3 below). Among boys for whom both ages at starting work and total numbers of siblings are known, only children appear to have had a signal advantage. The 30 only-children started work aged 11.92 while the 355 boys who had one or more siblings started work aged 10.61, a difference that is unlikely to have occurred by chance. Moreover advantage is also apparent comparing boys with only one sibling and boys with two or more. In fact as the table shows the advantages of children in smaller sibling groups persist until comparison is between boys with fewer than five and boys with five or more siblings. Even then the means continue to suggest disadvantage but it is not statistically significant. Total numbers of children in the family remains a statistically significant determinant of age at starting work, in a multivariate analysis (see Humphries, forthcoming).

Birth order, unfortunately not sufficiently frequently recorded in the autobiographies to support quantitative analysis, appears to have had ambiguous implications.[17] Eldest children sometimes appear to have obtained a head start, to have enjoyed some education and established strong ties with parents, before numbers of siblings arrived to strain the family exchequer and distract fathers and mothers. On the other hand, younger children often benefited from the contributions of working older siblings. Often children were marched into the labour force in rank order. In fact middle children seem anecdotally to have been at greatest risk, a view enunciated by Harry Carter (born 1749). 'My oldest and my youngest brothers were brought up to good country scolars (sic), but the rest of my brothers with myself, as soon as we were able, obliged to work in order to contribute a little to help to support a large family …' (Carter, 1900: 3). The youngest in the family appear to have fared best. For one anonymous writer (born 1825) his birth rank overrode a factor that usually blighted life chances: illegitimacy.

17 For the 174 boys whose position in their families is known although age at starting work first fell and then rose with rank the differences are not statistically significant.

Table 3. Age at Starting Work and Schooling Duration by Size of Sibling Group

Number of siblings	Age at starting work (sample size)		Difference of means (significance)	Schooling duration (sample size)		Difference of means (significance)
≥1	10.61	(355)	1.3	2.45	(374)	.426
=0	11.91	(30)	(.009)	2.88	(32)	(.066)
≥2	10.62	(319)	.55	2.44	(334)	.257
<2	11.17	(66)	(.089)	2.69	(72)	(.132)
≥3	10.50	(273)	.72	2.40	(291)	.309
<3	11.22	(112)	(.015)	2.69	(115)	(.033)
≥4	10.50	(228)	.51	2.36	(246)	.307
<4	11.01	(157)	(.063)	2.67	(160)	(.021)
≥5	10.51	(189)	.40	2.35	(201)	.266
<5	10.91	(196)	(.137)	2.62	(205)	(.041)
≥6	10.48	(153)	.39	2.32	(165)	.272
<6	10.86	(232)	(.162)	2.59	(241)	(.040)
≥7				2.34	(132)	.210
<7				2.55	(274)	(.131)

> I was, however, perhaps better situated than many illegitimate children are; for as the elder members of the family were all early obliged to go into service for their own livelihood, and also for the sake of assisting my mother, it was of course, natural that I should come in for an ordinary share of what was going (Anon., 1857).

Thus the famous family life cycle pressed down not on fathers, whose activity rate and work intensity was already high, or mothers who could rarely contribute much to their families' coffers by the kind of economic activities available to them. Instead the burden fell on the children, particularly the older children, of the household. They were forced to work early and hard and their burdens only diminished as their younger siblings joined the ranks. Thus Edward Davis (born 1828) significantly the oldest surviving son in his family, finally felt less pressure when he was about 15 and 'each member of the family grew old enough to work, they had to go, and this enabled us to fill our cupboard better than it had ever been before' (1898: 10).

In the eighteenth century, a variety of factors likely operated to disguise the bitter burden of younger on older children. Infant and child mortality remained high and in the cruelest possible way reduced dependency (Wrigley, et al., 1997). Schooling was not readily available and its effect on life time earnings uncertain (Mitch, 1992). Parents could be excused from thinking that a child's as well as their family's interests were best served by early work experience. But in the period under review, as well as marking each family's individual life cycle, intra-family dependency, like many of the other sources of pressure, experienced a climacteric. In the early nineteenth century population growth pushed the dependency rate to historically unprecedented levels. At the micro level this fed through to larger families and sibling groups. Even after 1860 when the numbers of children born in working families began to fall, child survival rates moved to offset this decline and maintain the pressures in many households (Stevenson, 1920). At the same time, the availability of and attitudes to education began to change. Children denied education by early working and family pressure were increasingly seen as deprived. In many mid-nineteenth century memoirs early working because of family need is seen as crowding out the education that mothers wanted for their sons and condemning them to a lifetime of toil and low productivity. An incident from a late autobiography illustrates a mother's regret.

Robert Watchorn's (born 1858) mother was a Derbyshire coal-miner's wife and as such enjoyed no opportunity to contribute to the family's income. Moreover as Robert recalled in 1869 there were six other children in his family, only one older than himself. His father worked hard but his wage was insufficient to 'provide ordinary comforts' especially as Watchorn senior did not forgo a breadwinner's levy, which he spent in the 'Swan and Salmon'. Robert's older brother, already at work, made a 'helpful' but on its own inadequate contribution. Mrs. Watchorn's 'painful reluctance' in withdrawing Robert from school to work in the pit was undoubtedly genuine. Her sobbing 'not only audible and deep, but terribly upsetting' was 'one of those incidents in one's life that are unforgettable'. In the set piece where Robert proudly gave her his first wages, the conflict between the family's needs and her aspirations for her cherished second son, along with resentment towards her insensitive husband all tumble together.

> She turned the coins over and over, time after time, like one playing a game of some sort of solitaire, but seriously pensive all the while; and the big, bright, pearl-like tears hung like dew drops from her eyelashes. Then quietly she rose and walked over to the table and, laying the five shillings down there, she just sobbed "Bobbie! This is like coining your body and soul painfully cheap". I had never before heard her utter a word of complaint about the failings of others, but she returned from my embrace to the coins on the table, and with a deep sign remarked, if your father had preferred to bring home his earnings in full, as you have now done, the "Swan and Salmon" might have prospered less, and you my darling Bobbie, might have been able to continue at school, as I so fondly desired (Watchorn, 1958: 18–19).

Robert Watchorn never opened his own pay packet until he was of legal age, became a member of the Band of Hope, sought to better his education at night school, and after emigrating continued to send remittances home to his mother, eventually moving his whole family to the US. When he married he had only two children.

Conclusions

The autobiographical recollections of working-class men shed light on hitherto unsatisfactory accounts of the fertility decline viewed through the lens of changes in the costs and benefits of children. Even before the beginning of the nineteenth century mothers and children constituted the core of the working-class family. Fathers were emotionally peripheral figures who straddled the family and a male world of work politics and religion. While their duty was to work as hard and long as possible to support their families, male responsibilities did not extend to stretching the wage to cover the variable demands of smaller or larger families. Moreover their own breadwinner share of the family's resources was immune to other claims. Thus they were ignorant of and insulated from the desperate redivision of scarce resources that additional children involved.

Mothers at the nub of this redivision were only too aware of the burden of additional mouths. Yet for them children were supports as well as burdens. Sons could not only earn more than their mothers, but surrendered their earnings willingly into their mothers' hands, motivated by ties of love as well as duty. The legitimacy of mothers' claims to these resources depended however on their scrupulous deployment in the interests of the family as a whole and more particularly in the interests of the children. In this way resources were transferred from older and stronger to younger and weaker siblings. Mothers managed these transfers and through them sought the survival of the family as a unit. Perhaps children's contributions to their families and support for their mothers took the edge off the latter's anxiety about family size. Nonetheless in cases where siblings were numerous and support from husbands and fathers uncertain the burden on children mounted. In the late eighteenth and early nineteenth centuries, population growth pushed the dependency rate to historically unprecedented levels. At the micro level this fed through to create a generation of ill-fed, unschooled and work-burdened children. In these relationships lie the clues to otherwise puzzling adverse trends in heights and to the (temporary) decline in literacy rates associated with industrialization.

These insights also illuminate the hitherto problematic chronology of fertility decline. The developing preference for smaller families did not depend on fathers' dawning recognition that late nineteenth-century children were increasingly burdensome bringing their views into congruence with their wives' long-standing preference. Instead it was based on the legacy of high fertility sharply experienced by mothers and children in the crucible of industrialization.

The autobiographers testify to mothers' attempts to protect children, to keep them in school or to try and obtain apprenticeships for them. But these attempts were hedged by familial needs and perhaps initially by the uncertainties about the returns to education. Moreover they often stopped short before the substitution of mothers for sons in the labour market, probably because mothers' comparative advantages remained in the home, especially where families were large. But the compact between mothers and their children rested on the former's abstemiousness, on mothers' sacrifice of consumption and leisure. In large families these sacrifices became oppressive. Although the voices of mothers are rarely directly heard, in the autobiographical evidence their sons speak for them. George Holyoke (born 1817) reflected.

> I had no business to be born at all, neither when I was, nor where I was, nor of whom I was – if without filial impiety I may say so […] My mother had many children; she reared eleven; but I soon came to see how much better it would have been for her – how much more enjoyment, peace, repose and freedom from anxiety would have fallen to her – had her family been limited to three or four children (Holyoke, 1896: 15).

As child labour disappeared and schooling became compulsory, the associated increased costs of children bore down not primarily on fathers whose efforts in breadwinning were already fully engaged but on mothers now bereft of their most important secondary source of support. Any perceived residual advantage of large families disappeared and pressures on mothers mounted as the stories that implicate them in attempts to evade child labour legislation suggest.[18]

Throughout the Industrial Revolution however it was not only mothers who felt the miseries of too many children. As the autobiographies show boys as well as girls in early-industrial families saw their own diets and schooling eroded by the appearance of additional children and, in the era before protective labour legislation, their own early entry into work prompted by the burden of dependency. It was as children that both men and women experienced first hand the miseries of large families. Their experiences as family members and child workers were recycled with a lag into new recognition of the costs of larger families and slowly and imperfectly into agreement about the preeminence of fertility control.

References

Acorn, George (1911), *One of the Multitude*, London, Heinemann.

Ammon, Charles George (n.d.), No Title, TS, Hull University Archive.

Anderson, Michael (1999), 'What Can the Mid-victorian Censuses Tell Us about Variations in Married Women's Employment?', *Local Population Studies*, 62, 9–30.

Anon. (1857), 'Life of a Blacksmith: Prize Autobiographies of Working Men', *The Commonwealth*, no. 7.

Anon. (1901), *The Life of a Chimney Boy: Written by Himself*, London, Charles H. Kelly.

Anon. (1982), *I walked by Night: By the King of the Norfolk Poachers*, edited by Lilias Rider Haggard, Oxford, Oxford University Press.

Arch, Joseph (1892), *Joseph Arch. The Story of His Life, told by Himself*, edited with a preface by Frances, the Countess of Warwick, London, Hutchinson and Co.

18 An analogous point is made by Robert Woods when he notes that the economic self interest of the household 'would be interpreted by the woman even if the level of its economic well-being was ultimately determined by the amount that could be earned by the man' (Woods, 1992: 206–7).

Arnold, William (1915), *Recollections of William Arnold*, with a preface by Henry Pickett and an introductory note by James Saxton, Northampton, privately printed.

Ashby, Joseph (1974), in Ashby, M. K., *Joseph Ashby of Tysoe, 1859–1919: A Study of English Village Life*, with an introduction by E. P. Thompson, London, The Merlin Press.

Bacon, Charles (1944–5), 'The Life Story of Charles Bacon (as told by himself)', TS, Leicester, Local Studies Library.

Bamford, Samuel (1967), *Early Days*, edited and with an introduction by W. H. Chaloner, London, Frank Cass & Co.

Barclay, Thomas Patrick (1934), *Memoirs and Medleys. The Autobiography of a Bottle-Washer*, edited by James K. Kelly, with a foreword by Sydney A. Gimson, Leicester, Edgar Backus.

Barr, David (1910), *Climbing the Ladder: the Struggles and Successes of a Village Lad*, London, Robert Culley.

Boot, H. M. and Maindonald, J. M. (2007), 'New Estimates of Age- and Sex-specific Earnings and the Male-Female Earnings Gap in the British Cotton Industry, 1833–1906', *Economic History Review*, forthcoming.

Brierley, Benjamin (1886), *Home Memories, and Recollections of a Life*, Manchester, Abel Heywood & Son.

Burgess, Joseph (1927), *A Potential Poet? His Autobiography and Verse*, Burgess Publications, Ilford.

Burn, James Dawson (1978), *The Autobiography of a Beggar Boy*, introduced by David Vincent, London, Europa.

Burnette, Joyce (2004), 'The Wages and Employment of Female day-Labourers in English Agriculture, 1740–1850', *Economic History Review*, 57, 664–690.

Carnegie, Andrew (1920), *Autobiography of Andrew Carnegie*, with a preface by John C. Van Dyke, London, Constable & Co. Ltd.

Carter, Harry (1894), *The Autobiography of a Cornish Smuggler (Captain Harry Carter, of Prussia Cove), 1749–1809*, edited with an introduction and notes by John B. Cornish, Joseph Pollard, Truro.

Chater, David (1950), 'Autobiography of Daniel Chater', TS, Hull, Brynmor Jones Library, Hull University.

Cooper, Thomas (1872), *The Life of Thomas Cooper. Written by Himself*, London, Hodder & Stroughton.

Cooper, George (1974), *George Cooper, Stockport's Last Town Crier, 1824–1895*, presented by Anne Swift.

Crittall, Francis Henry (1934), *Fifty Years of Work and Play*, London, Constable and Co.

Davenport, Allen (1986), *The Life and Literary Pursuits of Allen Davenport*, New York and London, Garland Publishing Inc.

Davis, Edward G. (1898), *Some Passages from My Life*, Birmingham, White & Pike Ltd.

Earle, Peter (1989), 'The Female Labour Market in London in the late Seventeenth and early Eighteenth Centuries', *Economic History Review*, 42, 328–54.

Emsley, J. W. (1901), *Social Questions and National Problems Their Evils and Remedies*, Bradford, Matthews and Brooke, Bradford.

Farish, William (1996), *The Autobiography of William Fairish. The Struggles of a Handloom Weaver. With Some of his Writings*, London, Caliban Books.

Freer, Walter (1929), *My Life and Memories*, Glasgow, Civic Press Ltd.

Forrest, Frank (1850), *Chapters in the Life of a Dundee Factory Boy. An Autobiography*, edited by James Myles, Edinburgh, Adam and Charles Black.

Galton, Frank Wallis (n.d.), 'Autobiography', MS., London, Department of Manuscripts, British Library of Political and Economic Science.

Gelles, Richard J. (1979), *Family Violence*, Beverley Hills, Sage.

Goring, Jack (n.d.), 'Autobiographical Notes', TS, London, Brunel University Library.

Greenwood, Major (1942), 'British Loss of Life in the Wars of 1794–1815 and in 1914–18', *Journal of the Royal Statistical Society*, 105, 1–11.

H--?---, Bill (1974), 'Autobiography of a Navvy', in Burnett, John (ed.), *Useful Toil. Autobiographies of Working People from the 1820s to the 1920s*, London, Allen Lane.

Hardy, Thomas (1985), *Jude the Obscure*, Harmondsworth, Penguin.

Hardy, Thomas (1832), *Memoir of Thomas Hardy, Founder of, and Secretary to, the London Corresponding Society, for Diffusing Useful Political Knowledge among the People of Great Britain and Ireland, and for Promoting Parliamentary Reform, From its Establishment, in Jan 1792, until his Arrest, on a False Charge of high Treason, On the 12th of May, 1794. Written by Himself*, London, James Ridgway.

Hardy, George (1956), *Those Stormy years. Memoirs of the Fight for Freedom on Five Continents*, London, Lawrence and Wishart.

Healey, James (1880), *Life and Remarkable Career of George Healey*, Birmingham, White and Pike.

Holroyd, Abraham (1892), 'Life of Abraham Holroyd', by William Scruton, from a manuscript provided by Mr. Holroyd to Mr. Scruton, in Forshaw, Charles F. (ed.), *Holroyd's Collection of Yorkshire Ballads*, London, George Bell and Sons., Ltd.

Holyoake, George Jacob (1907), *Sixty Years of an Agitator's Life*, London, T. Fisher Unwin.

Hopkinson, James (1968), *Victorian Cabinet maker: The Memoirs of James Hopkinson 1819–1894,* edited by Jocelyne Baty Goodman, London, Routledge and Kegan Paul.

Horrell, Sara and Humphries, Jane (1992), 'Old Questions, New Data, and Alternative Perspectives: Families' Living Standards in the Industrial Revolution', *Journal of Economic History*, 52, 849–90.

Horrell, Sara and Humphries, Jane (1995), 'Women's Labour Force Participation and the Transition to the Male-Breadwinner Family, 1790–1865', *Economic History Review*, 48, 89–117.

Horrell, Sara and Humphries, Jane (1997), 'The Origins and Expansion of the Male Breadwinner Family: The Case of Nineteenth-Century Britain', *International Review of Social History*, 42, 25–64.

Humphries, Jane (1990), 'Enclosures, Common Rights and Women: The Proletarianization of Families in Late Eighteenth and Early Nineteenth Century Britain', *Journal of Economic History*, 50, 17–42.

Humphries, Jane (1998), 'Female-headed Households in early Industrial Britain: The Vanguard of the Proletariat', *Labour History Review*, 63, 31–65.

Humphries, Jane (forthcoming), *Through the Mill: Child Labour in the British Industrial Revolution,* Cambridge, Cambridge University Press.

Kent, David A. (1990), '"Gone for a Soldier"; Family Breakdown and the Demography of Desertion in a London Parish, 1750–91', *Local Population Studies*, 45, 27–42.

Langdon, Roger (1909), *The Life of Roger Langdon, told by Himself. With Additions by his Daughter Ellen, with a preface by H. Clifton Lambert*, London, Elliot Stock.

Lovekin, Emmanuel (1994), 'Mining Butty' in Burnett, John (ed.), *Useful Toil. Autobiographies of Working People from the 1820s to the 1920s,* London, Routledge.

McKay, John (1998), 'Married Women and Work in Nineteenth Century Lancashire: The Evidence of the 1851 and 1861 Census Reports', *Local Population Studies*, 60, 25–37.

Marcroft, William (1886), *The Marcroft Family* Manchester, John Heywood.

Maynes, Mary Jo (1995), *Taking the Hard Road: Life Course in French and German Workers' Autobiographies in the Era of Industrialization*, Chapel Hill, University of North Carolina Press.

Mintz, Steven (1983), *A Prison of Expectations. The Family in Victorian Culture*, New York, New York University Press.

Mitch, David F. (1992), *The Rise of Popular Literacy in Victorian England: The Influence of Private Choice and Public Policy*, Philadelphia, University of Pennsylvania Press.

Outhwaite, B. R. (ed.) (1981), *Marriage and Society: Studies in the Social History of Marriage*, London, Europa.

Parkinson, Alison (2002), '"Marry – Stitch – Die or do Worse?" Female Self-employment and Small Business Proprietorship in London c. 1740–1880', Unpublished Phd Thesis, Oxford University, Oxford.

Place, Francis (1972), *The Autobiography of Francis Place, 1771–1854*, edited and with an introduction by Mary Thrale, Cambridge, Cambridge University Press, Cambridge.

Preston, Samuel H. (1976), 'Family Sizes of Children and Family Sizes of Women', *Demography*, 13, 105–114.

Price, Henry Edward (n.d.), 'My Diary', MS., Islington Public Library.

Rawstron, William L. (1954), 'Reminiscences', TS., Burnley and District Historical Society.

Reilly, Sarah A. (1931), *I Walk with the King. The Life Story of John Edward Reilly*, London, The Epworth Press.

Richards, E. (1974), 'Women in the British Economy since about 1700: An Interpretation', *History*, 59, 337–47.

Ricketts, Joseph (1965), 'Notes on the Life of Joseph Ricketts, Written by Himself c. 1858', *Wiltshire Archaeological and Natural History Magazine*, 60, 120–126.

Rymer, Edward Allen (1976), *The Martyrdom of the Mine, or 60 Years' Struggle for Life*, facsimilie reprint in 2 parts, edited and with an introduction by Robert G. Neville, *History Workshop Journal*, I and II, 220–244.

Seccombe, Wally (1990), 'Starting to Stop: Working-Class Fertility Decline in Britain', *Past and Present*, 126, 151–88.

Seccombe, Wally (1992), 'Reply', *Past and Present*, 134, 207–11.

Seccombe, Wally (1993), *Weathering the Storm. Working-Class Families from the Industrial Revolution to the Fertility Decline,* London, Verso.

Smith, Captain George (1870), *Won at Last or Memoirs of Captain George and Mrs. Hannah Smith of Bridlington Quay and York*, London, Elliot Stock.

Snell, K. D. M. (1985), *Annals of the Labouring Poor: Social Change and Agrarian England, 1660–1900*, Cambridge, Cambridge University Press.

Snell, Harry (Baron) (1936), *Men, Movements and Myself*, London, J.M. Dent and Sons, Ltd.

Stevenson, T. H. C. (1920), 'The Fertility of various Social Classes in England and Wales from the Middle of the Nineteenth Century to 1911', *Journal of the Royal Statistical Society*, 83, 401–32.

Stone, Lawrence (1977), *The Family, Sex and Marriage*, London, Weidenfeld and Nicholson.

Szreter, Simon (1996), *Fertility, Class and Gender in Britain, 1860–1940*, Cambridge, Cambridge University Press.

Tosh, John (1999), *A Man's Place: Masculinity and the Middle Class Home in Victorian England*, New Haven, Yale University Press.

Vincent, David (1981), *Bread, Knowledge and Freedom: A Study of Nineteenth-Century Working Class Autobiography*, London, Methuen.

Voth, Hans-Joachim (2000), *Time and Work in England, 1750–1830*, Oxford, Clarendon.

Wall, Richard (1994), 'Some Implications of the Earnings, Income and Expenditure Patterns of Married Women in the Populations in the Past', in Henderson, John and Wall, Richard (eds), *Poor Women and Children in the European Past*, London, Routledge, 312–35.

Wilson, John (1910), *Memories of a Labour Leader. The Autobiography of John Wilson JP MP*, with an introduction by the Dean of Durham and an appreciation by the Bishop of Durham, London, T. Fisher Unwin.

Woods, Robert (1992), 'Working Class Fertility Decline in Britain: Comment', *Past and Present*, 134, 200–07.

Wrigley, E. A. and Schofield, Roger (1981), *The Population History of England 1541–1871*, Cambridge, Cambridge University Press.

Wrigley, E. A., Davies, R. S., Oeppen, J. and Schofield, R. S. (1997), *English Population History from Family Reconstitution 1580–1837*, Cambridge, Cambridge University Press.

Education and Female Work Cultures in the Dutch Fertility Decline, 1880–1960

Angélique Janssens

Introduction

This article wants to contribute towards an examination of the role women played in shaping the demographic transition. It will in particular focus on the issue whether particular socio-economic groups of women were leading actors in changing fertility patterns. I assume that women, and especially working-class women, had specific interests in limiting fertility, given their responsibility for the family budget, and for feeding and clothing their children, and because of the heavy physical toll which large numbers of pregnancies and births exacted from their bodies and their health. The question then becomes under what circumstances women began to control and reshape their reproductive lives, and which historical circumstances or processes were leading women to adopt measures aimed at spacing or stopping births? In this contribution I will examine the claim that specific groups of working-class women through their experience in the paid labour market were better able to negotiate limitation of births and spousal cooperation. I will also look at the effect of female education on fertility behaviour. The effect of female education on fertility is well-known from contemporary demographic research in developing countries. The question is to what extent this effect can be determined for European countries in earlier periods as well.

Work Cultures and Education

A first set of hypotheses regarding women's role in the declining size of western families concerns the related issues of women's bargaining power within marriage and their access to information on sexuality and birth control strategies.

Limiting the size of one's family through either spacing or stopping presupposes not only a willingness to limit fertility and apply methods to space births or stop subsequent pregnancies once the required or maximum family size has been reached. It also requires contacts and knowledge about the means and about the places where these means might be bought and requested. According to the well-known thesis by Diana Gittins (1982), contraceptive knowledge amongst nineteenth- and early twentieth-century women was acquired and exchanged on shop floors and within factory walls. Unlike other women, more specifically those who did not have the opportunities for this type of intimate female exchanges before marriage, women working in industrial occupations or in office work would ultimately have smaller families. Gittins based her hypothesis on her oral history research amongst a group of English working-class women in the period 1900–1930.

However, the prevention of too many births, in addition, requires the cooperation of both husband and wife. In this respect Gittins suggested that the industrial work undertaken by the Lancashire female weavers in her study bolstered women's bargaining power vis-à-vis their husbands. Their industrial employment mostly brought women not only relatively high earnings but also the experience of working side by side with men. Thus, the absence of rigid gender divisions in the labour process would not only ensure a greater intimate bargaining power of women in marital relationships, but also engender the emergence of common goals and a common language between husbands and wives where it concerned family formation and the desired number of children. Gittins argued that women who had been working in isolated occupations before their marriage, for example as domestic servants, or women who did not have any experience in waged work, would remain not only ignorant of the means and methods to control fertility, they also would remain dependent upon their husbands' initiatives in this matter. The special position of the Lancashire female weavers and their families in the British fertility decline has recently been confirmed by Simon Szreter (1996).

The question however remains to what extent the 'Gittins thesis' may be generalised to other cohorts and to other historical contexts. In her book Gittins also argues that fertility outcomes are dependent upon a whole set of contextual and structural factors ranging from the structure of the local community, a husband's job security, the position of children and the interventions by state policies.

Serious disagreement exists concerning the question to what extent women at that time were aware of methods to regulate births and to what extent marital relationships allowed women to take an active lead in matters of sexuality. Recently, Kate Fisher (2000) has argued that English middle- and working-class women left their husbands in charge of sexual matters including the decision of when and how to use birth control. Moreover, methods to control births were mainly male methods, such as the use of condoms, abstinence, and withdrawal, so that male cooperation was a vital prerequisite. Fisher stresses the fact that any clear planning of births was wholly absent, and that matters of birth control were not at all discussed between couples. In the oral histories presented by Fisher, women appear to present themselves as largely ignorant where it concerns sexuality and birth control. The women interviewed by her all belonged to early twentieth-century birth cohorts and were forming their own families in the thirties and forties, or even fifties, of that century. A few important questions remain unclear however. First of all, we do not know to what extent these women were presenting themselves as they thought would fit in with the respectable, middle-class image of the good wife and mother without any sexual knowledge, rather than as an active partner in shaping their own families. Strong social norms and values of sexual prudishness for women in interwar Britain may have affected these particular cohorts of working-class women. Secondly, Fisher's work does not make it possible to decide to what extent ignorance and lack of female control in sexuality were equally impossible or difficult in earlier cohorts, in other social groups or geographical areas, or that her results are specific to English women in these particular cohorts.

Gittins' argument may be extended to include the differential effects of local male-dominated cultures in which women were kept away from the paid labour market. In that way, it might be argued, that widespread female participation in the paid labour market would produce local cultures in which birth control knowledge and contacts were likewise widespread and easy to access between family members, neighbours or old school friends. For the Netherlands, however, there is some unease concerning the Gittins thesis. Fertility levels remained very high in this country, primarily in the east and south of the country, which were also the regions where women participated in paid labour in larger numbers than in the west and north of the country. Industrialisation in the Netherlands came late, and was limited to specific towns in the south and the east of the country. Even compared to rural communities in the west and the north, the industrial towns in the south and east produced far higher birth rates right up to the 1960s. However, some differentials existed within and between the eastern and southern regions, both regarding fertility levels and the acceptability of industrial female labour. For, instance, the two major textile towns, Enschede (in the east) and Tilburg (in the south), had widely varying cultures in this respect. Whereas in Enschede single and married women alike were working in the textile mills in large numbers as weavers and in other textile occupations, both workers and the elite in Tilburg prided themselves upon a rigid gender division of the local labour market. Not only were married women completely banned from industrial work, textile occupations in Tilburg such as weaving and spinning were out of bounds for all women, married and single alike, as these occupations would bring them into contact with male workers. To what extent did these different local work cultures and gender systems promote different fertility regimes?

A second set of hypotheses concerns the effect of education on the propensity for women to limit the size of their families. The effect is well-known for late twentieth-century women: women with higher level educational attainment are the ones postponing child birth, they have smaller families and they are more often childless than women with lower level educational attainment (Janssens, 2003). The effect is also well-known for developing countries in the twentieth century. While more education for men increases fertility in some rural areas in the developing world – most notably in Africa –, more education for women lowers fertility in all regions of the world (Schultz, 1997). How does the effect work? Several interpretations are possible. Firstly, more education increases women's earning power in the paid labour market and the opportunity cost of women's time, and thus the costs of caring for children. In other words, with more education women give up more wage income when they care for children. In this model it is assumed that married women are allowed to engage in paid labour but that they give up working when they have children. Secondly, if women's educational levels increase relative to those of men, this will reduce their dependence on men and will further their emancipation. This will reinforce their position in the family and increase their bargaining power in marital relations. If, by contrast, men's education is increased while women's education remains the same, the effect on fertility is mostly positive. Several interpretations of this relationship are possible. First of all, higher levels of men's education will reinforce patriarchal tendencies and increase women's dependency on men. Furthermore, higher levels of male education will have a positive effect on male wages which will enable them to choose more children

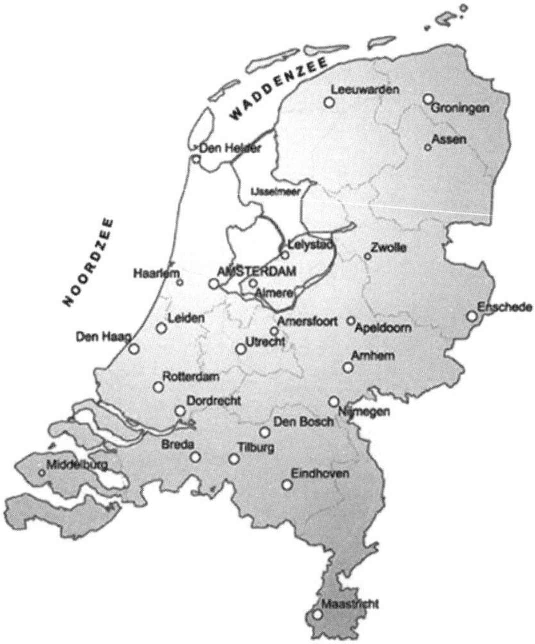

Figure 1. Map of the Netherlands.

as they would choose to buy more of other goods. The fact that men do not incur opportunity costs in the same way as women do when choosing more children makes an important difference here. It is therefore also probable that when women's educational attainment increases in step with men's, the effect on fertility may be absent. Robert Allen (2003: 123–131) has demonstrated the effect of this relative increase in female education for the rapid fertility decline in the Soviet Union in the twentieth century. His study also showed that the effect of education decreased as educational levels increased further. Thus, giving all women primary education was highly effective in reducing the Soviet birth rate.

In this paper I will examine the effect of labour market experience on the fertility patterns of two cohorts of women in two industrial towns in the Netherlands, Tilburg and Enschede. The two cohorts were born in 1881–1885 and 1911–1915 respectively; they could have been each other's mothers and daughters, so they may be seen as generations. However, I will first present some data on the Dutch fertility decline and the two local communities, before presenting the results from my analysis of fertility behaviour of these two generations of women.

The Context

Fertility rates in most countries of north-west Europe started to decline somewhere around the middle of the nineteenth century. Although the pattern of the fertility transition was remarkably similar, levels of fertility differed enormously. The Dutch fertility transition is rather late, with fertility falling for all provinces of the country only from around 1900 onwards. The table below illustrates the time lag of the Netherlands in comparison to surrounding countries (Engelen and Hillebrand, 1986). As in other countries, quite substantial differences in demographic patterns existed between the various regions. Roughly, the process took place along a south-west to north-east diagonal line. While the south-eastern provinces, such as North-Brabant, Limburg and Overijssel, still show rather traditional reproductive behaviour around the turn of the century, families in the north-western provinces of North- and South-Holland have already adopted modern reproductive practices.

Table 1. National Averages for Marital Fertility (as Measured by I_f), Selected Countries

Approximate date	Belgium	Germany	Netherlands
1880	0.751	0.735	0.848
1890	0.678	0.706	0.805
1900	0.596	0.659	0.763
1910	0.443	0.542	0.676
1930	0.280	0.264	0.482
1960	0.290	0.301	0.401

In the literature on the Dutch fertility decline economic modernization and attitudinal factors have figured prominently. Economic modernization is thought to have provided a motive for change in fertility behaviour whilst attitudinal factors are seen as determinants of the acceptability of this type of behaviour. The impact of economic modernization is largely regulated through cultural and above all religious opposition to any form of birth regulation. Acceptance of fertility limitation is low amongst orthodox Catholics and high amongst more liberal, secularized Protestant regions. In recent research economic modernization, mostly measured by levels of male population employed in agriculture and the percentage of women outside agriculture, is estimated to contribute most towards *change* over time in the development of marital fertility (Engelen and Hillebrand, 1986). Attitudinal factors, more specifically the proportion of Catholics and orthodox Protestants in the population, are held to account for the differences in *levels* of marital fertility.

The division between the north-west and the south-eastern parts of the Netherlands is reflected in the figures for marital fertility for four urban communities given below. Zaandam, one of the old industrial centres in the province of North-Holland, and much smaller than the nineteenth-century industrial towns Enschede and Tilburg, or the port city of Rotterdam, is undeniably the most 'modern' in fertility behaviour at the beginning of the twentieth century. Tilburg stands out as the most 'traditional' local culture with a level of fertility almost twice as high as for Zaandam. Both Rotterdam and Enschede challenge the north-west versus south-east divide within the country with quite similar levels of fertility. Within the period under discussion, a radical process of change took place. In all towns fertility fell, however, proportionally speaking change was most radical in Rotterdam and Tilburg. Nevertheless, even in 1960 fertility in Tilburg was still higher than elsewhere, although differences had become less pronounced.

Table 2. Marital Fertility in Selected Communities, Births 1908–1911 and 1959–1961*

	population in 1964	1908–1911	1959–1961
Rotterdam	731,525	251.6	126.2
Zaandam	52,583	184.1	144.5
Tilburg	142,968	337.8	174.8
Enschede	131,804	250.3	149.5

* Yearly average number of births per 1,000 married women <45 year of age
Source: figures taken from the *Bevolking der gemeenten van Nederland op 1 januari 1964*, CBS, 1964.

Tilburg and Enschede, again compared to Rotterdam and Zaandam, are clearly industrial towns with most of its female inhabitants employed in industry, as is shown in the table below. Both are textile towns, but in Tilburg the sector was fully concentrated on the production of woollen yarn and cloth, whereas the textile mills in Enschede were all cotton mills. Other significant differences existed. The pace of industrialization in Enschede was much faster than in Tilburg in which latter town cottage-weaving, mainly by male workers, continued to be of importance until the end of the nineteenth century.[1] Moreover, many women and girls worked at home for the textile factories as burlers and menders. This latter practice enabled factory owners to make use of cheap female labour without having to introduce them within their factory walls. Both (male) workers and entrepreneurs in Tilburg prided themselves upon the small numbers of unmarried women and girls in the factories, and certainly the total exclusion of married women from their industrial workforce. The local industrial labour market in Tilburg, therefore, was heavily segregated: women and girls working in textiles mills were a small minority, and those that did find employment in the textile sector were always segregated into separate work units, mostly employed as fluffers or winders. Married women, if they worked in textiles, they would always work at home, which practice continued as late as the 1940s.[2] In Enschede, however, the textile mills employed large numbers of women and girls. Sex-segregation on the shop floor was minimal: women could be weavers and spinners, and they did work side by side with male workers. This is probably the result of the continued pressure on the demand for labour in Enschede in the period between 1860 and 1930. There were not enough male weavers to fill all productive places. After 1930, however, when the number of looms per worker increased significantly, whilst production did not rise in a similar pace, female weavers could be discharged. They disappeared from the stage rapidly. In 1947 weaving had already become a male sector (Groot, 2001: 186).

From the above table it is also clear that female labour force participation in Enschede was considerably higher than in Tilburg. In 1930, four out of every ten women were active in the paid labour market in Enschede, as opposed to almost three out of every ten women in Tilburg. Given the rela-

1 In 1897 the number of cottage weavers still made out 55 percent of all weavers. After 1900, however, cottage weaving declined rapidly. In 1905 the proportion of cottage weavers had been reduced to 22 percent. See Gertjan de Groot (2001: 193).

2 In 1938 the proportion of women working at home in burling, mending, and fluffing, as opposed to within the factory walls, was still 38.5 percent. Home production by married women in Tilburg was vital for the textile entrepreneurs who therefore opposed all proposals aimed at total bans on married women's work. See Gertjan de Groot (2001: 205–206).

Table 3. Female Employment Structure by Sector in 1930, and Total Activity Rates in 1899 and 1930 */**

	I	II	III	IV	V	VI	VII
Rotterdam	0.0	29.9	29.0	27.2	13.6	28.6	31.0
Zaandam	0.2	24.0	20.0	41.7	13.8	19.0	24.1
Tilburg	2.2	50.1	15.2	18.7	12.4	29.0	37.4
Enschede	0.0	63.3	10.3	19.2	7.1	43.3	40.3

Columns:
I = employed in agriculture in 1930
II = employed in industry in 1930
III = employed in trade and financial services in 1930
IV = employed in domestic service in 1930
V = employed in professions and education in 1930
VI = total female activity rate in 1899
VII = total female activity rate in 1930

* female employment structure: % of women employed in selected economic sectors of all women aged 15–60
** activity rate: % of women employed of all women aged 15–60
Source: Census data taken from the *Dutch Historical-Ecological Databank*

tive distribution of female workers over the various economic sectors, this will have resulted in a female industrial workforce which was twice as large as in Tilburg. Given the comparable sizes of the two towns, female factory workers in Enschede were far more 'visible' than in Tilburg. Combined with the much stronger sex-segregation in Tilburg, we might speak of significantly different local work cultures.

In the following analysis I will be primarily looking at the effect these divergent work cultures may have had on the extent of birth limitation within marriage. For both towns two cohorts of women will be analysed, the first cohort of women is born in 1881–1885; the second cohort might be the daughters of the first cohort as they are born in the period 1911–1915. In addition, the effect of education may be examined in the life courses of those women who became teachers and office clerks and hence had benefitted from more years of education than their working-class counterparts.

The data used in this study are taken from the Population Registers and the Civil Registers of the towns of Enschede and Tilburg. Continuous population registers have existed in the Netherlands from 1849 onwards. The population registers enable the historian to follow the evolution of the family and the household on a day-to-day basis. It thus presents information on demographic events in an already linked format on the entire population, even the very mobile, and it facilitates the computation of a wide range of demographic rates.

The data concern two cohorts of women in each town, born between 1881 and 1885, and 1911 and 1915 respectively, resulting from four non-selective samples taken from the towns' birth registers. All women in these samples surviving until their 15th birthday were admitted into observation and followed through the Population Registers until they disappeared from observation. For all women the entire life course was reconstructed, including all information on their demographic and occupational careers. The data were analysed with the help of event history analysis techniques, which label covers a collection of statistical procedures which make possible complex analysis of duration data. Fertility behaviour is then analysed as the 'risk' for another birth to occur, whereby the effect of various independent variables may be examined. Work cultures and educational levels are of prime interest here. However, various other relevant socio-economic variables, such as social class of husband and religion will be taken into account as well. I will also be looking at the effect of a number of demographic variables such as age of the mother or the influence of child mortality.

Fertility Decline in Tilburg and Enschede: Results

The Dutch demographic transition took place in the course of these two generations of women born respectively in 1881–1885 and 1911–1915. But which women belonged to the group of innovators in this type of behaviour? The first issue we are interested in is the effect of the woman's own occupation. In order to categorise by occupation, I used the woman's first three occupational entries found in the Population Registers. In case the first entry stated 'no occupation', I used the second entry, but only if this stated a different occupation. Most occupational entries refer to occupations before marriage; unfortunately, married women's work was hardly ever registered.

In both cohorts women were found in only a few occupations, but there are important differences between the two local labour markets. First, com-

Table 4. Occupations of Cohort Members, Enschede and Tilburg

Enschede cohort 1	N=	%	*Enschede cohort 2*	N=	%
Teaching/retailing	11	3.8	Teaching/office work	40	13.8
Seamstresses/servants	44	15.3	Seamstresses/servants	74	25.5
Weavers/textile	163	56.8	Weavers/textile	129	44.5
No occupation	69	24.0	No occupation	47	16.2
Total	287	100	Total	290	100
Tilburg cohort 1	N=	%	*Tilburg cohort 2*	N=	%
Retailing/teaching	13	5.4	Retailing/office	38	12.4
Seamstresses/servants	72	29.9	Seamstresses/servants	75	24.6
Weavers/textile	52	21.6	Weavers/textile	76	24.9
No occupation	104	43.1	No occupation	116	38.0
Total	241	100	Total	305	100

pared to Enschede, a large proportion of young women in Tilburg did not have any occupational entry at all.[3] The difference is most pronounced in the first cohort, where four out of every ten Tilburg women went without occupation. It is expected that indeed this group was mostly not active in the labour market, either not at all or not in any formal way, even though considerable proportions of these women came from working-class backgrounds.[4] Given the fact that in both towns many working-class families still owned plots of land in the first half of the twentieth century, it is likely that working-class families still had ample opportunities to employ daughters gainfully within the family economy. Moreover, as we have seen, the Tilburg labour market provided ample opportunities for sweating in various textile jobs, for girls and

3 I also made use of the Marriage Registers to check for occupations for those who had no entry in the Population Registers. Only a very small number of additional occupations could be found.

4 The social background of cohort members who did not have any occupational entry: in the first Enschede cohort: 27 percent came from farming background and 53 percent from working-class background; Enschede cohort 2: 83 percent came from working-class background; Tilburg, for both cohort 1 and 2: about 75 percent came from working-class background.

married women alike. In the first Enschede cohort there were also quite a few farmers' daughters without their own occupational entry; we may assume that these young women were working on the family farm.

Secondly, working-class girls in Enschede went into textiles much more often than did girls in Tilburg. It is clear that in the first Enschede cohort weaving was the preferred occupation for young women. Given the fact that in both towns textiles dominated the local labour market more or less completely, the relatively low number of female textiles workers in the two Tilburg cohorts is remarkable and underlines the low visibility of women in the Tilburg textile industry already mentioned above. The other major occupations in both towns were in needlework and domestic service. Between the two cohorts the number of women in jobs requiring higher levels of education, such as teaching or office work, rose significantly. Women in these latter job categories will be our main possibility of looking at the effect of education on fertility.

As I already mentioned, only very few women had occupational entries after marriage. However, if they did have an entry for occupation after marriage, textile jobs predominated, both in Enschede and Tilburg: 50 to 80 percent of occupational entries after marriage gave an occupation in textiles. This shows that even in Enschede textile work, which was by definition factory work, was 'easier' to combine with marriage and children, probably because of the larger supply of this type of work, than were other trades and jobs. In Tilburg it is most likely that all married women working in textiles were actually working in the sweating sector of this industry.

In table 5 and 6 the results of the hazard analysis for another birth are summarized in a model which lumps all birth intervals together but includes the separate parities as independent variables. I will first discuss results for Enschede. We would expect the group of female textile workers and weavers, especially those in Enschede, to have taken the lead given the large labour force participation after marriage amongst this group. Few restrictions on the number of children would only seem to have been an obstacle in the case of continued factory work of mothers. But female textile workers in the first cohort do not seem to have been the most active group in limiting fertility, neither in spacing nor in stopping behaviour.[5] Rather the opposite, as their birth intervals were shorter than was the case for women who had been domestic servants and seamstresses, or for women who had had no registered occu-

5 As was shown in parity specific results.

pation at all. Textile workers almost seemed to have been maximising their fertility. This suggestion is further strengthened by the fact that textile workers were also marrying at much younger ages than other women, with a large proportion of them already pregnant when arriving at the altar. Those women we might be inclined to think of as belonging to the most 'traditional' group of women, servants and seamstresses, were actually exhibiting more 'modern' fertility behaviour. Moreover, the result for this group has the required statistical significance as well, while the effect can be seen as a strong one. Finally, it comes as a surprise to see that women teachers and retail workers were having shorter birth intervals than textile workers, or, for that matter, than any other occupational group of women. One would have expected, as a result of higher educational levels, a greater awareness in this group of the disadvantages of relatively large families. However, the reader should note that the result for this particular group is statistically of very low significance, whilst the number of observations for the group of teachers is quite small so that it is impossible to say anything definitive here.

The social group to which the husband belonged did not carry much weight in the case of the first Enschede cohort. None of the husbands' social status variables seem to be particularly strong or significant. Nevertheless, the results suggest that between the two cohorts the effect of the husband's social class variable changes from positive to negative. In the older generation, a higher social position increases the pace of childbearing, suggesting that the number of children was still a function of a family's economic resources. A husband's higher earnings translated itself into consumption patterns enabling the maintenance of larger families. Large numbers of children were a sign of wealth and social status. In the younger generation this was no longer the case; here the higher social classes began to limit their fertility through either spacing or stopping, or a combination of both. Large numbers of children were becoming a sign of poverty.

The occupational dividing lines between women are however overruled by religious distinctions. Around 1900 fertility seems to be mainly determined by religious denomination. Catholic women are having strong and highly significant risks of conceiving another child compared to any other group of women, regardless of the parity concerned.[6] Catholic women are having babies much

6 This latter result is not shown in the above table but was gained from parity specific analyses.

Table 5. Extended Cox-model for Fertility: All Parities Together, Including Parity Effect, Enschede Cohort 1 and 2

Variables	Cohort 1 Coeff	Signif	Cohort 2[7] Coeff	Signif
Occupation of woman (textiles omitted)				
Teaching-retailing-office[8]	0.1302	0.3702	0.1567	0.6073
Servants-seamstresses	-0.3463	0.9802*	0.0982	0.5315
No occupation	-0.0858	0.5111	0.1985	0.7526
Occupation of husband[9] (unskilled labourers omitted)				
Upper class	0.0623	0.2634	-0.6344	0.9249
Middle class[10]	–	–	-0.1645	0.6033
Farmers[11]	0.2037	0.6446	–	–
Skilled labourers	0.0054	0.2716	-0.0861	0.5492
Religion of woman[12] (Non-Catholic omitted)				
Roman-Catholic	0.6462	1.0000*	0.2776	0.9800*
No religion	–	–	0.0749	0.2283
Secularization	0.0731	0.3376	-0.3574	0.9560*
Migration status husband	0.1292	0.8260	-0.0648	0.4460
Age mother	-0.0043	0.9999*	-0.0053	1.0000*
Previous child dead	0.6527	0.9996*	0.3784	0.7803

7 Cases for which no husband was available have been excluded as these cases are likely to have incomplete or incorrect fertility histories.

8 For cohort 1 this group comprised primarily teachers and shopkeepers, whereas in cohort 2 this social group consisted predominantly of teachers and office workers.

9 Occupation unknown is included in category 'unskilled'.

10 For cohort 1 upper and middle classes have been taken together as one social group on account of the small number of observations for upper-class occupations.

11 For cohort 2 the number of farmers has become so small that they have been included in the group of skilled labourers.

12 The category 'other denominations' contained so few observations that analysis was impossible, therefore included with protestant denominations into 'non-catholic'. In the first cohort, none of the women started off their married lives as non-religious, therefore no estimation has been included for the category *no religion*. Some women however did switch over during their marriage into the registration *no religion*; these cases are captured by the variable *secularization*.

Variables	Cohort 1 Coeff	Signif	Cohort 2[7] Coeff	Signif
Any child dead	0.2189	0.8706	0.3176	0.8810
Parity effect (parity 2 omitted)				
Parity 3	-0.1577	0.7719	-0.3460	0.9871*
Parity 4	-0.0913	0.4190	-0.0600	0.2654
Parity 5	0.3793	0.9419	–	–
Parity 5+	–	–	0.4426	0.9846*
Parity 6	0.7302	0.9976*	–	–
Parity 7+	1.0534	1.0000*	–	–

Table 6. Extended Cox-model for Fertility: All Parities Together, Including Parity Effect, Tilburg Cohort 1 and 2

Variables	Cohort 1 Coeff	Signif	Cohort 2 Coeff	Signif
Occupation of woman (textiles omitted)				
Teaching-retailing-office[13]	0.0520	0.1770	0.3873	0.9904*
Servants-seamstresses	-0.0220	0.1713	-0.1230	0.7128
No occupation	-0.0869	0.6247	-0.0528	0.3765
Occupation of husband[14] (unskilled labourers omitted)				
Upper (middle) class[15]	-0.1128	0.4672	-0.1512	0.5429
Middle class	–	–	0.0321	0.1808
Farmers	–	–	–	–
Skilled labourers	-0.0690	0.5878	-0.2538	0.9911*

13 For cohort 1 this group comprised primarily teachers and shopkeepers, whereas in cohort 2 this social group consisted predominantly of teachers and office workers.

14 Husbands whose occupation is unknown are included in the category *unskilled labour*. The few farmers in both cohorts were all included in the group *skilled labour*. In this cohort only three husbands had no registered occupation.

15 Cohort 1 contained so few observations for upper-class husbands, that upper-class occupations were included with middle-class occupations for this cohort.

Variables	Cohort 1 Coeff	Signif	Cohort 2 Coeff	Signif
Religion of woman[16] (Non-Catholic omitted)				
Roman-Catholic	-	-	-	-
Secularization	-	-	-	-
Migration status husband	-0.3017	0.9927*	-0.0244	0.2106
Age mother	-0.0043	1.0000*	-0.0053	1.0000*
Previous child dead	0.2594	0.9394	-0.0063	0.0157
Any child dead	-0.0270	0.1900	0.1240	0.5253
Parity effect (Parity 2 omitted)				
Parity 3	-0.1893	0.8542	-0.2434	0.9604*
Parity 4	-0.3435	0.9741*	-0.0722	0.3945
Parity 5	0.0512	0.2255	0.1108	0.4983
Parity 6	0.5437	0.9942*	0.4770	0.9862*
Parity 7+	1.0100	1.0000*	0.9288	1.0000*

faster both in the early phases of family formation, up to and including the fourth child, as well as later on in this process. Family planning not only seems to be wholly absent, rather Catholic women seem to have been maximising the number of their children. It is important to add here that the effect of religion is not indirectly conveying the influence of income or social status. The social composition of the group of Catholic and Protestant women in the Enschede samples, as measured by their fathers'occupation, was more or less similar. The religious variable rather points in the direction of cultural factors, amongst which the subordinate role assigned to women in both family and society by the Catholic church and its doctrines is certainly highly relevant.

Given the importance of the religious factor, one would expect a significant contribution of the variable *secularisation*. This was not the case. But given the

16 Because of the mono-religious culture of the town analysis on religion was impossible. Nearly all women belonged to the Catholic church, and none of them switched over into being non-religious.

fact that all women who had switched over from being religious into being non-religious, had been members of the Dutch Reformed church, the most liberal of all Dutch denominations, this is perhaps less surprising. It testifies to the fact that the members of the Dutch Reformed church already had modern attitudes where it concerned family life, gender relations and birth control. For this group the process of secularisation did not lead to large differences in the acceptance of early demographic innovations between those who had left their church and the ones that stayed on.

Demographic variables were also important. As might be expected, increases in the age of the mother led to slightly longer birth intervals, but with a highly significant result. The death of the previous child also proved to have an important and significant effect: women experienced shorter birth intervals than would otherwise have been the case. Does this point towards conscious family planning in the sense that couples were aiming at a predetermined family size, and thus replacing the child they had lost? This hypothesis does not seem to be very convincing, as the effect is totally absent in the case of any of the previous children that were lost through death. It therefore seems more logical to assume that it was the result of breast feeding having stopped at the death of the previous child.

Clearly, women in the earlier cohort expected to be mothers. Motherhood was the standard trajectory of every married woman. And it was taken for granted that motherhood included more than just one or two children. As the parity variables suggest, it is not very likely that many women and their husbands were aiming for stopping behaviour in the early parities up to their fifth child. For all cohorts the results for these lower parities indicated that women had longer intervals compared to the interval between their second and third child, but coefficients here were rather small and above all mostly not significant. This may indicate that at least some women were trying to space the arrival of their children – thereby limiting the burden of a fast repetition of births –, whilst other women were probably not doing anything at all to prevent successive births. For the higher parities, those for the sixth child and over, results reveal a very different picture with birth intervals becoming strongly and significantly shorter. What had happened? It is likely that those women who were trying to create longer intervals between the births of their third, fourth or fifth child were also the ones who would ultimately switch over into stopping behaviour so that this particular group of 'spacers-and-eventually-stoppers' were not contributing to the observations for the higher parities. The results for the higher parities will thus have been determined predominantly or even exclusively by those women who were not in any way trying to limit the size of their family. Whilst they already had a large number of children born to them in a quick succession, they went on to have even more children, again with brief intervals, also in the higher parities. Although this type of hazard analysis cannot provide definitive and clearcut measures of whether spacing or rather stopping is going on in the various intervals, nevertheless, the results obtained here for the higher parities suggest a clear division between those women 'aiming' for a moderate number of children, and resorting to both spacing and (eventually) stopping, and a subgroup of women who were not regulating their fertility at all.[17]

While fertility limitation in the first cohort of women, was to some extent still an innovation and primarily practiced by specific subgroups, in the daughters' cohort women all seem to have changed over into more modern patterns of family formation. Social difference, specific occupational cultures, or even religious denomination are losing their influence in the second cohort of women. Limiting the number of children seems to have become a common pattern. The only exception are Catholic women. While for all parities taken together, the distinction between Catholic women and other women still stands out as important in the second cohort, as can be seen from the above table, this importance is limited to birth intervals in the lower parities. Up to and including the fourth child they do not seem to be aiming at postponement of another birth.[18] However, in the higher parities, this behaviour changes, so that Catholic women are changing over into behaviour highly similar to other women. It may be assumed that moral dilemma's prevented them from applying birth control measures in the earlier phases of family formation, so that they felt they could only begin to justify birth control after the birth of the fourth, fifth or even the sixth child.[19]

17 See the debate about the chronological importance of spacing versus stopping in: Szreter (1996: 432–439).

18 Again, results for separate parities are not shown here.

19 For the extensive control mechanisms exercised by the Catholic church and the moral dilemma's most Catholic women had to solve for themselves before they were able to decide in favour of birth control – even if this only meant abstaining from sexual intercourse – see: Schoonheim (2005).

While secularisation did not play any role in the first cohort, this became a relevant factor in the second cohort. Non-religious women, or women who had switched from being religious to non-religious, had longer birth intervals than religious women. This is surprising given the fact that in the earlier cohort there was no effect to be found of this process. It would seem more logical to expect stronger effects in the earlier phases, with clearer divides between those who had left the church and those who had stayed. Perhaps between the two cohorts a change occurred in the composition of the group that had left the church? Indeed, in the second cohort, secularisation also began to occur amongst Catholic women, albeit slowly and in small numbers. It is easy to assume that for Catholic women at that time a much larger discrepancy existed between those who had left the church and its pronatalist pressures and those who stayed behind and continued to conform in different ways to the rather traditional position of the Catholic church in the field of family limitation (Schoonheim, 2005).

Concerning the parity variables, interesting effects may be discerned. Results suggest that attempts to postpone or event prevent a new birth may have begun at much lower parities than before. The strong and significant result for parity three suggests as much, as do the results for the positive effects of parity five and higher. Apparently, in the second cohort the division came to lie between women who had had three or four children, and had been practicing spacing until then, and then stopped, and those women who had so far not done much to space their births and subsequently went on to have even more children.

Are we finding similar results for Tilburg? As Tilburg was a mono-religious town, with 98 percent of its population being Catholics, differences between denominations could not be included. Nor could the variable *secularisation* be included: in neither of the two cohorts did women turn away from the church. For the first cohort the coefficients for the female occupational variables have similar signs as for the first Enschede cohort, but they lack significance. In the first cohort, occupational experience of women does not seem to be related to their fertility behaviour. In the second cohort, we find again, that teachers and office workers have higher risks for another birth, than any of the other subgroups of women. However, unlike Enschede, this effect is highly significant in Tilburg. This is unexpected and most remarkable given the higher educational levels for this group.

As was the case in Enschede male occupational variables have no significant effect either, at least not for the first cohort. In the second cohort, the only significant result is the coefficient for skilled labourers. Contrary to the results found for Enschede, here all husband's social groups have negative signs, indicating that compared to unskilled workers higher social groups were all having larger birth intervals and thus fewer children. In the first Tilburg cohort, the only social variable of interest is the migration status of the husband. Women married to men born outside the town had significantly longer intervals than did women married to locals. To what extent is this the result of the innovative influence of 'outsiders' in a closed community such as Tilburg?[20] In the second generation, however, the effect has disappeared.

Of the demographic variables it is only the age of the mother that produces the expected effect. The higher the age, the longer her birth intervals are likely to be. The death of the previous child, or any of the previous children, does not have any significant effect. Nevertheless, the death of the previous child comes close to the required statistical significance, at least in the first generation, and suggests a relationship similar to the one found for Enschede. The death of the previous child shortens the birth interval for the next one. As is argued above, this might be the result of interrupted breast feeding. In the second cohort, the effect has disappeared, suggesting that overall more effective birth control is being applied and at the same time, that parents were not aiming for a specific family size. Otherwise, the death of any of their children, or their previous child, would have prompted them to replace the child they had lost. This would seem to suggest that women were still bearing more children than they would perhaps ideally have seen as optimal.

Interestingly, the parity effects are quite similar to the results found for the two Enschede cohorts. In the lower parities birth intervals are longer, the higher parities have intervals that are relatively brief. The effect in the lower parities is created by women spacing their intervals, after which they switch over into stopping behaviour. The women creating the effects in the higher parities are those women who were neither trying to space their births nor trying to stop after a particular family size had been reached.

20 Outsiders played a significant role in the rather closed Tilburg community between 1890 and 1920 in at least one respect: they were responsible for the introduction of socialist ideology and the establishment of socialist trade unions in Tilburg. See Wagemakers (1990).

Finally, to what extent did Tilburg women have higher fertility levels than Enschede women? It might be assumed that at least two factors may have prompted higher fertility levels in Tilburg. First of all, the town was homogeneously Catholic with a strongly autochthonous culture.[21] Outside influence and the introduction of new ideas, certainly where it concerned family, sexuality and childbearing, may therefore have been slow and difficult. The paternalistic influence of the local clergy and the elite class of factory owners was certainly aimed at banning outside influence to keep its mass of workers from being 'infected' with socialist ideology. Local Catholic workers unions were established by clergy members to strengthen the link between workers and traditional Catholic culture. Membership of 'outside' socialist unions could cost workers their job. Secondly, as was already mentioned above, the Tilburg labour market was strongly segregated by sex. Factories employed primarily male labour; female factory work was limited, and was certainly banned for married women. Female textile work, involving large numbers of women, went on in private homes and houses, invisible to the public eye. These rigid divisions by gender may have prevented change in the relationships between men and women, and may have made change in attitudes towards childbearing more difficult. The above model was therefore tested again with an additional variable for location (results are not shown here). The above speculations were however not confirmed. The location effect was small and far from significant. There is no reason to assume that Tilburg women were more strongly tied to high fertility behaviour than Enschede women. Of course, overall fertility in Tilburg was higher, but this was solely related to the effect of religion. There is thus no reason to believe that Catholic women in Tilburg were having larger families than Catholic women in Enschede.

21 In Tilburg the native born made up the majority of the population. Around 1900 about 75 percent of the population was born and bred in the town. For Enschede this applied to only 44 percent of the total population. See Janssens (1993: 46) and Janssens (2001).

Conclusions

What do the above results allow us to conclude? Quite contrary to what our theoretical presuppositions had led us to expect, participation in the modern industrial labour market did not lead women to introduce 'modern' reproductive behaviour. This was most evident in Enschede where female textile workers in Enschede were least inclined to space or stop births. As they had also married at relatively early ages, mostly prompted by a premarital pregnancy, they will ultimately have had a much larger number of children than any of the other social groups of women. The same effect appears to have existed in Tilburg, although results were not significant here. Rigid gender divisions in the labour market were absent in Enschede, thus the female textile workers in this study must have had experience of working side by side with men. They must have had the opportunity for exchanges on the work floor with other women, both single and married women, about intimate matters such as pregnancies and ways to limit them. And oral history evidence is indeed available, also for the Netherlands, that involvement in factory employment could act as a form of 'sex education' for young women and girls. Through contacts with older co-workers young people learned about the 'facts of life' or even gained some actual sexual experience themselves. This was even the case in the Tilburg textile factories where women and girls worked relatively segregated from male workers (Happel, Keune, Korremans and Rooij, 1980: 170).

Nevertheless, the potential advantage in information and experience that female textile workers may have had did not lead to changes in their reproductive behaviour. The results are remarkable as participation in the labour market after marriage was to all probability much higher in this group than in any other group. Whereas married textile workers in Tilburg could combine textile work with child care and other domestic duties in the family economy, this was not the case for women in Enschede. Sweating practices in textiles had been abandoned long before. Nevertheless, household economic considerations may have come into play in these textile families. The textile sector could still take up a large supply of child labour; moreover, child-workers were often recruited through their parents. Maximising the number of their children may have been a way of maximising total family income. Did women consider that reliance on their husband's wage as the main source of income in combination with their own probably intermittent wages was a less secure option than the one based on a large number of child and adolescent workers which might sustain parents – if they were lucky – up to and even through their old age? It is in any case significant that the effect disappeared more or less in the second cohort, at a time when the Enschede textile industry switched over to a more or less exclusive use of adult male labour, so that child labour – as well as female labour – became increasingly limited.

Domestic servants and seamstresses were in no way exhibiting traditional reproductive behaviour. In both towns, and in three of the four cohorts, they had smaller intervals between births than did textile workers, which result was highly significant in the first Enschede cohort. How can this be explained? Did servants and seamstresses by way of their contact with families in higher social strata change their family ideals and targets? It has also been suggested that this led domestic servants to aspire to socially mobile careers, if not for themselves, than at least for their children. Sociologists therefore coined the term 'bridging occupations' to denote all occupations in domestic service.[22] These occupations enabled those working in them to strive more or less successfully to higher social and occupational attainments by using the contacts and resources offered by their employers' higher social milieu. Similarly, limiting fertility may have been perceived as an important instrument in striving towards higher social goals. The research presented by Vanhaute and Matthys elsewhere in this volume presents a convincing case in support of the connections between domestic service, social mobility and the early adoption of fertility control.

The effect of education on the female life course patterns found in this study does not conform to our expectations. Women teachers and office workers were not at all leading the way in reduced fertility patterns. In both towns and all four cohorts they had even shorter birth intervals than had textile workers, although results were only significant for the second Tilburg cohort. Nevertheless, we would have expected these teachers and office workers to have longer intervals, rather than the other way around. This result is puzzling and difficult to explain, also given the fact that this occupational group had a tendency towards higher ages at marriage. Reduced fertility would then have been the effect. However, age at marriage was included in the above model, so that the occupational variable shows its independent effect. It might be

22 See for an extensive discussion on this: Bras (2002).

suggested, as is indeed done by Anne-Françoise Praz elsewhere in this volume, that these female teachers were quite specifically educated to transmit dominant Catholic values, and on top of that one might suggest that they served as examples to others. Nevertheless, as Boonstra (1993) demonstrated in his study of the – likewise very Catholic – Dutch town of Eindhoven, even education specifically based and focused on traditional norms and values did have a modernising influence on its participants and their fertility behaviour.

Religion proved to be of overriding importance. Sharp divisions existed between Enschede women in the first cohort according to religious denomination. Catholic women born in the 1880s had much higher risks at another birth; they were having much shorter birth intervals and will therefore ultimately have had much larger families than women of a different religious background. Their daughters however, born in the 1910s, although still tied to a high fertility regime in the earlier parities, began to space births after they had had their fourth or fifth child. It thus seems as if moral dilemma's and constraints prevented them from applying birth control measures in the earlier phases of family formation, so that they felt they could justify birth control only after the birth of the fourth, fifth or even the sixth child. The importance of traditional religious values as an obstacle in the fertility decline has of course played a prominent role in the older macro-historical approaches to the demographic transition. Already in Ansley Coale's attempts (1969) to provide causal explanations for the fertility decline in the western world religion was underlined as an important negative variable. Likewise, in the Lesthaeghe and Wilson model (1982) religion plays an important role. However, in these studies religion is presented as a gender-neutral effect preventing the adoption of rationalistic attitudes and individualistic perspectives. However, as Anne-Françoise Praz argues elsewhere in this volume, the effect of traditional Catholic cultures on the retarded adoption of birth control practices worked perhaps primarily through the specific gender relations enforced by the church and its priests. Traditional Catholic values not only promoted pronatalism but they also significantly weakened women's bargaining powers within marriage while failing to underline men's responsibility for the wellbeing and the sheer number of the couple's children.

Finally, the hazard analysis presented in this chapter did not suggest that the specific local cultures of the two towns had a significant independent effect on the fertility behaviour of the two cohorts of women. The much more closed and homogeneously Catholic culture of Tilburg, where in addition sex-segregation in the labour market must have been much stronger, did apparently not make it significantly more difficult for women to apply some form of birth control. Thus, Catholic women were in that respect not much better off in Enschede than in Tilburg.

References

Allen, Robert C. (2003), *Farm to Factory. A Reinterpretation of the Soviet Industrial Revolution*, Princeton, Princeton University Press.

Boonstra, Onno (1993), *De waardij van eene vroege opleiding. Een onderzoek naar de implicaties van het alfabetisme op het leven van inwoners van Eindhoven en omliggende gemeenten, 1800–1920*, Wageningen, Agricultural University Wageningen.

Bras, Hilde (2002), *Zeeuwse meiden. Dienen in de levensloop van vrouwen, ca. 1850–1950*, Amsterdam, Aksant.

Coale, A. J. (1969), 'The Decline of Fertility in Europe from the French Revolution to World War II', in Behrman, S. J., Corsa, Leslie and Freedman, Ronald (eds), *Fertility and Family Planning. A World View*, Ann Arbor, University of Michigan Press, 3–24.

Engelen, Th. and Hillebrand, J. (1986), 'Fertility and Nuptiality in the Netherlands, 1850–1960', *Population Studies*, 40, 487–503.

Fisher, Kate (2000), 'Uncertain Aims and Tacit Negotiation: Birth Control Practices in Britain, 1925–50', *Population and Development Review*, 26, 295–317.

Gittins, Diana (1982), *Fair Sex: Family Size and Structure 1900–1939*, London, Hutchinson.

Groot, Gertjan de (2001), *Fabricage van verschillen. Mannenwerk, vrouwenwerk in de Nederlandse industrie (1850–1940)*, Amsterdam, Aksant.

Happel, Hans, Keune, Lou, Korremans, Tom and Rooij, Ad de (1980), *De ondergang van de Tilburgse textielindustrie*, volume 3, Tilburg, Instituut voor Ontwikkelingsvraagstukken.

Janssens, Angélique (1993), *Family and social change. The household as a process in an industrializing community*, Cambridge, Cambridge University Press.

Janssens, Angélique (2001), '"Eens door de wol geverfd, nu door de wol getekend ..." De 'trage' ramp van de ondergang van de Tilburgse textielindustrie, 1900–1980', *Ex Tempore*, 20, 87–105.

Janssens, Angélique (2003), 'Economic Transformation, Women's Work and Family Life', in Kertzer, David I. and Barbagli, Marzio (eds), *The History of the European Family, Family Life in the Twentieth Century*, vol. 3, New Haven/London, Yale University Press, 55–110.

Lesthaeghe, R. and Wilson, Ch. (1982), 'Les modes de production, la laïcisation et le rythme de la baisse de la fecondité en Europe de l'ouest de 1870 à 1930', *Population*, 37, 623–645.

Schoonheim, Marloes (2005), *Mixing Ovaries and Rosaries. Catholic Religion and Reproduction in the Netherlands, 1870–1970*, Amsterdam, Aksant.

Schultz, T. Paul (1997), 'Demand for Children in Low Income Countries', in Rosenzweig, Mark R. and Stark, Oded (eds), *Handbook of Population and Family Economics*, Amsterdam, Elsevier, 349–430.

Szreter, Simon (1996), *Fertility, Class, and Gender in Britain 1860–1940*, Cambridge, Cambridge University Press.

Wagemakers, A. J. M. (1990), *Buitenstaanders in actie. Socialisten en neutraal-georganiseerden in confrontatie met de gesloten Tilburgse samenleving*, Tilburg, Stichting Zuidelijk Historisch Contact.

'I Think I'd Rather Die than Go through with a Pregnancy Again.' Experiences of Childbearing and Birth Control in Sweden in the 1930s

Sofia Kling

Introduction

Sara Nilsson was thirty years old and living in Norrköping when she gave birth to a boy in May, 1935. It was her first child and she was quite determined that it would also be her last. She had several reasons for her decision. She had rheumatic fever once and suffered twice from stomach ulcers. Both her pregnancy and the subsequent delivery had been difficult. Her husband was a textile worker and Sara described him as sober and conscientious in every way. Unfortunately his income was low and this meant that Sara also had to work, 35 hours a week. She returned to work less than a month after her delivery, leaving her son with relatives. She feared that a second pregnancy would cause her to lose her job. Her husband seems to have agreed with her that they would not have any more children.

A month after the birth of her son, Sara made contact with the *Riksförbundet för sexuell upplysning* (RFSU) to receive reliable contraceptive information.[1] She was not the only one doing this; hundreds and hundreds of people – men and women – turned to the same organisation relating the same problems. They were tired, their bodies were tired, they lacked money, and they already had too many children. They did not want any more babies and, therefore, they needed the help offered by the RFSU.

The birth of Sara's son occurred during a period of very low birth rates in Sweden. Fertility had declined constantly since the 1880s, reaching its

1 Labour Movement Archives and Library, RFSU Archive, E:2, letter 432. Sara Nilsson's name is fictive. The letters quoted in this paper have all been anonymised in order to protect the correspondents' identities.

lowest point of 1.3 children per woman in 1933 (Bernhardt, 1971: 5).[2] Sara's relatively high age at the birth of her child, and her determination to avoid future pregnancies can be seen as representative of a larger trend in society: women increasingly stopped having children at an early age, and often after having only one or two children (Stanfors, 2003: 17). This development, from large families with five or six children to smaller families with only one or two children, is one of the most important changes in modern times, but also one of the least understood, despite a large body of research.

Research on the Swedish fertility decline has, however, been sparse. Fertility started to drop in the 1890s and reached its lowest point in 1933 (1.3 children per woman). In an early study of fertility patterns in Stockholm, Karl Edin and Edward Hutchinson showed that the number of children correlated positively with income. Families with low income presented the lowest number of children (Edin and Hutchinson, 1935). Later studies have connected high fertility with rural areas, preferably characterised with a high level of religiousity (Lockridge, 1983; Larsson, 1984). In Sweden, as in other countries, research on the fertility decline has relied mainly on macro-theoretical analysis, linking the reproductive behaviour of women to structural changes such as industrialisation, secularisation, and mass-education (Szreter, 1994: 9). This approach has its benefits – for example, it does make it possible to analyse rather large aggregate data – but it also creates problems. Most relevant in this case is its tendency to obscure the rather basic fact that all reproductive decisions are made at the individual level by women and men such as Sara Nilsson and her husband. When fertility is linked directly to structural changes it is easy to create an impression that female reproductive organs are directly affected by social forces such as industrialisation or the modernisation process. This impression is, of course, a false one. There is no automatic connection between societal change and fertility because fertility is always and ultimately determined by individual behaviour. Karen Mason points to the fact that even though fertility decline, by definition, takes place at the aggregate level 'the processes that result in that change occur […] through changes in individual behaviour' (Mason, 1997: 160). This is important to remember.

This is why the connection between structural changes and low birth rates cannot be of the automatic kind as is suggested by much previous research.

2 See also Statistics Sweden (SCB), available on-line: www.scb.se.

Between structures and fertility stands the individual. It is her reactions to structural processes and cultural changes that eventually will affect fertility patterns. 'Industrialisation' did not affect the frequency with which couples had sex, or whether they employed any kind of contraception. It did affect people and as a result they may have chosen to adapt their sexual behaviour in order to restrict their reproduction (Townsend, 1997: 96–100; Watkins, 1993: 559–560). If we want to understand fertility decline, and not merely describe it, we need to attempt to understand how men and women experienced societal changes, and how this affected their reproductive decision-making (Bledsoe, Guyer, Lerner, 2000: 1). We need to know that it was experiences, like those of Sara Nilsson who had stomach ulcers and a low income, that made people choose effective methods of birth control rather than relying on the practices known from earlier generations. But we also need to know that these experiences were part of a greater, general pattern. As already pointed out, Sara Nilsson was not alone in experiencing health as a problem, nor was she alone in taking action to avoid future pregnancies. We need to find out how individual experiences relate to the general pattern.

A Collection of Letters

It was ambitions like these that sent me looking for the personal voices of 'ordinary' contracepting people. I found them in a collection of almost 500 letters, written between 1929 and 1940, and addressed to the RFSU, a Swedish organisation working for sexual education. Most of the letters come from ordinary working-class people and they contain questions related to contraception, abortion, and other forms of birth control.

What can be said about these five hundred correspondents? Who were they? What, if anything, did they have in common? Firstly, most of the correspondents were of working-class origin. Actual occupation is mentioned in only 30 percent of all cases, but among these working-class occupations are in an overwhelming majority. The 70 percent without occupation can, to a very large degree, still be labelled working class. The social and economic circumstances described in these letters reveal the correspondents as most likely belonging to this category. The same holds true for those letters which mention the occupation of the spouse, but not of the correspondent him-/herself. One important aspect is the fact that married women only rarely mentioned an occupation of their own.[3] None of the letters written by married men mention female work outside the home. Rather than seeing this as faithful descriptions of how work was organised within the families I would like to interpret the silence concerning female work as a result of the ideal of the male breadwinner. It is unlikely that almost no married women worked outside the home, nevertheless this was how they wanted things to appear, in a letter written to doctors and other experts. This is a matter I will return to later.

The over-representation of working-class correspondents is not very surprising. The RFSU worked closely with the labour movement and members of local unions and local socialist clubs were collectively affiliated to the RFSU. This meant that the politically active part of the working class was probably familiar with it. It might also indicate that quite a few of the correspondents were politically conscious. Furthermore, the RFSU regularly advertised in socialist papers which was how most correspondents claimed to have learned about it. Most of the correspondents were thus part of a literate segment of the population. This indicates that they only rarely came from very poor backgrounds, a fact which was also clear from the letters. Very few letters contain descriptions of pure poverty. A vast majority is also fairly well-written.

Secondly, the letters came from men as well as women; almost half of the letters (44 percent) were written by men. However, men and women often differed about what they wrote and the type of help they sought. Men were more interested in sexual matters and methods of contraception – they might for instance want to change a sexually unsatisfactory contraceptive (usually condoms) for something less disturbing (usually diaphragms). Women were more interested in security and avoiding pregnancy at all costs. It was also more common for women to ask for help with an abortion.

Thirdly, a majority of the correspondents lived in the countryside. This is not very surprising considering that only one third of the Swedish population lived in urban areas in 1930 (Rogers, 1995: 177). Still, it says something about the possibilities of the correspondents to gain sexual or contraceptive knowledge at the local level. Doctors were usually unwilling to discuss sexual

3 Only four married women stated that they had an occupation of their own.

matters and the same holds true for other authorities, such as representatives of the local churches.

I have chosen to restrict this study to include primarily the motives for birth control among the 270 correspondents who were *married*. Nonetheless, the correspondence also contains 129 letters from unmarried, but usually engaged, people.[4] A majority of these (57 percent) are men. The rationale for birth control usually mentioned by these correspondents is not further explored in this paper. Other information revealed by these correspondents, such as the gendered areas of responsibility connected with sexuality and contraception, is however of further interest.

Specifying the Problem

The focus of this work is on the men and women present in the RFSU correspondence. I wish to find out what childbearing and birth control meant to married people in this period. Why did they choose to restrict their fertility and how did they accomplish this? The answers to these questions will also help us find some of the driving forces behind the shift from large to small families that took place between 1870 and 1930 – the pattern scholars refer to as the fertility transition.

I believe that at the individual level reproductive decisions are closely related to both personal experiences and to the formation of personal identities. When people make reproductive decisions they do not merely respond to the outer world; they also try to create something for themselves. I think reproductive decisions are (unconsciously) related to questions such as *Who am I? Who do I want to be? How do I want other people to see me?* – rather than being (automatic) responses to structural changes. I also believe that the personal experiences of giving birth and bringing up children, or maybe the experience of growing up with too many siblings, plays an important role in active reproductive decisions. Of course this does not mean that I deny the importance of structural change. Structures and structural changes are important but do

4 The remaining letters are from correspondents who were single, divorced or widowed. In addition, the civil status of sixty correspondents remained unknown.

not automatically affect fertility. Structures affect people; people affect fertility. I think it is crucial to remember this if we want to understand changes in reproductive behaviour.

Gender as an Important Analytical Tool

A growing body of research has emphasised the importance of seeing the contracepting couple as a constellation of *two* people, not always in agreement and not always able to reach workable compromises. Women take all the physical risks connected with childbirth and they are the ones primarily responsible for raising the children. This means that women's relation to the decision to restrict fertility inevitably differs from that of their partners (Mackinnon, 1995: 7; Gittins, 1982: 12–18; Seccombe, 1993: 157; Greenhalgh, 1995: 14). It does not, however, mean that men have no personal interest in controlling fertility. I believe that it is important to include both mothers and fathers when fertility is analysed mainly because both of them are parts of the reproductive unit, despite the fact that their experiences differ but also because female experiences are best understood *in relation to* male experiences (Greene and Biddlecom, 2000: 104). This is why I find it important to analyse the letters from a clear gender perspective.

What do I mean by gender perspective? I understand gender as something fluent and constantly under construction rather than something stable and grounded in biology. Gender is a process intertwined with the construction of identity. It offers meaning to the biological sex: through acting, dressing and moving in a 'feminine' manner I communicate to the surrounding society that I belong to a certain biological gender – the one with two x-chromosomes. The fact that gender is a process implies continuity and repetition: theorists have argued that gender is *produced* through the constant repetition of specific gendered actions (Butler, 1999: 178–79). A decent woman living at the end of the nineteenth century should, for example, be unaware of sex. The fact that she was likely to have gained sexual knowledge through married life was something that needed to be concealed, since sexual expression was considered either a male characteristic or a symptom of illness. For men, on the other hand, gender identity required that their actions signalled sexual knowledge and experience, no matter how limited these experiences actually were. Thus sexual ignorance was demonstrated again and again by 'feminine women', and sexual knowledge by 'masculine men' – and gender was produced. Thereby they shaped their own gendered identities since gender results from the constant performance of specific, regulated and compelling actions. In other words, gender should not be understood as a motive for action but as a consequence of action. In this case women did not demonstrate sexual ignorance because they *were* women, but they *became* women by behaving in ways that were understood as naturally feminine (Butler, 1999: 178–79). This is what makes the production of gender an important aspect in the construction of personal identities.

Gender and Class

Women did not only demarcate themselves from men when demonstrating sexual ignorance but also from *other women*. Gender contains an important class aspect without which the formation of gender cannot be understood. This is what makes certain constructions of womanliness or manliness more worth striving for than others. There exists an idealised version of being female or male that appears as the most *natural* and *normal* one. This means that when women demonstrated sexual ignorance they did this to distance themselves not only from men, but also from those subordinate forms of femininity exhibited by the irresponsible or lecherous woman who made sexual experience visible. The demonstration of sexual ignorance can therefore be said to include a claim for respectability (Seccombe, 1993: 178).

I understand class in much the same way as I understand gender, namely as a process, as something accomplished through active practices, and not as an abstract structure or hierarchy into which people are inserted. Gender and class are formed through the repetition of specific actions. When gender is produced, so is class; when class is produced, so is gender (Acker, 1999: 53–54). The sociologist Beverley Skeggs illustrates how working-class women demonstrate respectability to avoid the official picture of what it means to be working class; acting respectably becomes a characteristic signalling that one is *not* working class (Skeggs, 1999: 78). This means that they actively try to act in accordance with bourgeois norms regarding femininity. In this manner, by following gendered and principally middle-class norms, the upper segments of the working classes distance themselves from 'the disorderly working class' and thus construct themselves as respectable, as not working class. This does not mean that they want to *become* middle class, but should rather be understood as a process through which the working classes form their *own* identity.

While it is true that the working classes adopt bourgeois norms, it is equally true that they attach new meanings to them (Horgby, 1993: 284–91; Tosh, 1999: 17; Finch, 1993: 2).

It is time to return to the contracepting couples of this study. I wish to show not only how earlier experiences of childbearing and childrearing affected the willingness of parents to have more children, but also how their reproductive behaviour became strategies for forming both their personal identities as men and women, and their collective identities as *respectable* working-class people.

Arguments for Birth Control: Voices from the 1930s

The arguments for birth control given by the correspondents can roughly be divided into either health-related or childrearing concerns. The first group consists of 91 letters written by men and women who worried about the general health of the mother or feared the risks of pregnancy and delivery. The latter category contains 180 letters from individuals who claimed that they could not afford to have more babies and those who said they were unable to take care of additional children. However, the correspondents only seldom mentioned just one argument for adopting birth control. Instead they delivered a whole list of reasons thereby giving the impression that *everything* in their situation made it impossible to have another child. Presumably this was also how they experienced the situation. I have not, however, been able to do full justice to this aspect of the correspondence. In categorising the letters I have given priority to the one motive most fervently pursued in each letter. Since this inevitably is a matter of interpretation, all numbers mentioned in the following should be considered with care.

Childbearing and Health

The connection between maternal health and birth control is perhaps the most obvious one when it comes to linking personal experiences to reproductive decisions but it is a connection little noticed by scholars. The fact that childbearing exposed women to serious health risks is of course acknowledged by most scholars, but seldom by those exploring the causes behind fertility decline (Riley, 2003: 6). This is perhaps not so strange. Maternal health improved during the nineteenth century and significantly fewer women were likely to die in childbirth in the 1930s than a hundred years earlier. Moreover, general improvements within the area of medicine had made not only childbirth, but life afterwards, a much less risky affair. So how can maternal health be a motive for birth control in the early twentieth century when it had actually much improved from the beginning of the nineteenth century? The answer is that there was a cultural change that paralleled the medical one. The *experience* of childbearing and disease changed and this is what made people want to stop having babies.

That maternal health was an important argument for not wanting more children is clear from the correspondence. About one third of the men asking for contraceptive advice, and one fifth of the women, referred to the health of the mother. The proportions are more or less the same when it comes to pleas for abortion. The fact that men were more likely than women to write to the RFSU with concerns for the woman's health is somewhat surprising. Since the letters exclusively referred to the health of the mother, one might expect that women were the ones mainly concerned about how an additional pregnancy would affect them. However, this does not seem to have been the case.

The unexpected pattern can probably be easily explained by considering the affection that family members usually had for one another. It is important to remember that reproductive decisions were always made within a relationship and that this relationship normally was characterised by affection. The correspondence reveals plenty of evidence that husbands generally took great personal responsibility for the physical wellbeing of their wives. It is also likely, because contraception was usually a male responsibility,[5] that men recognised

5 Whether birth control was a male or female area of responsibility is a debated question. The correspondence analysed in this study shows that birth control was a male responsibility in Sweden in the 1930s. I have very little information about earlier periods. I agree with Kate Fisher, who claims that birth control was a male responsibility because it concerned sex, sexuality and the sex life of the spouses. The correspondence gives plenty of evidence of the fact that birth control (with the exception of abortion) was inseparable from sexuality. This fact made it difficult, or even impossible, for women to suggest new contraceptive methods etc., since this inevitably would be equal to taking a sexual initiative, and this was something that most women were unable to do.
Some scholars, for instance Sune Åkerman and Kate Fisher, conclude that contraception was a mainly male area of knowledge and responsibility, while others, for example David

the active role they played in exposing their wives to health risks. Therefore, they saw birth control as a means through which they themselves could affect the health of their wives in a positive direction.

Preventing poor Health

Some correspondents wanted to stop childbearing because they worried about the risks of another pregnancy and delivery, while others worried more about their current level of health and how this condition might be worsened by the additional burden of a pregnancy. The women of the latter category mentioned all kinds of different diseases and conditions: diabetes, heart problems, eye problems, the after-effects of polio, tuberculosis, bad legs, varicose veins, and so on. Some of the conditions described may have been the result of a long childbearing history although the correspondents themselves did not draw this conclusion. Other conditions are of a kind that could be drastically worsened by an additional pregnancy. There are also conditions unrelated to childbearing (Riley, 2003: 18). The following quotations illustrate this.

> I suffer from chlorosis it can't be cured said doctor Berg but we have to eat iron. And I've had catarr in my womb with bleedings every fourteenth day and sometimes more all because of weakness the doctors say and so a year ago I had a miscarriage also because of weakness this can't go on said doctor Jonsson, this is how it goes when she's so weak the anaemic shouldn't have babies he said the mother gets ill and the child gets ill and it shows on the girl she's been sick since the day she was born. *(Married mother of three, from Västmanland, 1938)* [6]

> She's been treated for tuberculosis in her left lung 1928–1929 then she got water in her lungs got well 1932. Convalescent til 1934. [...] I fear that her nerves won't stand the burden of always having to think about her first period of illness if it would break out again. *(Industrial worker with one child, married to 37-year-old woman, from Värmland, 1940)* [7]

Levine, argue that birth control was a female responsibility. According to Levine, birth control was a female responsibility since it was 'an area of domestic life'. Levine argues that the ideology of separate spheres, which dictated that men were responsible for supporting the family while women were responsible for everything connected with domestic life, made birth control a female responsibility. The correspondence analysed in the present study offers no support for such an interpretation. See Fisher, 2000; Åkerman, 1981; Levine, 1987.

6 Letter 295.

7 Letter 355.

Motives for birth control connected to the general health of mothers are best understood in relation to the intense public health work that took place during the first decades of the twentieth century. The new public health agenda had its ideological roots in the new field of bacteriology. By identifying disease as something not only present within bodies but also between them, attention was transferred from sick people to potentially sick people, and the goal became to prevent rather than just cure diseases. This agenda quickly received political legitimacy and improving medical services became an important socio-political issue. A whole new field for social reform was opened. Numerous health campaigns emerged and they reached people through a web of school doctors, teachers, health care inspectors, nurses and travelling informants from different social organisations such as the RFSU (Johannisson, 1997: ch.6; Ross, 1992: 48–51). Women, as carriers of future generations, were often the focus of the campaigns and improving the health of women became a strategy for strengthening the nation as a whole (Johannisson, 1995: 90–92).

This shift in the way health was perceived was also connected to the process of secularisation. Swedish historian Eva Hamberg reveals how the secularisation process changed the way people perceived and valued health. When people began to see themselves as responsible for their own wellbeing they also started to attach new values to health itself. It became important to maintain health not only to be able to work, but also because good health was considered important in itself (Hamberg, 2003: 54–55; Kvåle, 1981: 104–112; Blom, 1980: 92). Very few of the correspondents mentioned any personal connections with the church, and those who did mention religion or the church did this in order to distance themselves from values they perceived as religious (such as negative attitudes to contraception, or premarital sex). This scepticism towards religion should be seen in relation to what has been said earlier about the political aspect of the RFSU and its members. The closeness of the RFSU to socialism and the labour movement made it difficult to reach faithful church-goers. The correspondents may therefore have been more sceptical towards religion than the larger population, but they may be seen as part of a general and far-reaching process of secularisation. As a result of this process, health and disease was increasingly perceived as something over which humans had some degree of control rather than depending on fate or the will of God (Seccombe, 1993: 179). Public health campaigns offered rational means for fighting disease and for maintaining good health by supplying information about cleanliness and personal hygiene. This quotation may illuminate the result of this process: 'My wife has diabetes, we have two children, doctors have told us it's enough with these children.'[8] In this letter, birth control is seen as a way to improve, or at least avoid worsening, the health of the mother. The correspondent also emphasised the role the doctor played in the decision-making process, an aspect to which I will return.

To prove these changes with the information given in the letters is difficult but some indications are still to be found. One such indication is that those who considered themselves to be in poor health rarely suffered from any serious diseases. They might have had a bad leg or suffered the after-effects of polio, or they might simply refer to themselves as weak.[9] One of the letters that reached the Counselling Clinic was written in 1938 by a 34-year-old mother of three. Her letter included the following complaints:

> The thing is I suspect I'm pregnant. [...] Oh, and now my backache is getting unbearable, and therefore I fear the worst. For the thing is that my back, which always pains me even under normal circumstances, is a sheer inferno during pregnancy with its additional burdens. I feel completely worn down, and think that I'd rather die than go through with a pregnancy again. [...] My body and my nerves aren't of a kind that can take more.[10]

This woman did not wish to terminate her pregnancy because she feared it would end her life, although this surely was the case for many other women writing to the RFSU. Instead she wanted to terminate her pregnancy because she could not stand the back pain. This attitude to physical suffering indicates a new attitude to health and suggests that good health was seen as a valuable commodity with a legitimacy of its own. Terminating a pregnancy – which was illegal – became a legitimate action for maintaining good health.

The fact that people appear to have visited the doctor with a surprisingly large number of physical problems is another indication. Many visited the doctor to be cured from a stomach ache or some other relatively minor problem that might not have required a consultation with a doctor only a couple of decades earlier. Furthermore, people attached great weight to what doctors said. Every warning against having more children was taken very seriously. The correspondents reveal a familiarity with medical language and a great awareness of health and illness. Different diseases were described in detail and the correspondents often used medical language. Perhaps they did so to emphasise

8 Letter 165. *Married man with two children, from a village in Norrbotten, 1938.*

9 For instance letters 329, 332, 408.

10 Letter 337.

the gravity of their condition but presumably also because they had adopted the vocabulary of medical experts. This also implies an increasing trust in science, and confirms that the number of people holding the belief that God or fate controlled their health and wellbeing was decreasing. The increased presence of doctors and medical experts in local society also contributed to the changing perceptions of sickness and death. Indeed, the mere presence of doctors in the local community showed people that conditions of health could be influenced.

Taken together, these behaviours show that people increasingly considered it possible to be in control of their own physical bodies. Preventing future pregnancies became one way of doing this (Danielsen, 2000: 32).

The Fear Of Another Pregnancy

Some women, and their male partners, were more worried about the actual pregnancy and the delivery. These correspondents usually had had rather bad experiences during earlier childbirths. Such was the case for the two women quoted below.

> I'm expecting since little over a month […] Have had 8 children (and 2 miscarriages). I'm in despair, don't know what to do. I'm sick from the first day to the last. And after the delivery (which is always difficult) I become so very weak a doctor has to be there. I got a little boy two years ago, but had to go to the hospital before, got eclampsia etc. My nature is very nervous. *(37-year-old woman with eight children, from Norrbotten, 1936)*[11]

> I think a new baby would be a disaster. I'm very weak during pregnancy must eat iron supplement, and additional iron and calcium while breastfeeding. *(Married woman with two children, from Medelpad, 1938)*[12]

> I'm 25 years old and pregnant for the fifth time since I was 18. When I was 18 the 'circumstances' forced me to marry a man I had nothing in common with but the child. One year later I had a miscarriage (3½ months) after another year a child that had to be cut in pieces at birth and a warning from the doctor against future pregnancies since I had such difficulties having them and probably wouldn't be able to give birth to a living child again. […] I gave birth to a girl about a year ago. The child was alive and still is but it was very hard for me and I'm still not recovered. My opinion is that the doctor who told me that I shouldn't have more babies also should have told me how to prevent this. *(25-year-old married woman with two children from Västergötland, 1934)*[13]

11 Letter 425.
12 Letter 496.
13 Letter 343.

These letters may be considered in at least two different ways: they either come from a specific group of women with particularly traumatic childbearing experiences, or they are symptoms of a more radical change in how childbearing was experienced by all, or at least most, women. The first interpretation implies that this group of women is constant; the only reason why women with these kinds of experiences did not refuse to have more babies during earlier decades was that they simply were not able to do so. However, the many women (and male partners) who wrote to the RFSU because they feared a future pregnancy makes me inclined to rely more on the second interpretation i.e. that there was a change in how the childbearing process was experienced by women in general.

The experience of childbearing changed partly for the same reasons as attitudes toward health in general had changed, and partly for reasons exclusive to the experience of childbirth. The most important aspect here is the cultural understanding of pain. Anaesthetics did not become widely used in Swedish hospitals until the 1960s which means that there were no real changes in the amount of pain a woman had to bear during childbirth before this time (Milton, 2001: 157). However, it seems likely that the experience of this pain underwent crucial changes during the nineteenth century. This change accompanied the process of secularisation.

In most pre-industrial societies, pain was a more or less normal condition. Swedish historian Karin Johannisson has written about pain as an integral part of everyday life: pain was, in one form or another, always present (Johannisson, 1997: 83). The most important force in helping people to cope with it was religion, which in the case of Sweden means Lutheran Christianity.

Pain has never been far from salvation in Christianity: history is full of martyrs and monks who suffered and gained access to heaven. Jesus himself suffered a painful death on the cross. There is also a clear connection between pain and sin: pain can be seen as a reminder of our sinfulness (Caton, 1999: 96). The pain of childbirth is explicitly connected to Eve's fall from grace, of which we can read in Genesis: 'I will greatly multiply thy sorrow and thy conception; in sorrow thou shall bring forth children; and thy desire shall be to thy husband, and he shall rule over thee.'[14] The Christian faith supplied women with an interpreting framework which gave their suffering meaning.

14 King James Bible, Genesis, ch. 3, verse 16.

Pain during childbirth was laid upon women by God. This made pain meaningful and therefore bearable.

Christianity was not the only belief that invested pain and suffering with special meaning but it was probably the most pervasive one. This makes the process of secularisation most interesting. This was a process that Sweden had largely already witnessed by the beginning of the twentieth century. That this had an impact on people's values and attitudes seems clear (Hamberg, 2003: 54–55). That it also affected women's experiences of pain and illness in connection with the childbearing process is rather obvious considering the function religion played in investing pain and suffering with meaning (Caton, 1999: 102). With the decline of religion the meaning disappeared and only pain remained.

One final aspect of the changing experience of the childbearing process should be considered and this is the growth of the women's movement. The emancipation of Swedish women started in the 1850s and gradually gave women legal and economic rights. Questions about masculinity, femininity, marriage and love were discussed regularly from the end of the 1870s and traditional gender regimes were changing, albeit slowly. Although this hardly changed the childbearing experience as such, it most probably changed society's attitudes to specifically female experiences. It might have made society (including doctors) more willing to listen to women and, most importantly, it might have made men more likely to listen to their wives (Jejeebhoy, 2002: 193). It is for instance possible that the attitudes and actions of these two men resulted from such a process:

> We're both 35 years old and married since 1929. We got a child in 1930 and the delivery was extremely difficult for my wife. Ever since, the thought of a new pregnancy has terrified her. [...] I feel that I have a responsibility and therefore I use condoms and also 'withdrawal' to be absolutely sure. In spite of this my wife gets very distressed every time her period is late. She even has symptoms etc. This is getting on the nerves for both of us and I've therefore decided to send you a letter. *(35-year-old man from Västerbotten, 1934)* [15]

> My wife, who is 19, had a boy a couple of months ago, but he only lived for one day. [...] The delivery lasted for 4 days, so the sufferings were difficult for my wife. [...] We're now wondering if she can expect the same pains the next time and if the child will die again. [...] Whatever the outcome I must absolutely do something, so that I don't bring her into pregnancy again, at least the coming year, since she's both physically and mentally worn down. *(25-year-old man from Västmanland, 1936)*[16]

15 Letter 438.
16 Letter 426.

Furthermore, the emancipation process might have helped women to trust their physical experiences and to listen to their bodily signals (Anderson, 1999: 259). The fact that husbands and doctors actually listened to women relating their childbearing experiences most probably encouraged wives and female patients to speak out in a way they might not have done fifty years earlier.

In summary, birth control motives related to the health of the mother indicate that the experience of childbearing and disease had changed, and that people increasingly considered themselves to be in control of their own physical wellbeing. An important aspect of this change was the secularisation process which offered people a more rational attitude to health and changed the cultural understanding of pain. Public health campaigns during the beginning of the twentieth century that provided information about cleanliness, personal hygiene and nutrition offered rational means by which people could affect their own health. Birth control became another strategy for doing this. By using contraception (or contraceptive methods) men and women actively pursued strategies that would improve, or would at least avoid worsening, the health of women. By so doing they also shaped their mutual future.

Parenthood and Respectability

It was not only the experience of childbearing that underwent changes during this period; this happened also to the experience of child*rearing*. This experience was mainly influenced by two factors: the financial situation of the family, and the number of children present in it. Consequently, these were two of the most commonly mentioned arguments for birth control by the correspondents.

Economic Considerations for Adopting Birth Control

The most commonly mentioned motive for not wanting more children was the financial situation of the family. When not put forward as the main motive it was still mentioned as at least a contributing concern, indicating that economic considerations were never far away when couples reflected on the children they had and the children they might have in the future.

Previous research has often pictured the husband as more likely than the wife to act upon economic calculations (Gittins, 1982: 161; Thomas and Williams, 1998: 284). The male breadwinner ideal pervaded all levels of society, from the political, through social and administrative institutions, and to the minds of ordinary men and women. It would, therefore, have come as no surprise if men were the ones mainly concerned about the economic burden of a new child (Johansson, 2002). However, this study offers no support for such an interpretation. Twenty-two percent of the women asking for contraceptive advice do so for economic reasons compared to 14 percent of the men. The same is true for about one fifth of those asking for an abortion, regardless of sex. This indicates that men were less focused on economic questions than one might have assumed considering the great impact of the breadwinner ideal. Of course, one did not have to be the main breadwinner to assume responsibility for the financial situation of the family.

That people wanted to avoid having more children for economic reasons did not mean that they lived on the border of starvation or that they referred to themselves as poor. Rather, this decision was made because they wanted to maintain their present standard of living. It was in the light of this rather humble ambition that the prospect of more babies became problematic as the following letters illustrate.

> I have two children and the youngest is only one year old. My husband works at the factory and is badly paid and so we can't raise any more children properly. *(Woman from Skåne, 1936)*[17]

> It's not because we don't like children that we don't want any, but because we live under such bad and insecure circumstances and have such an insecure existence. I work at the ironwork here, low salary but the worst is I don't know for how long I have a job at all. *(30-year-old man from Värmland, 1935)*[18]

> Now the thing is we don't want any more children […] because I'm a plumber and the work is very seasonal. *(Man from Dalarna, 1937)*[19]

These letters suggest that it was not an economic *necessity* for most families to stop having babies. Instead, the correspondents seem to have found themselves barely maintaining what they considered to be an acceptable standard of living

17 Letter 374.
18 Letter 428.
19 Letter 222.

and feared that an additional child might force them to endure a standard of living inferior to their expectations (Seccombe, 1993: 177). This is perhaps best illustrated by the first of the letters quoted above in which the woman expresses her concern about being able to raise the children *properly*. First and foremost parents think of the children they already have when they discuss birth control from an economic perspective; it is *their* standard of living that is the principal matter of concern. This is further illustrated by the following quotations:

> We don't want any more children under any circumstances since we already have three boys and it's often hard enough to find food and clothes for them. *(27-year-old mother of three from Östergötland, 1936)*[20]

> … and you're responsible for the children you bring to the world […] Sure I've loved and cared for the ones I have already, but I've also wept a lot, thinking about their future. *(Married woman with five children, from Norrbotten, year unknown)*[21]

Thus, parents took action to avoid future pregnancies to guarantee the already existing children a good upbringing.

Scholars have often singled out the economic incentives for birth control as being particularly important. They claim both that the economic transformation of society – linked to different modes of production – shaped a new attitude towards children, and that childrearing gradually became more expensive during the course of the nineteenth century (Becker, 1960: 210). I do not deny the importance of the first development but the second is of more relevance to the present study. General economic improvements during the end of the nineteenth and the beginning of the twentieth century seem to have increased people's expectations of life. It changed their image of what constituted a good living and made people strive for more than mere survival (Sogner, 2003: 80). The correspondents wanted to be able to offer their children a better childhood than the one they had experienced themselves. One man hinted at his childhood of shortage and deprivation when he wrote: 'I'm the oldest of 12 siblings I don't have to say anymore since it was a working-class home I think you'll understand anyway.'[22] Parents did not consider themselves capable of supporting the same number of children as the older generation

20 Letter 419.
21 Letter 476.
22 Letter 467. *Man, engaged to be married, from Östergötland, 1933.*

had done indicating that the perceived costs of raising children had increased. It is important to remember that this was the result of a cultural, and not an economic, change. In other words, it was not the actual price of clothes that changed in relation to incomes, but rather the perception of how many clothes a child needed and of what kind. Parents probably believed the costs of raising children to be beyond their control and that they had little choice but to conform to the established materialistic norms of their social context (Alter, 1992: 16). It is from this perspective that parents, despite the fact that they were not actually fighting poverty, still found it economically impossible to raise another child.

These materialistic ambitions of the correspondents can also be seen as part of their efforts to construct themselves as respectable. Swedish research has shown how the family's standard of living became an important social asset during the first half of the twentieth century (Frykman and Löfgren, 1979: 125–27). Being able to keep a room with no real practical function, exchange an old sofa for something new and fashionable and, of course, to keep it all clean and tidy became important when working-class families constructed their identities as respectable men and women. This required a sufficient income, but also a limited number of children. An official report from 1941 concluded that women with many children probably were less interested in the material aspects of their home; they did not care much about dust in the corners and it did not matter to them if the tea cups were broken (Åkerman, 1941: 238). A clean and tidy home was thus acknowledged to go hand in hand with fewer children.

The gendered division of labour between husband and wife is something that makes these materialistic ambitions, as well as their effects on reproduction, particularly interesting. While the wife was primarily responsible for the surface of the home – its interiors, cleanliness, and the clothes of the children – the economic prerequisites for this were mainly supplied by her husband. These separate areas of work were grounded in ideas about what it meant to be a man or a woman. Femininity was increasingly produced through the ability to present a tidy home as well as by creating a harmonious family unit. Masculinity was produced through the ability to support the family but also through qualities such as sobriety and education (Horgby, 1993: 368). These norms meant that both wife and husband had an interest in upholding the ideals of the female housewife and the male breadwinner. The respectability of the woman depended on the amount of time she was able to spend at home, and the housewife became, during the first decades of the twentieth century, a strong symbol of relative prosperity (Frykman and Löfgren, 1979: 126). Since women were the ones particularly responsible for presenting a nice home, and healthy and well-dressed children, it is likely that their involvement in the financial situation of the family was fairly strong. Their participation is confirmed by the many women who wrote to the RFSU for economic reasons.

It can be concluded that the need for birth control somewhat paradoxically resulted from improved economic circumstances during the first decades of the twentieth century. The improved standard of living gave rise to new materialistic expectations. Parents wanted to create a materially secure environment for their children at the same time as they strove to construct themselves as respectable men and women. This process of identity formation meant different things for men and women but for both a sufficient income was crucial. While the size of income was out of control for most individual working-class men, most realised that they were able to control their fertility. Thus, efficient birth control became a means through which the working-class population improved the living conditions of both their children and themselves while constructing themselves as respectable men and women.

The Experience of Parenthood

Respectable childrearing was not only about creating a materialistically safe childhood for one's children; it was also about creating an emotionally safe home. This aspect of childrearing which was more about love, care and intimacy than about money and physical environments, was becoming increasingly important during the first decades of the twentieth century. It also was almost exclusively considered a female domain.

During this period a new concept of motherhood evolved making childrearing a more important, and more time-consuming, task for women in all social classes. It became crucial for mothers to raise their children in *a proper manner*, in a clean and proper home, and to care not only about the children's nutrition and physical wellbeing, but also about their emotional and psychological development (Reiger, 1985: ch. 6–7; Giddens, 1992: 45). The success of this project often depended on how many children the woman had: it was no doubt easier to be responsible for the emotional development of two children than it was for six especially when women were equally responsible for presenting a perfectly clean home (Ross, 1992: 49).

The many responsibilities of the housewife are described in a Swedish report from 1941. The report concluded, among other things, that women spent about two and a half hours every day preparing meals and doing the dishes, and almost two hours every day cleaning (Åkerman, 1941: 95). The additional work created by a second or third child was also described. Each child created its own mess, had a bed that needed to be made, produced more laundry, more clothes to patch, more food to prepare, and more dishes to do. The report also pointed to the constant interruptions of the every-day routines which came with more children; they had to be looked after, comforted, helped to the toilet, and so on (Åkerman, 1941: 95).

This was work that inevitably followed with each child and it is therefore not very surprising that many of the women who wrote to the Counselling Clinic were quite satisfied with the two or three children they already had and eager to find means to avoid future pregnancies. As many as 40 percent of the women writing to RFSU for contraceptive advice, and 23 percent of those trying to get an abortion, supported their request by referring to the number of children they already had. Nearly 50 percent of these women had four children or less. The letters of two women discuss this.

> I have 2 children 6–4 years old now I wouldn't like to have any more if it could be avoided in some way that is good for me. My husband is an industrial worker and I feel I can't be responsible for more children.[23]

> I've got 3 children the youngest is 6 years, I'm 34 and my husband will soon be 50. With today's demands on childcare and upbringing […] everything seems hopeless.[24]

Obviously, this sense of already having enough children was very subjective and often grounded on ideas about how many children the parents considered themselves able to raise in a manner they thought proper. This was not solely an economic question but also a matter of how much time the mother could spend on each child. This is quite clear in the letters quoted above. The 1930s, more than any earlier period, was the decade when the norm of the housewife was established in all social classes. It was a period when the mother's central role in securing the wellbeing of the children was more strongly emphasised than earlier, and when new norms for cleanliness and nutrition were established (Hirdman, 1989: 153–58; Ohrlander, 1992: 115, 271–75;

23 Letter 484, written in 1934, by a married woman in the Stockholm area.

24 Letter 337, written in 1938.

Danielsen, 2000: 93; Kvåle, 1981: 147–49). As a consequence, the upbringing of children became a much greater responsibility than it had been during earlier decades.

This emphasis on *how* mothers raised their children was a clear shift from earlier periods. John Gillis describes how mothers and children became family icons with symbolic functions during the second half of the nineteenth century. With the separation of work from home, men became more and more dissociated from family life, while women and children became increasingly associated with it in a manner that made them almost synonymous (Gillis, 1996: 72–73). The concept of motherhood also assumed new dimensions as it became a full-time, lifelong commitment (Gillis, 1996: ch. 8; Reiger, 1985: 117). Paradoxically, this natural maternalism was something that many women, particularly working-class women, had to *learn*. A complex web of organisations, childcare centres and social workers took it upon their shoulders to communicate the ideology of true motherhood to working-class women. This essentially bourgeois ideology included norms regarding cleanliness and nutrition, but also characteristics such as maternity and femininity.

Skeggs explains working-class women's acceptance of bourgeois norms as a way for them to gain respectability. By adopting these norms, 'respectable' working-class women confirmed not only their gender but also their superior form of womanliness. The realisation of ideals concerning home and family thus became a means for 'respectable' women from the upper strata of the working classes to differentiate themselves from 'the boldness and dirtiness' thought to characterise lower segments of the working classes (Skeggs, 1999: 78; Levine, 1987: 187; Horgby, 1993: 368).

Skeggs's analysis refers to present-day England but a similar argument can be applied to Sweden in the 1930s. Several Swedish studies have shown how principally bourgeois norms regarding women's domestic duties were used by various social institutions such as the poor relief board, the child welfare board and different charity organisations to separate respectable women from those who were considered not respectable. In doing this, they both contributed to the diffusion of bourgeois norms and controlled their implementation. 'Respectable' women were generally more likely to receive poor relief or other kinds of assistance, while those women who lacked desirable traits became objects of corrective action (Plymoth, 2002: 126–30; Hatje, 1999: 55; Bergman, 2003: 74–76; Horgby, 1993: 410–11). Other institutions such as schools also contributed to the implementation of bourgeois norms in working-class families in two ways. They put the parents under economic pressure and it was in schools where children, and the efforts of their mothers, were presented, appraised and maybe even corrected (Ross, 1986: 74–75). Taking care of children *properly* thus became an important factor in the identity formation process. This, too, demanded that there be not too many children.

It can be stated that one important argument for not wanting more children was the care for the children already present in the family. The creation of new domestic norms made childrearing a greater responsibility than it had been during earlier decades. As a result, fewer children did not mean that the family saved money or that the mother had more time for herself. Rather, more money and more time could be spent on each child. This was how *respectable* families would distribute their resources. Still, it must be emphasised that working-class families, though adopting certain bourgeois ideals concerning the division of labour, family life, and childcare, did not actually want to *become* middle class. They constructed their own identity by adopting specific norms whilst filling them with new meanings which were grounded in the circumstances of their own lives. Their goal was usually to be good and respectable parents, and active birth control was one way they could make this happen.

Conclusions

This paper has examined the Swedish fertility decline by analysing almost 500 letters written by men and women during the 1930s. Source materials of this kind have been accused of failing to shed light on the generality of fertility decline. It has been argued that mass behaviour needs to be explained by large-scale processes such as industrialisation or mass-education that had a crucial impact on the masses (Woods, 1992: 134). These objections should be taken seriously but my conviction remains that fertility research needs sources like this. These personal letters cover a gap in a field crowded with numbers. More importantly, they offer information on how structural changes were *experienced* at the individual level and, in turn, how this influenced the contraceptive practices among ordinary men and women. These letters do tell us something important about which changes at the structural level really mattered at the level where reproductive decisions were actually made. This study shows that the experiences women had of carrying and delivering babies decisively influenced their willingness, and that of their husbands, to have more children. What this indicates is that changes at the structural level, which in some way affected these individual experiences, might also be seen to have affected birth rates at the aggregate level. I have emphasised how the perception of pain underwent important changes during the nineteenth century and how improvements in the area of medicine resulted in new attitudes to physical suffering. Both of these aspects can be linked to the greater process of secularisation. Not only the physical experiences of childbearing mattered when couples decided against having more babies, equally important were the experiences of raising children. Maternity (and to some extent paternity) was an experience that created frustrations of different kinds. The love for the children already present in the family, combined with difficulties in offering them an emotionally as well as materially secure childhood, often led to the decision to avoid future pregnancies.

An increasing number of children decreased the woman's chance to become what she considered to be a good mother. The 'good mother' represented a superior form of womanliness defined by respectability, purity and femininity. Thus, the project of gaining reproductive control can also be seen as a project through which women constructed themselves as respectable women. By having a reasonable number of children she distinguished herself from sexually decadent women with their too numerous (and dirty) children living in crowded and untidy homes.

More or less the same can be said about men. The ideal of the male breadwinner effectively separated the respectable man from the unrespectable. A man who financially supported his wife and children and had a responsible attitude towards sex and contraception distinguished himself from those who brought too many children into the world without being able to properly support them. Thus, birth control became both a strategy for restricting fertility and a means through which men and women constructed themselves as respectable members of a desirable masculinity or femininity. What this also indicates is that any process at the structural level influencing how parents experienced their parental responsibilities, is important towards an understanding of patterns of fertility. This text has underlined the importance of gender ideals such as the female housewife and the male breadwinner. These matters shaped people's experiences and affected their everyday life. They formed the ways in which they perceived themselves as a family, their own role within the family, their identities as men and women, and as mothers and fathers. And it decisively affected their reproductive behaviour.

References

Acker, Joan (1999), 'Rewriting Class, Race, and Gender: Problems in Feminist Rethinking', in Marx Ferree, Myra, Lorber, Judith and Hess, Beth B. (eds), *Revisioning Gender*, Thousand Oaks Calif., Sage, 44–69.

Alter, George (1992), 'Theories of Fertility Decline: A Non-specialist's Guide to the Current Debate', in Gillis, John R., Tilly, Louise A. and Levine, David (eds), *The European Experience of Declining Fertility, 1850–1970. A Quiet Revolution*, Cambridge Mass. and Oxford, Blackwell, 13–27.

Åkerman, Brita (1941), *Familjen som växte ur sitt hem,* Stockholm.

Åkerman, Sune (1981), 'How did the Great Decline in Fertility Start?', in Brändström, Anders and Sundin, Jan (eds), *Tradition and Transition. Studies in Microdemography and Social Change,* Umeå, The Demographic Database, 187–240.

Anderson, Margaret (1999), 'No Sex Please We're Demographers: Nineteenth Century Fertility Decline Revisited', in Damousi, Joy and Ellinghaus, Katherine (eds), *Citizenship, Women and Social Justice: International Historical Perspectives*, Melbourne, The University of Melbourne, 251–262.

Becker, Gary S. (1960), *Demography and Economic Change in Developed Countries*, Princeton, Princeton University Press.

Bergman, Helena (2003), *Att fostra till föräldraskap: Barnavårdsmän, genuspolitik och välfärdsstat 1900–1950*, Stockholm, Stockholm Studies in History.

Bernhardt, Eva (1971), *Trends and Variations in Swedish Fertility: A Cohort Study*, Stockholm, Statistiska Centralbyrån.

Bledsoe, Caroline, Guyer, Jane I. and Lerner, Susana (2000), 'Introduction', in Bledsoe, Caroline et al. (eds), *Fertility and the Male Life Cycle in the Era of Fertility Decline*, Oxford, Oxford University Press, 1–26.

Blom, Ida (1980), *Barnebegrensning – synd eller sunn fornuft*, Bergen, Universitetsforlaget.

Butler, Judith, (1999), *Gender Trouble: Feminism and the Subversion of Identity*, New York, Routledge.

Caton, Donald (1999), *What a Blessing She Had Chloroform: The Medical and Social Response to the Pain of Childbirth from 1800 to the Present*, New Haven, Conn., Yale University Press.

Danielsen, Hilde (2000), *Dei moderne kvinnene i Odda: Ein studie av mødrehygiene og barneavgrensing i mellomkrigstida*, Bergen, Norsk Vassskraft-og Industristadmuseum.

Edin, Karl Arvid and Hutchinson, Edward (1935), *Studies of Differential Fertility in Sweden*. London, P.S. King.

Finch, Lynette (1993), *The Classing Gaze: Sexuality, Class and Surveillance*, St Leonards, NSW, Australia, Allen & Unwin.

Fisher, Kate (2000), '"She Was Quite Satisfied with the Arrangement I Made": Gender and birth control in Britain 1920–1950', *Past and Present*, 169, 161–193.

Frykman, Jonas and Löfgren, Orvar (1979), *Den kultiverade människan*, Malmö, Gleerups förlag.

Giddens, Anthony (1992), *The Transformation of Intimacy: Sexuality, Love and Eroticism in Modern Societies*, Cambridge, Polity Press.

Gillis, John R. (1996), *A World of Their Own Making: Myth, Ritual, and the Quest for Family Values*, New York, Basic Books.

Gittins, Diana (1982), *Fair Sex. Family Size and Structure, 1900–1939*, London, Hutchinson.

Greene, Margaret E. and Biddlecom, Ann E. (2000), 'Absent and Problematic Men: Demographic Accounts of Male Reproductive Roles', *Population and Development Review*, 26, 81–115.

Greenhalgh, Susan (1995), 'Anthropology Theorizes Reproduction: Integrating Practice, Political, Economic, and Feminist Perspectives' in Greenhalgh, Susan (ed.), *Situating Fertility. Anthropology and Demographic Inquiry*, Cambridge, Cambridge University Press, 3–28.

Hamberg, Eva M. (2003), 'Christendom in Decline: The Swedish case', in McLeod, Hugh and Ustorf, Werner (eds), *The Decline of Christendom in Western Europe, 1750–2000*, Cambridge, Cambridge University Press, 47–62.

Hatje, Ann-Katrin (1999), *Från treklang till triangeldrama: Barnträdgården som ett kvinnligt samhällsprojekt under 1880–1940-talen*, Lund, Historiska Media.

Hirdman, Yvonne (1989), *Att lägga livet till rätta. Studier i svensk folkhemspolitik*, Stockholm, Carlssons förlag.

Horgby, Björn (1993), *Egensinne och skötsamhet: Arbetarkulturen i Norrköping 1850–1940*, Carlssons bokförlag, Stockholm.

Jejeebhoy, Shireen J. (2002), 'Convergence and Divergence in Spouses' Perspectives on Women's Autonomy in Rural India', *Studies in Family Planning*, 4, 299–308.

Johannisson, Karin (1995), *Den mörka kontinenten: Kvinnan, medicinen och fin-de-Siècle*, Norstedts förlag, Stockholm.

Johannisson, Karin (1997), *Kroppens tunna skal: Sex essäer om kropp, historia och Kultur*, Norstedts bokförlag, Stockholm.

Johansson, Peter (2002), 'Moderskapspolitiken och den manlige familjeförsörjaren: Politik, administration och synen på kvinnors rätt till ersättning vid födsel 1924–1931', in Bergman, Helena and Johansson, Peter (eds), *Familjeangelägenheter: Modern historisk forskning om välfärdsstat, genus och politik*, Stockholm, Symposium, 21–51.

Kvåle, Ingrid (1981), *Alt hva mødrene har kjempet ... Barnebegrensning i et lokalsamfunn 1910–1940: utbredelse, metoder og motiv*, Oslo, Universitetet i Oslo.

Larsson, Margareta (1984), *Fruktsamhetsmönster, produktionsstruktur och sekularisering. En jämförelse mellan 69 härader vid 1800-talets slut,* Stockholm.

Levine, David (1987), *Reproducing Families: The Political Economy of English Population History*, Cambridge, Cambridge University Press.

Lockridge, Kenneth A. (1983), *The Fertility Transition in Sweden. A Preliminary Look at Smaller Geographical Units, 1855–1890,* Umeå, The Demographic Data Base.

Mackinnon, Alison (1995), 'Were Women Present at the Demographic Transition? Questions from a Feminist Historian to Historical Demographers', *Gender & History*, 7, 222–240.

Mason, Karen O. (1997). 'Gender and Demographic Change: What Do We Know?', in Jones, G. W., Douglas, R. M., Caldwell, J. C. and D'Souza, R. M. (eds), *The Continuing Demographic Transition*, Oxford, Clarendon Press, 158–182.

Milton, Lena (2001), *Folkhemmets barnmorskor: Den svenska barnmorskekårens professionalisering under mellan- och efterkrigstid*, Uppsala, Acta Universitatis Upsaliensis.

Ohrlander, Kajsa (1992), *I barnens och nationens intresse: Socialliberal reformpolitik 1903–1930*, Stockholm, Almqvist & Wiksell.

Plymoth, Birgitta (2002), *Fostrande försörjning: Fattigvård, filantropi och genus i fabriksstaden Norrköping 1872–1914*, Stockholm, Almkvist och Wicksell.

Reiger, Karreen M. (1985), *The Disenchantment of the Home: Modernizing the Australian Family 1880–1940*, Oxford, Oxford University Press.

Riley, James C. (2003), 'Did mothers Begin with an Advantage? A Study of Childbirth and Maternal Health in England and Wales, 1778–1929', *Population Studies*, 57, 5–20.

Rogers, John (1995), 'Social Differentials and Fertility Decline in Uppsala and Västerås 1870–1930: A Contribution to the Understanding of the Fertility Transition', in Brändström, Anders and Tedebrand, Lars-Göran (eds), *Swedish Urban Demography During Industrialization,* Umeå, Report no. 10 from the The Demographic Database.

Ross, Ellen (1986), 'Labour and Love: Rediscovering London's Working-Class Mothers, 1870–1918', in Jane Lewis (ed.), *Labour and Love: Women's Experience of Home and Family, 1850–1940*, Oxford, Blackwell, 73–96.

Ross, Ellen (1992), 'Mothers and the State in Britain, 1904–1914', in Gillis, John R., Tilly, Louise A. and Levine, David (eds), *The European Experience of Declining Fertility, 1850–1970. A quiet revolution*, Cambridge Mass.and Oxford, Blackwell, 48–65.

Seccombe, Wally (1993), *Weathering the Storm. Working-Class Families from the Industrial Revolution to the Fertility Decline*, London, Verso.

Skeggs, Beverley (1999), *Att bli respektabel: Konstruktioner av klass och kön*, Bokförlaget Daidalos, Göteborg.

Stanfors, Maria (2003), *Education, Labor Force Participation and Changing Fertility Patterns: A Study of Women and Socioeconomic Change in Twentieth Century Sweden*, Stockholm, Almqvist & Wiksell International.

Sogner, Sølvi (2003), 'Abortion, Birth Control, and Contraception: Fertility Decline in Norway', *Journal of Interdisciplinary History*, 34, 209–234.

Szreter, Simon (1994), *Fertility, Class and Gender in Britain 1860–1940*, Cambridge, Cambridge University Press.

Thomas, James and Williams, A. Susan (1998), 'Women and Abortion in 1930s Britain: A Survey and its Data', *Social History of* Medicine, 2, 283–309.

Tosh, John (1999), *A Man's Place: Masculinity and the Middle-Class Home in Victorian England*, New Haven, Conn., Yale University Press.

Townsend, Nicholas (1997), 'Reproduction in Anthropology and Demography', in Kertzer, David I. and Fricke, Tom (eds), *Anthropological Demography: Toward a New Synthesis*, Chicago, The University of Chicago Press.

Watkins, Susan Cotts (1993), 'If All We Knew About Women was What We Read in *Demography*, What Would We Know?', *Demography*, 30, 551–577.

Woods, Robert (1992), 'Debate: Working-Class Fertility Decline in Britain', *Past and Present*, 134, 200–207.

'... But I'm so Embarrassed, I Said, if It's Another Baby!' Schooling, Girls and Declining Fertility in Urban South Australia in the Late Nineteenth and Early Twentieth Century

ALISON MACKINNON, CAZ BATSON, and JULIE PETERSEN-GRAY

Introduction

Caldwell's assertion that 'the fertility transition has a claim to be the most important happening of our time' (Caldwell and Caldwell, 1997: 15) is hardly surprising, given his significant input into the development of related theory. And the transition's importance continues since, rather than stopping at replacement levels as many anticipated, western fertility rates continue to plummet (see Golini, 1998). Notwithstanding the importance of the fertility decline in *our* time, it undoubtedly also had salience for the women who vociferously fought for control of their reproductive lives in print and public debates in the late nineteenth and early twentieth centuries. Some of the earliest cohorts of women to experience both those debates and the fertility transition were those in white settler societies of European origin, such as South Australia.

Fertility transitions have been explored in different ways by demographers, historians and anthropologists and quite diverse explanations and theories have been postulated as a consequence. Whilst teams of historical demographers (Coale and Watkins, 1986) have usefully mapped the contours of macro-demographic change, however, the poverty of major explanatory frameworks has often been noted (Cleland and Wilson, 1984; Alter, 1992). Eschewing purely economic explanations and theories of modernisation, demographers have somewhat 'complicated' the picture by turning to culture as an explanatory device; a device that offers great scope to the historian. In this context, Kertzer (1995) has suggested two different, but often interwoven, strands of thought. The first views culture as 'a grab-bag of non-demographic, non-economic characteristics that influence behaviour without themselves being susceptible to economic or demographic explanation' (Kertzer, 1995: 29). The second, emerging from within anthropological demography, is integrative and has a distinct political economic flavour. Here, culture is conceptualised as part of 'a model of the interaction of political, economic and cultural processes […] designed to produce a better understanding of the determinants of demographic behaviour' (Kertzer, 1995: 29). The latter, multi-faceted approach to explanation has much to recommend it (cf. Greenhalgh, 1995; Gillis, Tilly and Levine, 1992) and is the approach preferred here.

Working within a political economic framework, feminist economist Nancy Folbre has argued that the bargaining power of women in families increased as the transition to capitalism diminished patriarchal control over adult children and reduced the economic benefits of large families (Folbre, 1983; see also Mosk, 1983: 40). Bringing a gender relations perspective to bear on fertility change, the question might then be posed: 'Did women's bargaining power within partnerships increase in the latter part of the nineteenth century and, if so, what factors made a difference?'

Feminists are centrally concerned with cultural explanations of reproductive and social change. Australian philosopher Moira Gatens (1998: 4) has contended, for example, that gender can be understood as a set of regulatory norms that function to constrain the forms of conduct of men and women, as well as restricting their options for social action.[1] Arguably, for norms to be effective, they must be impartially and universally applied. However, drawing on the work of Ullmann-Margalit (1977), Gatens has proposed that gender norms are best understood as 'norms of partiality'; that is, norms that perpetuate inequality by promoting the interests of the party (or group) the inequality favours:

> Gender norms support a *status quo* in which one party is placed in a position of advantage and power in relation to the other party and this situation is itself presented as the 'natural order of things' rather than an exercise of power. (Gatens, 1998: 5)

1 The concept of 'gender norms' bears comparison with Karen Mason's (1997) 'gender systems'.

Norms are perpetuated by customs and habits, by various discourses and practices, and by institutions. Yet at times, not least during periods of rapid social change, they may also shift in quite significant ways. When norms begin to shift and the 'natural order of things' comes under challenge, power relations are likely to be contested. One might speculate, then, that the norms surrounding fertility and family formation changed in the late nineteenth and early twentieth centuries, a period of dramatic fertility decline, and thus pose the question 'Did changing norms subtly influence the power balances in gender relations at this time?'

Finally, in recognising the utility of an integrative approach to culture in investigations of fertility change, Hammel's (1990) contention that 'culture does not exist in some autonomous sense, but rather [...] is constituted' (cited in Kertzer, 1995: 47) is noteworthy. Can we observe culture and cultural change in the process of constitution and reconstitution in particular situations, in particular times? Perhaps a useful place to start is through a focus on education, a key element of culture making.

Education and Fertility Decline

Although the concepts of 'education', 'schooling' and 'literacy' have often been blurred (Lutz, Goujon and Doblhammer-Reiter, 1998), education as a lever of change has attracted considerable attention in past and present attempts to explain fertility transitions. Indeed, as evidenced in the work of Malthus (1803) the notion that education and knowledge might lead to control of population growth has a long history. Caldwell (1998: 681) notes Malthus' view that 'the diffusion of education and knowledge' might bring into force 'the preventive check, the delay of marriage' and Lees (1992: 313) further reminds that he advocated public schooling 'to teach citizens the true cause of their misery and to encourage them to adopt self-restraint and later marriage'.

Without doubt, the broadening of educational opportunity in the last quarter of the nineteenth century was one of the most potent socio-cultural change factors in western societies. In his classic formulation, John Caldwell (1980) made several important claims for the centrality of mass compulsory schooling as a change agent and, in so doing, emphasised that *breadth of education* (proportion receiving some schooling) was more influential than *depth of education* (average duration of schooling).[2] First, Caldwell maintained, that mass schooling reduced the time children were able or willing to spend working on behalf of the family and, concurrently, increased the costs of children both directly, in relation to school costs, and, indirectly, in foregone labour or income (the well-known intergenerational wealth flows theory). Second, mass schooling created new social norms about childhood as a time of dependency. Third, it accelerated cultural change, the creation of new cultures and, related to this, the propagation of western middle-class values within less developed countries.

Significantly, whilst acknowledging the economic impact of mass schooling through decreased child labour and increased consumption, Caldwell argued the *cultural influence of education* was most important. Education identified the child as a future, not a present, worker; it imposed middle-class values and stressed universal values rather than the particularistic ones of the family. As the cost of having children soared, Caldwell (1980: 28) argues, parents begrudgingly gave them up to the new state school systems whose teachings liberated them from the superstition and exploitation of their parents.

Did increased schooling *for girls* liberate them from the superstition and exploitation of their parents? Australian historian Ann Larson (1994), in a study of two Melbourne suburbs in the late nineteenth century which found that differentials between girls' and boys' schooling decreased with compulsory schooling, argues precisely this:

> Liberation, albeit quiet and subtle, is not too strong a word to use for the benefits to working class girls […] suddenly, unexpectedly, their schooling was treated as seriously as their brothers'. (Larson, 1994: 93)

Did education shift the gender norms of the time, particularly in relation to women as subjects, and their relative power within relationships? Can evidence of such shifts be found within their fertility patterns? On leaving school, girls were certainly more likely to find employment in factories than in domestic service, as had been the case before the advent of mass education, and such work experience may have contributed to family limitation. Diana Gittins

2 Caldwell (1980: 486), citing Coale (1969), defined mass schooling as 90 percent of children of primary school age attending school.

(1982), writing of the United Kingdom for example, claims that work experience before marriage in office or factory settings 'was very likely to equip the future working-class wife with knowledge of effective contraceptive techniques through discussion with workmates' (cited in Szreter, 1996: 53). Further support for the importance of schooling for girls and its influence on fertility patterns comes from Daniel Scott Smith's (1996) investigation of education and marital fertility in early twentieth-century Iowa, United States of America. Observing that 'something happened to girls who went to school that helped them, as married women, in setting or attaining lower fertility goals' (1996: 388), Scott Smith posited their fertility behaviour was 'altered by their contact with longer, and/or a more modern form of schooling'. Could that alteration have been in the norms of gender; in the acknowledgement that girls, too, could benefit from intellectual activity and from rational planning of their lives?

Interestingly, in the research discussed above, it is schooling rather than literacy *per se* that seems to be the driver of change and this may explain, in part, why countries such as Sweden, with a long history of female literacy, did not record a measurable decrease in fertility until the latter part of the nineteenth century (Mosk, 1983; Rogers, 1995). Accepting the premise that schooling was critical, then, the South Australian Family Formation Project (SAFFP) was designed to tease out constituent factors and contribute further to the debate.[3] The central aim of the SAFFP is to explore the pattern of falling fertility in South Australia at the micro level, looking for evidence of the impact of institutional factors such as class and education on individual decision-makers. More broadly, the SAFFP aims to further test Caldwell's thesis that mass education was an important factor in fertility decline and also extend his work by focusing attention on the place of women in this picture rather than that of 'the family'.

Covering the period, 1870–1930, the SAFFP is an interdisciplinary study within which both quantitative and qualitative methods are being applied to

3 The South Australian Family Formation project (SAFFP) was funded by the Australian Research Council (ARC) from 1996 to 1998. We wish to acknowledge the vital support of the ARC. The chief investigators, Alison Mackinnon and Ian Davey, were joined by PhD student Julie Petersen-Gray and Research Associate Caz Batson. The University of South Australia and the Research School of Social Sciences, ANU, also provided project support to Alison Mackinnon in 1999.

the phenomenon of fertility decline. Specifically designed to meet the challenge of large aggregate studies by including broad institutional contexts and the impacts of those contexts on individuals, the role of elementary education, which became 'free, compulsory and secular' in South Australia in, 1875, is of central interest. Consistent with Mackinnon's (1997) earlier work on the fertility patterns of highly educated women in South Australia, and Larson's (1994) on schooling and work in Melbourne, the SAFFP makes central a gender perspective, asking how certain changes in women's lives shaped their life chances. The nature of the relationship between access to schooling and falling fertility is of particular interest, as it was for Mackinnon and Larson.

The South Australian Family Formation Project

In 1870, when this story begins, South Australia was a thirty-four-year-old colonial settlement, its society bound, in the main, by the norms and traditions of its parent society, Britain. These were tempered, however, by a very different physical environment and contained a particular 'slice' of the originating society, a 'slice' that did not contain the same extreme class and religious elements. In fact it contained a larger proportion of dissenters, of radical Protestants; those who looked for greater freedom of religious expression and were wary of an established church. South Australia prided itself on its foundation as a free colony, one based on the Wakefield system, which not only envisaged a balance of labour, capital and land, but also of the sexes.[4]

As in the parent country, Britain, and in all other Australian colonies, fertility in South Australia declined rapidly in the late nineteenth century, although not always with the same patterns or the same timetable. By 1892, fertility had declined by 10 percent in Britain (Knodel and Van de Walle, 1979: 220), with different classes, occupations/ occupational groupings, and counties declining at different rates at different times (Szreter, 1996). It is estimated the decline in Britain was complete by about 1911.

4 In Edward Gibbon Wakefield's scheme of colonisation, equal numbers of men and women were to form the new colony, allowing for the growth of families and avoiding imbalances of the sexes, often blamed for prostitution and other ills in the more eastern colonies.

In contrast, evidence suggests many Australian families, formed by young couples who were immigrants, were nuclear from the start – perhaps because the absence of close kin made partners more reliant on each other, more 'modern' (Caldwell in Quiggan, 1988: iii; Grimshaw and Willett, 1981). As well, the fertility decline clearly manifested earlier in Australia, a 10 percent decline being recorded in 1881, and was also more rapidly completed, falling a further 30 percent by 1901 (Caldwell and Caldwell, 2001: 94).

In the South Australian context, fertility was apparently well into transition by about 1885 (Anderson, 1999) and almost complete by 1901 (Stevenson, 1982). As depicted in figure 1, the average number of children per married woman declined from a peak of 7.28 in the period 1831 to 1836 (a figure higher than the Australian average: Linford, 1950) and moved steadily down to 2.6 in the period 1897 to 1902 (Caldwell and Ruzicka, 1977). The average number of children per married women rose slightly in the period 1916 to 1936 but remained below an average of three for the rest of the twentieth century

In his 1903 annual report, the South Australian Registrar of Births, Deaths and Marriages speculated the 'serious' decline in birth rates (1886 being identified as the year it 'set in') might be attributed in no small part to increased age at marriage and 'changing, smaller family preferences'. In relation to the latter, he commented:

> it is believed, though this department can offer no undoubted proof [...] that in recent years some – perhaps a good many – of the married people of the state have preferred to have small or, at any rate, not large families, and have in consequence had recourse to various means to restrict the number of their offspring. (South Australia, Parliament, 1904)

For what reasons and with what techniques did that restriction occur? Was the Registrar correct in suspecting changing preferences?

Figure 1. Average Number of Children, all South Australian Marriages 1831–1902

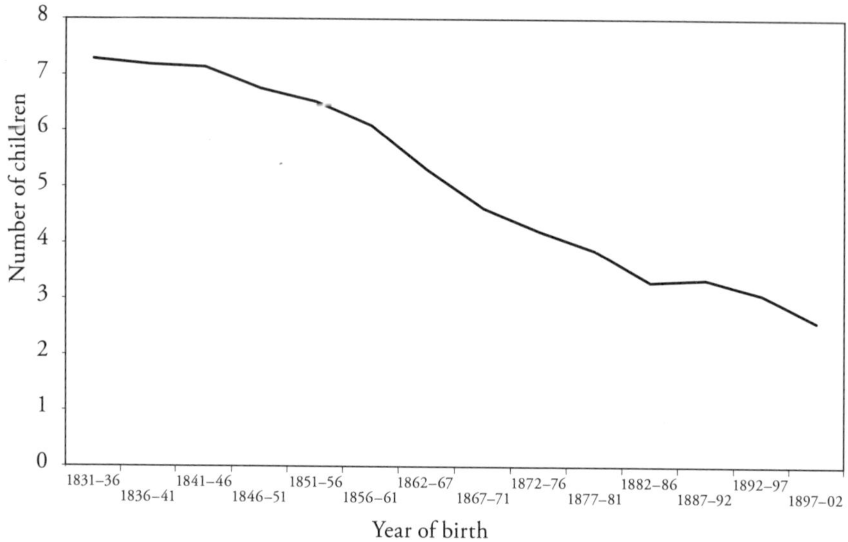

The SAFFP Database

Drawing on school attendance records, vital statistics and other literary and oral sources, the SAFFP database substantially charts education, life course and fertility records for a total of 447 South Australian females born between 1880 to 1899. To construct the SAFFP database, a computerised random sample of girls was initially drawn from Ian Davey's education database, which contains Hindmarsh Primary School attendance records in the late nineteenth and early twentieth centuries (Davey, 1981; Davey and Wimshurst, 1992: 158–171, particularly fn 5, p. 170).[5] This school was located in a predominantly

5 The Hindmarsh education database is a computerised data set of attendance and related records for Hindmarsh Primary School students collected by Ian Davey, one of the Chief Investigators of this project. This database was converted from Fortran into SPSS language/information and extensive manual checks were then carried out to ensure data accuracy and integrity. The Microsoft Access software program was used to categorise and store data collected in the SAFFP project.

working-class area of the city of Adelaide. The data drawn from attendance records permitted identification of the level of education potential subjects had attained (from Infant level to Grade 5, with satisfactory completion of Grade 4 signifying passing of the Compulsory Standard), as well as their parents' occupations.

Six cohorts of girls were then established on the basis of the broad 'class' groupings previously developed by Mackinnon and Davey (see Mackinnon, 1997) with reference to fathers' occupational data (unskilled workers, skilled workers and white collar workers) and two birth periods (1880 to 1889 and 1890 to 1899).[6] In order to increase the overall sample size and address the under-representation of certain groups of girls in the Hindmarsh database – particularly daughters of white collar workers – additional education records were subsequently sourced from Mitcham and from East Adelaide Primary School, both more middle class than working-class Hindmarsh. With this mix a sample representative of Adelaide as a whole was assembled. Family reconstitution was then used to link subjects' school attendance records to routinely generated official records, with death certificates serving as the starting point for tracing.[7] All information from a potential subject's death, birth and marriage (if applicable) certificates, as well as her children's birth certificates and applicable divorce or adoption records was obtained and cross-checked before any decision to include or exclude a subject was taken. Death certificates served as the primary source of information concerning the subjects' mothers' ages at marriage and death, occupation and birth issue. The final database, a rich and valuable record of school attendance and family formation in South Australia, is yet to be fully explored.

Of the 447 female subjects ultimately selected for inclusion in the SAFFP database, there is no record of marriage for 49 subjects (11 percent) and

6 Given that 1886 was identified as the year in which the South Australian fertility decline set in (SA Registrar of B, D, M: South Australia, Parliament 1904), the researchers selected subjects who attended school in the 1880s and 1890s in the hope that the impact of dramatic change in a short period would be captured.

7 The authors gratefully acknowledge the assistance of the Registrar of Births, Deaths and Marriages in South Australia without whose friendly cooperation the project could not have proceeded, and research assistant Ann Riddle who undertook much record linking work in the archives.

103 subjects (23 percent) apparently did not bear children.[8] Evidence of illegitimate children is scarce, there being only one subject who never married but bore three children, and another who gave birth to a child (father unknown) prior to her first marriage. In both instances, these children were included in relevant analyses. Five subjects who did not bear children are recorded as having adopted, fostered or assumed responsibility for parenting stepchildren; such children were excluded from analyses.

In view of the comparatively high number of childless women – 56 of whom were born in the 1880s and 47 in the 1890s – the extent to which the early death of subjects and spouses may have jeopardised or artificially truncated reproductive spans was investigated. A total of 34 women were identified as having died before reaching the age of 50, nine of whom were aged 24 or less ($\bar{x}$ birth issue = 0.11) and six aged 40 and above ($\bar{x}$ birth issue = 3.66). The 35–39 age bracket accounted for the highest number of deaths, with the mean number of children born for the nine women it contained being 1.6. Additionally, six spouse deaths that may have adversely impacted the reproductive life of their partners were identified, none of which occurred during war time. One subject re-married the following year and produced three children and two re-married eight to ten years later, one bearing her fifth child and the other her third and fourth. The remaining subjects who lost husbands through early death either did not re-marry or married late in life. Finally, the database records a total of five divorces, three of which occurred later in life when the women were aged 50 and over.

In terms of grade level of education achieved, the SAFFP database contains intact information for a total of 367 or 82 percent of subjects. Of these, 15.5 percent achieved Junior/Infant, 12.5 percent achieved Grade 1, 11 percent achieved Grade 2 and 26 percent achieved Grade 3. Of the 35 percent (109 subjects) who achieved Grade 4 or higher, five moved beyond elementary school to attend high school. Information concerning the Compulsory Standard, available for a total of 342 or 76.5 percent of subjects, indicates that 35.4 percent achieved the Compulsory Standard and 64.6 percent did not.

8 Stillbirths were not recorded at this time so 'childlessness' cannot always be assumed to be voluntary. It is also possible that some early infant deaths were treated as stillbirths and not registered as live births.

Whilst the two birth cohorts (1880s n = 251; 1890s n = 196) do not capture the beginning of the fertility decline in South Australia, they reflect a time when a substantial proportion of children were attending school following the 1875 introduction of 'compulsory' primary education. In this context, the availability of extensive education records obviously facilitates closer consideration of Caldwell's contention that *breadth*, rather than *depth*, of education was the more potent force for change. As well, the decision to study a sample of girls born in the later part of the nineteenth century attends to McDonald's (2000: 430) suggestion that 'more value may be obtained from studying why fertility continues to decline to low levels after it has commenced to fall'.

Findings: Intergenerational Changes in Fertility Patterns

After initially calculating the median age at marriage and the mean number of children (refer table 1) for all subjects in the unskilled, skilled and white collar categories, those recorded as bearing no children were excluded and generational differences in birthrates and marriage ages were then examined for daughter-mother pairs. Acknowledging the considerable diversity of experience reflected in the size of standard deviations reported in table 1, a downward trend in fertility patterns from the mothers' generation, born in the period 1840–1879, to that of their daughters, is nonetheless clearly evident. Of particular note is the overall decline in the average number of children born to women in the 1880s cohort ($\bar{x} = 3.78$, sd = 2.41) compared to their mothers ($\bar{x} = 7.49$, sd = 2.83), and also for the women in the 1890s cohort ($\bar{x} = 2.93$, sd = 2.14) compared to their mothers ($\bar{x} = 7.07$, sd = 2.97). Further to this, a comparison of mean numbers of children born across class categories reveals that, overall, the skilled category accounts for the largest daughter-mother difference, with an average number for women in both cohorts taken together of 3.00 (sd 2.15) compared to 7.44 (sd 3.05) for their mothers. The skilled category also accounts for the largest differential between the daughters and their mothers within the two birth cohorts.

Further to these intergenerational differences, and as might be expected, table 1 points to some interesting differences between the daughters who became mothers. Not only is the overall mean number of children born to

Table 1. Age at Marriage and Mean Number of Children by Occupational Status, for Two Cohorts of Daughters and Their Mothers

Marriage Age	(all daughters)		(daughters became mothers)		(mothers)	
	N	Median	N	Median	N	Median
1880s Cohort						
Unskilled	84	22.0	72	21.5	58	21.0
Skilled	76	24.0	67	24.0	70	21.0
White Collar	66	25.0	56	25.0	68	21.5
Total	226	24.0	195	23.0	196	21.0
1890s Cohort						
Unskilled	57	24.0	47	23.0	47	21.0
Skilled	81	22.0	74	22.0	73	21.0
White Collar	35	24.0	28	24.0	23	24.0
Total	173	23.0	149	23.0	143	21.0
All						
Unskilled	141	23.0	119	22.0	105	21.0
Skilled	157	23.0	141	23.0	143	21.0
White Collar	101	25.0	84	25.0	91	22.0
Total	399	23.0	344	23.0	339	21.0

such women in the 1890s cohort ($\overline{x} = 2.93$, sd = 2.14) appreciably lower than that for women in the 1880s cohort ($\overline{x} = 3.78$, sd = 2.41), the mean issue for the 1890s cohort within each social class category is consistently lower than that of the 1880s cohort. In the unskilled category, women in the 1890s cohort had 0.6 children fewer than their counterparts born in the 1880s, those in the skilled category had 0.8 fewer children and those in the white collar category, 1.1 fewer. A pattern of declining fertility between social class categories is also discernible within the 1890s birth cohort where the women in the skilled category had, on average, 1.0 children fewer than those in the unskilled, and women in the white collar category had 0.1 less than those in the skilled. The period studied, then, was one of substantial change in fertility patterns.

Table 1 (continued).

Number of children	(all daughters)			(daughters became mothers)			(mothers)		
	N	Mean	St. dev	N	Mean	St. dev	N	Mean	St. dev
1880s Cohort									
Unskilled	84	3.63	2.83	72	4.24	2.60	60	7.42	2.96
Skilled	85	2.69	2.62	67	3.42	2.49	73	7.84	3.00
White Collar	82	2.48	2.35	56	3.63	1.98	78	7.22	2.54
Total	251	2.94	2.65	195	3.78	2.41	211	7.49	2.83
1890s Cohort									
Unskilled	66	2.59	2.99	47	3.64	2.95	51	7.25	3.06
Skilled	91	2.13	1.86	74	2.62	1.72	85	7.09	3.04
White Collar	39	1.85	1.42	28	2.57	0.96	32	6.72	2.57
Total	196	2.23	2.24	149	2.93	2.14	168	7.07	2.97
All									
Unskilled	150	3.17	2.93	119	4.00	2.75	111	7.34	3.00
Skilled	176	2.40	2.27	141	3.00	2.15	158	7.44	3.05
White Collar	121	2.27	2.11	84	3.27	1.77	110	7.07	2.54
Total	447	2.63	2.50	344	3.41	2.33	379	7.30	2.89

Notes:
1. A total of 65 mothers had more than one daughter attending the schools from which education records were sourced.
2. A total of 14 subjects were included in the database despite there being no information available for their mothers.

Source: SAFFP database and SA Registry of Births, Deaths and Marriages.

Changing ages of marriage obviously warrant attention but South Australia's unique historical position must first be recognised. Whilst South Australia was peopled in the main by British settlers, the median age at marriage for women in the colony nonetheless sat some distance below that for England and Wales in the period 1866 to 1876, with parity not evidenced until as late as 1901. The significance of the younger median age at marriage for South

Australian women in the 1866–1876 period is highlighted by McDonald (1974: 107), who cites it as 'the only instance, for either sex, in all the colonies, when age at marriage was significantly earlier than England and Wales'. By way of explanation, it is considered likely that the commitment to achieve a balance of the sexes in South Australia's 'Wakefieldian' system of settlement exerted a downward influence on age at marriage.

Median ages at marriage for all subjects, and their mothers, are reported in table 1. As might be expected, given that the median age at marriage for all South Australian women moved slowly up from 21.6 in 1866, to 21.8 in 1871 and then to 22.5 in 1881 (McDonald, 1974: 105, 140), the subjects' mothers had a median age at marriage of 21.0. In contrast, the median for the subjects overall, as well as for those who became mothers themselves, was two years higher (23.0). Further to this, table 1 records differences in the median ages of marriage for the daughter-mother pairs within social class categories. Of these, the overall median ages at marriage for the white collar cohort subjects who became mothers (25.0), and their mothers (22.0), stand in notable contrast to those associated with the unskilled cohort (median = 22.0 and 21.0 respectively).

Bearing in mind that age at marriage can only partly explain the dramatic intergenerational differences in fertility reported above, and Caldwell's (1980) assertion that mass compulsory schooling altered fertility in measurable ways, the influence of education variables was considered next. Could higher levels of schooling per se have led to a family limitation? Or, as Gittins' (1982, cited in Szreter, 1996) theorising about the relationship between workplace settings and availability of accurate contraceptive knowledge suggests, could occupation at marriage have been influential? Attention thus turned to a closer investigation of factors such as level of education achieved, age on leaving school and post-school occupations.

Data obtained about the grade level of education subjects achieved, their median ages on leaving school and mean birth issue for the two cohorts taken together is reported in table 2. Looking first at level of education, the consistent downward trend in mean issue for all subjects (daughters), apparent from Grade 1 upwards, provided a tantalising hint that higher levels of education might be linked to lower birth issue as contemporary cross-country econometric studies have demonstrated (UNDP, 1995: 110). Thus the apparent anomaly at the Junior/Infant level was investigated further. It was found that whilst there was nothing particularly unusual about this group of women, in terms of ages at marriage, school leaving ages, urban/rural residency and so on, the mean issue for the two birth cohorts was substantially different: 4.1 for the 1880s cohort (n = 14) and 2.7 for the 1890s cohort (n = 30). Further investigation of the original records of the women in the 1890s cohort not only revealed that a high proportion did not bear children but also that a disproportionately high number suffered from chronic illnesses such as tuberculosis and diabetes.

Table 2. Age at Leaving School and Mean Number of Children by Level of Education, Cohorts 1880 and 1890 Taken Together

	Age left school				Mean number of children					
	Daughters		Daughters (became mothers)		Daughters			Daughters (became mothers)		
	N	Median	N	Median	N	Mean	St dev	N	Mean	St dev
Level of Education										
Junior/ infant	57	12.9	44	12.9	57	2.42	2.26	44	3.14	2.09
Grade 1	45	11.8	38	11.7	45	3.00	2.33	38	3.55	2.10
Grade 2	40	12.0	30	12.7	40	2.78	2.92	30	3.70	2.82
Grade 3	96	13.0	68	13.0	96	2.51	2.68	68	3.54	2.54
Grade 4 or higher	127	13.0	98	13.2	129	2.40	2.23	99	3.12	2.06
Total	365	13.0	278	13.0	367	2.54	2.45	279	3.35	2.28

Source: SAFFP database and SA Registry of Births, Deaths and Marriages.

Subsequently, a quite different picture emerged when all subjects who did not produce children were excluded from the analysis; the consistent downward trend transforming into a bell curve. Women who achieved Grade 3 or higher produced fewer children than those who achieved a Grade 2 education, but the mean issue for those with a Grade 4 or higher education ($\bar{x} = 3.12$, sd = 2.06) is only marginally less than for those who did not move beyond the Junior/Infant level ($\bar{x} = 3.14$, sd = 2.09) and, similarly, the mean number of children produced by those who achieved a Grade 3 education ($\bar{x} = 3.54$, sd = 2.54) bears comparison with that for women who left school after Grade 1 $\bar{x} = 3.55$, sd = 2.10).

Whilst the data reported in table 2 provides no compelling evidence that the level of education achieved markedly influenced the number of children produced, the SAFFP database continues to provoke thought around this seminal question. Interestingly, for example, it is apparent that the women in the cohort overall who later produced four or more children were generally more likely to have only completed Grades 1, 2 or 3, whilst those who produced two or three were much more likely to have completed Grade 4.

Returning to table 2, it can be seen that the range in the girls' school leaving age is very narrow, the lower boundary being set by those who achieved Grade 1 (11.7 years) and went on to become mothers, and the upper by those who achieved Grade 4 or above (13.2 years) and who also went on to become mothers. On investigation of school attendance profiles in the data set, the narrowness of the range was judged to be largely attributable to the sporadic nature of attendance at school, with many girls simply not attending regularly enough to progress to higher grades. In so far as it was not uncommon for girls in this era to be kept at home to assist with laundry, housework and illness or childbirth – despite the introduction of 'compulsory' schooling – this finding did not surprise.

In further examining the potential role of education variables, some evidence to support the contention that higher educational attainment led to a higher marital age was found. Of those who married at ages 16 to 20, for example, 50 percent had only completed Grade 2 or below whilst 75 percent of those who married at ages 23 to 24, and 69 percent of those at ages 25–27, had completed Grade 3 or 4. Thus although, as previously noted, there was not a huge differential in the median school leaving age (one and a half years) across education levels, the number of years that individual girls attended school may well have been influential in determining their age at marriage. On the other hand, there may have been something qualitatively different about the experiences and personal goals of those who moved beyond the lower grades.

Finally, in order to draw the threads of analysis together, a standard multiple regression was performed with the number of children born to the women in the SAFFP as the dependent variable.[9] The decision to focus on years in attendance at school, in this context, rather than grade level achieved or age on

9 Whilst occupation at marriage was not utilised in the regression due to the very high number of missing cases, it warrants further investigation via other methods.

leaving school was taken in light of the results reported above and the obvious assumption that those who achieved higher grades would have attended school for longer and left school at an older age. The results obtained (see table 3) indicated that the overall regression model was significant F (3, 382) = 30.97, $p = .000$ with the three predictor variables in combination accounting for 18.9 percent (adjusted $R^2 = .196$) of the variance in the number of children born. Thus the regression shows that, consistent with Caldwell's explanation, depth of education played a role although other variables were clearly at play.

Table 3. Number of Children, Regression Model for Two Cohorts

Variables	β	*Sig*
Age at marriage	-0.399	.000
Born in the 1890s	-0.139	.003
Years attended school	-0.116	.013

Note: $R^2 = 0.196$, F (3,382) = 30.97, $p = .000$.

Deliberate efforts to space births beyond normal biological expectations are usually seen as a major means of birth control and evidence of some use of family limitation. Rogers (1995), drawing on Livi-Bacci, points out that 'generally the interval [in a society with natural fertility] falls between 24 and 36 months'. With this in mind, some preliminary investigations of relationships between birth intervals and level of education were undertaken. Data pertaining to birth intervals between marriage and the first child was excluded from analysis, this interval being generally regarded as qualitatively different from others, as was that for birth intervals beyond the eighth child due to small sample size.

The overall birth interval (mean months) for women in the 1880s cohort was 32.3 (n = 167) and for all women in the 1890s cohort, 34.5 (n = 112). Within the 1880s cohort, a steady decline in the overall birth interval (mean months) was evidenced as the level of education achieved increased, from 36.0 for those who did not progress beyond a Junior/ Infant education (n = 36), to 33.1 for those who achieved Grade 2 or 3 (n = 86) and 27.6 for those who achieved Grade 4 or above (n = 45). Within the 1890s cohort, those who reached Grade 4 or above also showed a noticeably lower overall birth interval

Table 4. Mean Birth Intervals by Level of Woman's Education and by Birth Cohort

	1st–2nd		2nd–3rd		3rd–4th		4th–5th		5th–6th	
Level of education	1880s	1890s	1880s	1890s	1880s	1890s	1880s	1890s	1880s	1890s
Junior/ Infant and Grade 1	36.90	36.43	43.07	41.95	35.95	39.20	39.51	48.64	42.04	39.00
Grade 2 and 3	37.99	42.07	36.35	42.56	33.12	49.83	32.94	63.7	32.38	48.90
Grade 4 and above	40.56	36.59	35.79	42.87	33.85	48.74	30.10	32.97	32.38	22.76
Total	38.46	37.15	37.90	42.45	34.04	43.86	34.12	43.00	34.00	34.15

(mean months = 30.6; n = 54) than did those who completed Grade 2 or 3 (mean months = 39.4; n = 12) or Junior/ Infant education (mean months = 37.9; n = 46). It is noteworthy that the overall birth intervals for women in the 1890s cohort who received less education fall outside of Livi-Bacci's proposed boundaries.

A more detailed comparison of individual birth intervals (mean months) by level of education achieved is contained in table 4. Amongst the variable patterning evident at the different education levels, the overall between cohort differences in birth intervals for the second and third (4.6 mean months), third and fourth (9.8 mean months) and fourth and fifth children (8.9 months) immediately attract the eye. It seems there was at least some increase in spacing across the two cohorts. It also appears that in lower parities women spaced their births more than at higher parities. Could it be that those who had very large families (say five or six children) were not either using spacing or stopping behaviours? It is hard to be precise about this issue as the numbers of women who reached the higher level of education and had several children were very small, confounding numerical analysis.

Perhaps, an exploratory analysis of total reproductive years might be more productive. As table 5 shows, there was an overall downward shift of approximately 22.5 months between decades in terms of total reproductive years (measured in mean months), from 114.6 to 92.0. In fact, a comparison between the 1880s and 1890s at all levels of education reveals downward shifts

Table 5. Female Reproductive Period in Mean Number of Months by Level of Education

	1880s birth cohort			1890s birth cohort		
	Age at marriage (median)	Age at last birth (median)	Total reproductive period	Age at marriage (median)	Age at last birth (median)	Total reproductive period
Level of education						
Junior/ Infant and Grade 1	22.00	35.00	134.11	23.00	31.00	89.75
Grades 2 and 3	24.50	33.00	110.60	23.00	32.00	93.05
Grade 4 and above	24.00	34.00	106.50	24.00	32.00	86.63
Total	24.00	34.00	114.56	24.00	32.00	92.03

in terms of total reproductive years. Within the 1880s cohort, women who achieved a grade 4 and above level of education clearly had a shorter reproductive span (106.5 months) than those with junior, infant and grade 1 (134.1) but, within the 1890s cohort, the reproductive span for women who achieved these education levels was comparable. Shortening of the reproductive span could obviously account, in part, for the differential discussed earlier – that of fewer children by level of education attained – since years spent in reproduction will clearly influence the number of children born. Such a finding would be consistent with the results of another South Australian study which led the author to conclude that 'the most significant factor overall is a substantial reduction in the period spent bearing children' (Anderson, 1999: 254). Here, then, is Malthus' preventive check, albeit in a slightly different form.

Table 5 also facilitates the exploration of a possible relationship between level of education and age at birth of last child, drawing on the notion that this might reveal the use of family limitation. Overall, the observed differences within and between cohorts are interesting and perhaps warrant further investigation. Of particular interest is the fact that last births occurred, on average, almost two years earlier for those in the 1890s cohort (32 years of age) than for those in the 1880s cohort (34 years of age). As ages of marriage were similar clearly some 'stopping' behaviour was apparent. Completed families were achieved at an earlier age. For those who married later and who 'stopped' childbearing earlier, the number of reproductive years was limited. Young South Australian women were completing family formation, with smaller families, by their early thirties, with obvious health and social benefits. Their lives were qualitatively different from the generations before. Those who worked before marriage, then bore two or three children within about eight years, had many years beyond that childbearing stage, allowing opportunities for work or community involvement.

The results show that level of education attained influences age at marriage and indirectly total years available for reproduction. The precise manner in which those reproductive years contracted for girls with Grade 4 and above education who were born in the 1880s is unclear but we can see that they married later, if not always appreciably so, possibly spending more years in paid work before marriage, a situation for which their education prepared them.

In the sample overall, 35 percent completed the Compulsory Standard or above, qualifying them for significant work opportunities at that time. Another 26.2 percent completed Standard 3, qualifying over 60 percent in all for work beyond the very basics. The period in which women in the sample left school and sought jobs (mainly from the early 1890s to the 1910s) was one in which work opportunities outside the home opened up dramatically for South Australian women, in spite of the depression that affected much of the colony in the 1890s (Magarey, 1993: 95). Many were rejecting domestic service, as they did in Melbourne (Larson, 1994: 188). Helen Jones points out that the participation of all women aged fifteen to sixty years in the workforce rose from 24.9 percent in 1871 to 32.9 percent in 1891. By 1891, therefore, almost a third of all women were employed (Jones, 1986: 65). In 1900 over 2000 women worked in factories (much preferred to the restrictions of domestic service), rising by 1904 to 4000 and to 6000 in 1919–20. Between 1900 and 1920 women's share of the manufacturing labour force increased from 15 to 20 percent. For those who passed the Compulsory Standard, possibilities in clerical work and teaching opened up. Ann Larson points out that, of non-agriculturally employed women in Victoria in 1901, 70 percent were in service or working in a factory or workroom (Larson, 1994: 112). This was a shift downward from 79 percent in 1871. Presumably some of the missing 9 percent were able, due to their education, to move into the emerging areas of clerical or retail work or even into teaching through the pupil teacher route, a scheme that enabled promising students to undertake a type of teaching apprenticeship. In neighbouring South Australia a similar pattern existed.

Opportunities in education and the workplace were significantly reshaping women's life chances in this period, of that there is no doubt. But did these opportunities alter women's position within marriages and other consensual unions? Knowing that the reproductive years were shortened does not tell us very much about the significance of such a major life transformation. Nor does it tell us why women ceased childbearing earlier. What difference did those years at school, those years in the workplace, possibly enjoying a modicum of independence, make to the way in which women communicated with their husbands when they did marry? Were new values, new desires, inculcated by their schooling, by their work, or both? Did they gain a small shift in bargaining power with their partners? Did they reshape the gender norms of the period?

Increasing Bargaining Power?

Caldwell claims that the pre-transitional family survives the early period of capitalist development in a two-tiered system of a capitalist economy and a pre-capitalist family, supporting high fertility until the traditional family morality and culture is undermined. Was the traditional family morality and culture undermined by the nature of schooling, particularly by its more individualistic and secular character? Importantly, he argues *that mass education dissolved this traditional familial culture*. While acknowledging the economic impact of mass schooling, Caldwell argues, as has been seen, that it was *the cultural influence of education that was most important*. Also, the previous section has shown that the numbers of years immersed in familial culture in their homes of origin could contract for many who tallied up several years of school attendance.

Were these Australian young women the *modern* precursors of the contemporary pattern, of late marriage and fewer children? A fascinating attempt to link postmodern approaches to values, and the resulting attitudinal change to fertility preferences, was made by Dirk Van de Kaa (1998). He specifies, in the contemporary context, the existence of 'mental' cohorts intent on increasing the freedom of choice of individuals, supportive of pluralistic ideas and seeking gender equity and the emancipation of minority sections of the population'. These cohorts, he believes, exert 'considerable influence on demographic preferences' (1998: 11). Can Van de Kaa's work on contemporary society be applied to the historical situation? Were young educated women in the late nineteenth century a different 'mental cohort' in that their life patterns could include some notions of life beyond the round of childbearing and rearing: a period, albeit short for many, of economic independence? Perhaps their state schooling nurtured a more secular approach (Lockridge, 1983) and a sense that girls and women could succeed as well as boys in the tasks set by the school.

Here historical demography needs assistance from women's historians and historians of gender relations (Mackinnon, 1995). Elsewhere one of us has written about the major gender issues under broad discussion in the period, a time when 'the woman question' dominated popular culture (Mackinnon, 2000; see also Quiggin, 1988; Anderson, 1999). Newspapers and pamphlets of the time questioning women's role could hardly have escaped the eyes of young female readers. And, as Caldwell points out, 'women's movements exerted influences far beyond the circle of feminist activists' (Caldwell, 1999: 502). Women's suffrage was granted in South Australia in 1894, far earlier than all European societies, and the wide debates before and after that historic legislation could scarcely be ignored. Girls who completed significant levels of education (in Australia the Compulsory Standard) were often taught by young female teachers and aspired to paid work themselves. The active debates in the popular press about 'the marriage question' and 'the woman question' might also have led them to question the ways in which their mothers and grandmothers had lived and the inevitability of childbearing (see Bacchi, 1986).

How did Fertility Decline? The Question of Family Limitation

The way in which South Australian women limited their families is not a major focus of this essay. However, as it bears upon the argument on changing values and subjectivities it will be briefly considered. A pattern of stopping rather than spacing most likely characterised the fertility transition in South Australia. Yet most discussions of the nineteenth-century Australian fertility decline include references to 'innovative' (Quiggin, 1988: 119), 'increasingly effective' (Caldwell and Ruzicka, 1978: 90), and more 'informed' (Larson, 1994: 57) fertility control methods. Evidence in Australia about knowledge, distribution and use of these new methods is scant, and many authors refer to the evidence given in the New South Wales 1903 Royal Commission into the Decline of the Birthrate (RCDB) to support their claims. Neville Hicks and Kerreen Reiger, amongst others, question this evidence and their findings (Hicks, 1978: 157; Reiger, 1985: 114). Evidence as to information about and effectiveness and availability of birth control methods in South Australia from 1860 until the 1930s is correspondingly difficult to find, although birth control almost certainly existed. Perhaps what was 'innovative' and 'more informed' was the attitude of young women to themselves, to their futures and to the possibilities of limiting families.

Overall it seems that abstinence and withdrawal, with a final option of resort to abortion, were the most likely means by which the fertility decline, so obvious in the cohort of girls studied here, was achieved. If such age-old methods were the methods of choice then some new way of thinking about themselves, some shifts in the 'gender norms' or patterns of bargaining power, must have characterised the young women of South Australia. Anderson reminds us that the 1903 Royal Commission into the Decline of the Birthrate accepted that the idea that family limitation was spreading was 'common knowledge':

> During the last quarter of the nineteenth century, a wave of popular feeling spread over a great part of the civilized world, favourable to the individual control of the size of families; and with it there has been a general diffusion of the knowledge of methods by which restriction might be accomplished which previously was wanting. The history of this movement is a matter of common knowledge. (RCDB, 1903: 17, cited in Anderson, 1999: 256)

And, if abstinence and withdrawal were common women must have had the cooperation of their husbands. As Quiggin says of the neighbouring colony of Victoria at a not dissimilar time, wives were now expected to be companions to their husbands. Quiggin claims 'they should have been in a position to talk about the physical and emotional pressures of frequent childbearing and large families and to suggest that measures be taken to ease their burdens' (Quiggin, 1988: 74). 'This was important', she continues, 'because, although abortion and some forms of contraception could be used without their husband's knowledge, women needed a cooperative husband if they were to space or curtail their pregnancies by the use of *coitus interruptus* or by periodic or total abstinence' (1988: 74).

'Everything Was a Secret in Those Days'

Can one identify those cultural factors that might have reshaped gender norms: the sense of movement, of negotiation, of the ongoing reconstitution of relations between social actors in a constantly changing social context which is central to understanding the changes in reproductive decision making? Can one detect a sense of the subjectivities of the women involved? Two brief extracts from interviews with elderly South Australian women reveal some telling contradictions.[10] While many women of this generation strongly denied any knowledge of birth control, even of birth processes, it is clear that they were not totally ignorant, but were more likely reflecting prevailing taboos on speaking about reproduction (see also Caldwell, 1999; Fisher, 2000).

'Mrs M', born in 1903, had lived most of her life in urban Adelaide. Her father was a tram driver, and she was the second eldest of 10 siblings. She had had two years of night school education after leaving primary school at thirteen, worked as a doctor's receptionist before marriage, and married at twenty-one a man who later became a bank officer. Mrs M had one surviving child, and had strong Presbyterian religious affiliations.

> No! I did not know anything. Green as grass. They didn't tell you anything. Everything was secret in those days.

> No! I'd been with my mother [...] right up until the [...] midwife came. My father came home from work that day. I'd been home all day mopping up water and I didn't know where it was coming from, and, my mother said, you get something and wipe that up, and I did that [...] The doctor had to come [...] and I sung out to the women next door, I said, Mrs Neagle, could you come in here, I said I think my mother is going to have another baby (in a surprised voice). So this is right up to half past six, seven o'clock at night. And my father said to me You mind what you are saying, my girl [...] I was so disgusted, my husband, husband to be, was coming through the gate, and I said to him, I said if you think that I'm going to go through what I've been through today, and seen my mother go through, I said you're mistaken. I'm not going to get married, well he said, It's manners to wait you're asked (laughs) and then my father said, well everything is alright, you've looked after your mother well. Well, I said, I know this country needs population, Dad, but nobody expected you to do it on your own (laughs). Don't you speak to me like that, he says.

10 These interviews were conducted by Julie Petersen-Gray.

Interviewer: You can remember that your mother was in pain?

> Oh yes, I didn't know what was going on at the time. I said to my sister Amy, Amy was married at the time, and I said you know Mum is getting so fat, I said and I'm so embarrassed when Stan [husband to be] comes. She said Mum's not fat, I was that green. She said to me, look, Stan's been around the world, she said, and he's not stupid. I said, but I'm so embarrassed, I said, if it's another baby! My sister didn't tell me much, but my girlfriend from night school told me […] Children come out the same way that they go in, I couldn't work that out. And I said don't be ridiculous, that's an impossibility, they cut them across the stomach, that's how they get them out. Oh! She said, they do not.

Later, speaking of her own marriage Mrs M referred to birth control: 'They were called French Letters in those days […] Because my husband was a returned man, he knew all about them …'

These passages are helpful in their complex interweaving of a pride in ignorance and a defiant refusal of childbearing. A number of times Mrs M talked of her ignorance – 'I was that green' – and said that she 'didn't know anything' about birth control. Her father's words reinforce the need to be silent on such matters: 'you mind what you are saying my girl'. She claimed her mother did not tell her anything, but later in the interview said that her mother-in-law had told her that when she missed a period it was time to see a doctor. Nevertheless she registered a strong feeling of disgust at the notion of her mother's continual childbearing, telling her future husband that she was not going to go through 'what her mother went through'.

This sense of unease at constant childbearing suggests, perhaps, a different set of expectations from one who had achieved a certain level of education and enjoyed a period in the workforce. Perhaps these women did come to see 'the true cause of their misery' in Malthus's terms. Is this the sense of gender inequity that McDonald discusses? He claims that 'in high-fertility contexts, gender inequity within the family may be experienced as, *inter alia*, a generalized dissatisfaction with the rigors and dangers of a constant round of childbearing and child rearing imposed by spousal, familial and societal expectations' (McDonald, 2000: 428). Mrs M had enjoyed two years of night school and had worked as a doctor's receptionist: conditions, one might expect, for a greater knowledge of the body than she admitted. Bearing out Diana Gittins' (1982) notion of sharing knowledge, Mrs M also admits that her friend from night school told her about childbirth – not her mother or her sister. Had the doctor made comments about too frequent childbirths, we wonder, following Seccombe's argument that doctors, while not usually giving women information about contraception, often made it clear that constant childbearing was bad for health (Seccombe, 1990).

'Mrs K' was born in 1898 in the country town where she lived for most of her life. Her father was an odd job man, and she was the youngest of 11 siblings. She had had seven years of formal education before working as a nurse's assistant, marrying a salesman at the age of nineteen. She had three children. Mrs K had been christened as a Lutheran but was opposed to formal religion.

> No! I did not want any children. (loudly) […] I'd had enough of kids, don't worry. I never wanted them. But I got them. All's the same. Play around you must get caught! I got them.

Mrs K's ideas of birth control seem to have relied on traditional beliefs.

> 'Cause people told us in those days, while you're feeding a baby, you'll never get pregnant again. That's a lie! (laughs)
>
> [I had] No information from mother or sister! But, but what my sister did tell me, and that's sister Rose who had those ten children, she said to me one time, and this was when I was having Patty, so she said I'll tell you something. Oh I thought to myself, she must know what to do, well, if I could get rid of this baby I would, I had two, two babies, both of them only two years between the two of them, I didn't want any more. So, she said to me, one of these nights, she said you get in and have a real hot bath, as hot as you can bear it, and she said after that you've got to drink some washing soda. Washing soda! Did you ever hear of such a thing in all your life? And I was fool enough to drink it. I don't know how much I took. I have no idea. I couldn't tell, she must have told me how much to take. Oh! It was terrible stuff. Terrible stuff!
>
> After Patty was born there was something wrong with me […] Whether it was the washing soda, washed them all away or not, I don't know (laughing). I had no idea. I mean those things you never discussed. Everything was a secret in those days, your whole life.

What do these extracts tell us that remains hidden (secret?) in the statistical data? Were these women 'liberated from the superstition and exploitation of their parents', as Caldwell and Larson suggest? Both excerpts tell seemingly contradictory stories of women negotiating sexuality and childbirth. Mrs K and Mrs M both reinforce a number of times that they had no knowledge about contraception, about their sexuality; they 'knew nothing'. This was as much a reflection of the prevailing expectations of 'decent' women, as Houghton found: 'in the Victorian home sex was a secret […] no-one mentioned it … [and] at the bottom it sprang from a feeling of personal revulsion' (cited in Caldwell, 1999: 501).

On the other hand they tell stories about contraceptive methods (prolonging breastfeeding), abortion attempts (taking hot baths) and birthing. Their experiences tell a different story of shared confidences about childbirth and attempted abortion, much of which could be termed superstition. Crucially, in both instances the women tell of a lack of desire for the large families of their youth. Both women married young yet avoided the constant childbearing that might have accompanied long marriages. Both worked before marriage, one as a nurse's assistant, the other as a doctor's receptionist. Some knowledge of the body was inevitable. Of course one cannot generalise from two brief extracts. One can, however, see two women who imagined themselves differently in spite of their often frustrated attempts to bring their desires to fruition.

Behind those frustrations, failures and disappointments lies part of the explanation for the fertility decline, a decline brought about by many Mrs Ms and Mrs Ks determined to be different from their mothers and grandmothers. Their husbands had changed too. Mrs M's husband had 'been around the world', was 'a returned man' (i.e. from the war), where in common with many soldiers he had learned about 'French letters' (condoms). A clearer engagement with the broader changes in women's lives at this time, their greater involvement in mass education and in the paid labour market, their later age at marriage, for example, is part of the context for their changing motivation.

Conclusions

And what part did education play in this subtle transformation? Had the Malthusian concern that schools should teach citizens self-restraint been all too successful? It is argued here that schooling for girls contributed to that broad unraveling of gender norms, of the taken-for-granted nature of immersion in family, of constant childbearing. In South Australian elementary schools where girls spent increasing numbers of years they could be treated as boys were, albeit within the standards of their day. Within school systems some norms could be impartially applied. They could spend long periods out of the household, see themselves as individuals, and envisage, briefly, a time of independence in the labour market. Within the context of changing social and economic circumstances, young women, beneficiaries of compulsory schooling and new work opportunities, began to refuse a life of constant childbearing. They could 'reimagine' themselves ('I'm not going to get married'; 'I'm not going to have children') and their ability to shape their social worlds, worlds which included their perceptions of themselves as social actors as well as reproducers.

References

Alter, George (1992), 'Theories of Fertility Decline: A Non-specialist's Guide to the Current Debate', in Gillis, John, Tilly, Louise and Levine, David (eds), *The European Experience of Declining Fertility. A Quiet Revolution, 1850–1970*, Cambridge, Mass., Blackwell, 13–27.

Anderson, Margaret (1999), 'No Sex Please We're Demographers: Nineteenth-Century Fertility Decline Revisited', in Damousi, Joy and Ellinghaus, Katherine (eds), *Citizenship, Women and Social Justice*, Melbourne, University of Melbourne Press, 251–262.

Bacchi, Carol (1986), 'The "Women Question"', in Richards, Eric (ed.), *The Flinders History of South Australia: Social History*, Adelaide, Wakefield Press, 403–432.

Caldwell, John (1980), 'Mass Education as a Determinant of the Timing of Fertility Decline', *Population and Development Review*, 6(2), 225–255.

Caldwell, John (1998), 'Malthus and the Less Developed World: The Pivotal Role of India', *Population and Development Review*, 24(4), 675–681.

Caldwell, John (1999), 'The Delayed Western Fertility Decline in English-Speaking Countries', *Population and Development Review*, 25(3), 479–513.

Caldwell, John and Caldwell, Pat (1997), 'What do we Know about Fertility Transition?', in Jones, G. W. et al. (eds), *The Continuing Demographic Transition*, Oxford, Clarendon Press, 15–25.

Caldwell, John and Caldwell, Pat (2001), 'Regional Paths to Fertility Transition', *Journal of Population Research*, 18(2), 91–118.

Caldwell, John and Ruzicka, Lado (1977), *The End of Demographic Transition in Australia*, Department of Demography, Australian Family Formation Project, Monograph no. 5, Canberra, Australian National University.

Caldwell, John and Ruzicka, Lado (1978), 'The Australian Fertility Transition: An Analysis', *Population and Development Review*, 4(1), 81–103.

Cleland, John and Wilson, Christopher (1984), 'Demand Theories of the Fertility Transition: An Iconoclastic View', *Population Studies*, 41(1), 5–30.

Coale, Ansley (1969), 'The decline in fertility in Europe from the French Revolution to World War 11', in Behrman, S. J., Corsa, Leslie and Freedman, Ronald (eds), *Fertility and Family Planning: a world view*, Ann Arbor, University of Michigan Press.

Coale, Ansley and Watkins, Susan (eds) (1986), *The Decline of Fertility in Europe*, Princeton, Princeton University Press.

Davey, Ian (1981), 'Patterns of Inequality: School Attendance and Social Structure in the Nineteenth Century, Canada and Australia', in Hurt, John (ed.), *Childhood Youth and Education in the Late Nineteenth Century,* proceedings of the 1980 Annual Conference of the History of Education Society of Great Britain, History of Education Society, 1–30.

Davey, Ian and Wimshurst, Kerry (1992), 'Understanding irregular school attendance: beyond the rural-urban dichotomy', in Goodenow, Ronald K. and Marsden, William E. (eds), *The City and Education in Four Nations*, Cambridge University Press, Cambridge U.K.

Fisher, Kate (2000), 'Uncertain Aims and Tacit Negotiation: Birth Control Practices in Britain, 1925–55', *Population and Development Review*, 26(2), 295–317.

Folbre, Nancy (1983), 'Of Patriarchy Born: The Political Economy of Fertility Decisions', *Feminist Studies*, 9(2), 261–284.

Gatens, Moira (1998), 'Institutions, Embodiment and Sexual Difference', in Gatens, Moira and Mackinnon, Alison (eds), *Gender and Institutions: Welfare, Work and Citizenship*, Cambridge, Cambridge University Press, 1–15.

Gillis, John, Tilly, Louise and Levine, David (eds) (1992), *The European Experience of Declining Fertility. A Quiet Revolution, 1850–1970*, Cambridge, Mass., Blackwell.

Gittins, Diana (1982), *Fair Sex: Family Size and Structure, 1900–1939*, London, Hutchinson.

Golini, Antonio (1998), 'How Low can Fertility Be? An Empirical Exploration', *Population and Development Review*, 24(1), 59–73.

Greenhalgh, Susan (1995), *Situating Fertility: Anthropology and Demographic Inquiry*, Cambridge: Cambridge University Press.

Grimshaw, Patricia and Willett, G. (1981), 'Women's History and Family History: An Exploration of Colonial Family Structure', in Grieve, N. and Grimshaw, P. (eds), *Australian Women: Feminist Perspectives*, Melbourne, Melbourne University Press, 134–155.

Hammel, E. A. (1990), 'Theory of culture for demography', *Population and Development Review*, 16, no. 3, 455–485

Hicks, N. (1978), *This Sin and Scandal: Australia's Population Debate, 1891–1911*, Canberra, Australian National University Press.

Jones, Helen (1986), *In Her Own Name: Women in South Australian History*, Adelaide, Wakefield Press.

Kertzer, David (1995), 'Political-Economic and Cultural Explanations of Demographic Behaviour', in Greenhalgh, Susan (ed.), *Situating Fertility: Anthropology and Demographic Inquiry*, Cambridge, Cambridge University Press, 29–52.

Knodel, John and Van de Walle, Etienne (1979), 'Lessons from the Past: Policy Implications of Historical Fertility Studies', *Population and Development Review*, 5(2), 217–245.

Larson, Ann (1994), *Growing up in Melbourne: Family Life in the Late Nineteenth Century*, Canberra, Australian National University.

Lees, Lynn Hollen (1992), 'Safety in Numbers: Social Welfare Legislation and Fertility Decline in Western Europe', in Gillis, John, Tilly, Louise and Levine, David (eds), *The European Experience of Declining Fertility: A Quiet Revolution, 1850–1970*, Cambridge, Mass., Blackwell.

Linford, R. (1950), 'Interstate Differentials in Human Fertility in Australia', *The Economic Record*, June, 87–97.

Lockridge, Kenneth (1983), *The Fertility Transition in Sweden*, Report no. 3 from the Demographic Database, Umeå, Sweden, University of Umeå.

Lutz, Wolfgang, Goujon, Anne and Doblhammer-Reiter, Gabriele (1998), 'Demographic Dimensions in Forecasting: Adding Education to Age and Sex', *Frontiers of Population Forecasting*, supplement to *Population and Development Review*, 24, 42–58.

McDonald, Peter (1974), *Marriage in Australia: Age at First Marriage and Proportions Marrying, 1860–1971*, Department of Demography, Australian Family Formation Project, Monograph no. 2, Canberra, Australian National University.

McDonald, Peter (2000), 'Gender Equity in Theories of Fertility Transition', *Population and Development Review*, 26(3), 427–439

Mackinnon, Alison (1995), 'Were Women Present at the Demographic Transition? Questions from a Feminist Historian to Historical Demographers', *Gender and History*, 7(2), 222–240.

Mackinnon, Alison (1997), *Love and Freedom: Professional Women and the Reshaping of Personal Life*, Cambridge and Melbourne, Cambridge University Press.

Mackinnon, Alison (2000), 'Statistics and Social Imaginaries', in Tedebrand, L.-G. (ed.), *Sex, State and Society: Comparative Perspectives on the History of Sexuality*, Umeå, Sweden, Almqvist and Wiksell International, 209–231.

Magarey, Susan (1993), 'Sexual Labour, Australia 1880–1910', in Magarey, S., Rowley, S. and Sheridan, S. (eds), *Debutante Nation: Feminism Contests the 1890s*, St Leonards, Allen and Unwin, 91–99.

Malthus, T. R. (1803, republished 1992), *An Essay on the Principle of Population*, Cambridge, Cambridge University Press.

Mason, Karen Oppenheim (1997), 'Gender and Demographic Change: What do we Know?', in Jones, G. W. et al. (eds), *The Continuing Demographic Transition*, Oxford, Clarendon Press, 159–182.

Mosk, Carl (1983), *Patriarchy and Fertility: Japan and Sweden, 1880–1960*, New York and London, Academic Press.

Quiggin, Pat (1988), *No Rising Generation: Women and Fertility in Late Nineteenth-Century Australia*, Canberra, Department of Demography, RSSS, Australian National University.

Reiger, Kerreen (1985), *The Disenchantment of the Home: Modernizing the Australian Family*, Melbourne, Oxford University Press.

Rogers, John (1995), 'Social Differentials and Fertility Decline in Uppsala and Västerås, 1870–1930', in Brändström, Anders and Tedebrand, Lars-Göran (eds), *Swedish Urban Demography During Industrialization*, Report no. 10 from the Demographic Database, Umeå, Sweden, Umeå University, 175–218.

Seccombe, Wally (1990), 'Starting to stop: working class fertility decline in Britain', *Past and Present*, 126, 151–188.

Smith, Daniel Scott (1996), '"The Number and Quality of Children": Education and Marital Fertility in Early Twentieth-Century Iowa', *Journal of Social History*, 50(2), 367–392.

South Australia, Parliament (1904), *Proceedings*, Paper no. 19.

Stevenson, Thomas L. (1982), *South Australia in Transition: A Geographical Interpretation of the Beginning of Fertility Decline, 1836–1901*, Ph.D thesis, Flinders University of South Australia, Adelaide.

Szreter, S. (1996), *Fertility, Class and Gender in Britain, 1860–1940*, Cambridge, Cambridge University Press.

Ullmann-Margalit, E. (1977), *The Emergence of Norms*, Oxford, Oxford University Press.

United Nations Development Program (UNDP) (1995), *Human Development Report 1995*, New York and Oxford, Oxford University Press.
Van de Kaa, Dirk (1998), *Postmodern Fertility Preferences: From Changing Value Orientation to New Behaviour*, Working Papers in Demography no. 74, Canberra, Australian National University.

Women's Influence on Fertility and Mortality during Industrialisation, Stuttgart, 1830–1910

RITA MÜLLER and SYLVIA SCHRAUT

The population development in nineteenth- and twentieth-century Europe is characterised by the gradual decline of birth and death rates. The model of the demographic transition describes a process which, starting from traditional demographic behaviour, via the decline of mortality in the first half of the nineteenth century, leads to a remarkable population growth. A decline in birth rates – which occurred not gradually but in several steps – since the end of the nineteenth century first caused a reduced population growth, then its stagnation, and finally the natural decline of population in many contemporary Western industrialised countries.[1] Although this model deals with elementary human behaviour and human experiences such as marriage, giving birth, and dying, it seems to be, in a strange way, 'without gender' (Mackinnon, 1995; as an exception see: Gillis, Tilly, Levine, 1992; Szreter, 1996).

In the social sciences it is generally accepted that the decline in the numbers of children born in the 'second demographic transition' is due to a mixture of factors which are by no means gender-neutral, namely, the change in the cost-benefit-relation of children as well as the impacts of mental value changes such as, for example, the emotionalisation of the relations between parents and children following the decline of birth rates, the emancipation of women, and finally, the general trend towards individualisation and the diminishing importance of marriage and family (Lesthaege, 1992). But social-scientific explanations dealing with the demographic transition are primarily aimed at explaining current population developments and are mainly based on social

1 In recent decades the model of the demographic transition has been examined in several respects. In particular its explanatory power and its geographical and cultural range have been questioned. In this article, however, we do not want to take up again these debates (see for example Khalatbari, 1999: 29–45 or Mackensen, 1999: 5–28).

development processes which can be observed since the second half, if not since only the last third of the twentieth century. Therefore, these explanatory patterns are not really useful for the interpretation of the role of women in the second and third phase of the demographic transition – during the decline of mortality since the first half of the nineteenth century and the first decline in birth numbers at the end of that century. Constructing a model of the demographic transition which takes into account gender, it is necessary to combine this model with findings from social history, gender history and cultural history with regard to the processes of change in the transition from a feudal society to the nineteenth- and twentieth-century bourgeois world. Demographic developments in this period were not only influenced by structural changes in the economy, in the health system or in health concepts, but also by the rise of a bourgeois middle class whose members were increasingly concerned with questions of health, family forms and population. This list is not intended to be exhaustive. In the following only some aspects will be outlined.

The impact of industrialisation on the organisation of work within and outside the family: Attempts to explain the demographic transition in general include economic development. Above all, the impact of a rise in agricultural productivity and the increase of jobs in other economic sectors are emphasised. Both developments allowed demographic behaviour to become gradually independent from the ups and downs of the agricultural economy (Livi-Bacci, 1999: 165ff.). However, what is often ignored in discussions of the demographic transition is the process of change from the traditional to the modern organisation of work and family. It is assumed that in pre-industrial Europe two-thirds to three-quarters of the gainfully employed population maintained themselves and their families by agricultural work; only about 10 to 20 percent of the population worked in the traditional trades. Since the middle of the nineteenth century at the latest, a considerable shift occurred in the structure of the economy, away from agriculture towards the industrial and service sector.

In addition to the rise of the modern class of factory workers, it was especially the rise of the new class of white-collar workers that characterised the developing new organisation of work. What is of importance in our context is the impact of the above mentioned processes on the organisation of work within the family. Characteristic of the majority of pre-industrial households in agriculture and trade was the intersection between gainful employment and the family economy (Mitterauer, 1992a and Mitterauer, 1992b). Based on a gender-specific division of labour, both women and men in farming and artisinal households were responsible for their share in ensuring the family's economic survival. There was no separation of work and residence, work and family life were closely linked, and the care for and education of children took place in the framework of the family's trade or business; this means that the care for children was subordinate to economic demands (Scott and Tilly, 1984). If, for example, business required the participation of the craftsman's wife in selling the goods on the market, then other members of the household had to take care of toddlers. If, in agriculture, harvest time had come, all female and male household members had to participate in the work process, and siblings not old enough to be included in harvesting, had to take over the care for the infants. Heide Wunder coined the apt term 'work couple' [Arbeitspaar] to characterise the couple of the early modern period which in this way had to maintain the family and guarantee its income (Wunder, 1992).

In pre-industrial society there is only one small group to which the organisation of the household and the organisation of work described above did not apply: the early modern educated civil servants in the vicinity of courts, public administrations, law courts, and universities – the core of what was to become the modern educated middle class. It is characteristic of this group that gainful employment was defined as predominantly male employment. The work of an educated specialist required studies which were, in general, a prerequisite for men and led to careers exclusively accessible by men. In this, before 1800, numerically very small circle of the population we may observe at an early stage the gender-specific division of work into paid male work outside the family's home and unpaid female work within the family's household. As the husband's work was separated from family life, the female family members could devote their time to childrearing. The size of this social group grew considerably in the process of the professionalisation of administration and public services during the nineteenth century. Finally, it was joined by the new class of white-collar workers created by industrialisation. Both groups developed the household forms and the 'bourgeois' life-style which, in the course of the nineteenth century, became a model for other groups within the population.[2] Seen from the perspective of the demographic transition it is significant that the decline of mortality in the first half of the nineteenth century runs parallel

2 As for the lifestyles of these groups see for example: Davidoff, Hall, 1987 or Habermas, 2000.

to the growth of a social group in which wives were increasingly released from the task of gainful employment in order to concentrate on family tasks.

The development of the bourgeois gender model: It is not accidental that this early modern educated middle class of civil servants and white-collar workers forms the core of that social group which, in the course of Enlightenment and Romanticism, conceived the bourgeois gender model which later on captured the entire middle class and developed great attraction for other social groups as well (Frevert, 1988). The early bourgeois programme comprised the incorporation of the gender roles Rousseau had been able to convey successfully to his audience in *Emile*: the definition of sense and activity as male characteristics, and of sensibility, eroticism, and motherly love as female ones (Schmid, 1992 and Schmid, 2000). Further milestones on the way to the bourgeois gender model were decisions taken during the French Revolution, such as the definition of politics as a male field of action and the assignment of the social task of educating good republicans to the female citizen (Opitz, 1998), and the classification of male fields of activity as activities belonging to the 'public sphere', whereas the domestic sphere of the family, which was defined as private, was assigned to the 'female gender' (Hausen, 1976). These restrictions of the female scope of action, however, were linked to an up to then unknown enhancement of 'female' characteristics and abilities, which may have considerably sweetened the change in gender roles for many bourgeois women. Here we can only touch upon these cultural developments, for which research in gender history has presented ample evidence. We assume that these developments also had an impact on mortality and fertility. If the early bourgeois image of femininity met with the main task of women in everyday life – the rearing and education of children – then it can be expected that women made considerable investments in these predominantly 'female' tasks. If in the context of these investments the survival chances of infants increased, then – in view of the high costs of child rearing for the educated middle classes – the question of population control was on the agenda. Because 'a growing number of surviving children requires – when fertility remains the same – greater efforts in child care and is prerequisite to a reduction of the number of children' (Livi-Bacci, 1999: 192).

The Demographic Transition in Stuttgart

In the following our hypothesis will be examined based on the example of Stuttgart. The capital of Württemberg, which developed into an industrial town and finally into a big city, only provides the historical framework so that we will limit ourselves to a brief description of the town's development. Stuttgart was hurled into the industrial age after having been connected to the railways in the 1840s. In 1800 the town counted 21,000 inhabitants. In 1910, Stuttgart, with a total population of 286,000, ranked fifteenth among the big cities of the *Reich*. The fact that despite the growth of the working-class population every fifteenth inhabitant worked in public service refers to Stuttgart's vital function as a capital and seat of numerous central administrations. As early as the beginning of the nineteenth century these bourgeois dignitaries, who combined their pride as burghers with the loyalty of Württemberg subordinates, were committed to the solution of the city's social and medical problems.

What primarily qualifies Stuttgart for a research into the questions mentioned above is the existence of a demographic database on 5,000 nineteenth-century families containing data on marriage behaviour, births, and mortality, as well as numerous other data.[3]

3 The data were collected in the DFG-financed research project 'Sozialer Wandel im Großraum Stuttgart' [Social change in the region of Stuttgart] directed by Prof. Wolfgang von Hippel, University of Mannheim. The following reflections refer to the data of adults and their children collected in the Stuttgart database. The source from which these data were drawn only registers men and women who married in Stuttgart and founded a family of their own or married persons or widows and widowers who moved to Stuttgart with their family. It does not register singles who stayed only for a short time in Stuttgart and did not found a family there (the 'drifting sand' of industrialisation). Therefore, we assume that the database shows a slightly distorted picture of the mortality of adults. Our analyses are however representative for the vast majority of persons who settled down in Stuttgart for a certain period.

The Development of Mortality in Stuttgart

According to the model of the demographic transition the change in demographic behaviour was initiated by a decline in mortality. As can be expected, mortality in Stuttgart declined in the course of the nineteenth century. A comparison with other big cities, with Prussia and the *Reich*, shows some typical developments. In cities such as Stuttgart, which were well-equipped with medical facilities, mortality declined earlier than in rural Württemberg. For a short time, health risks arising from urbanisation inverted this trend, but after 1870 mortality in Stuttgart started off on a definitive decline.

Figure 1. Development of Mortality 1816–1913

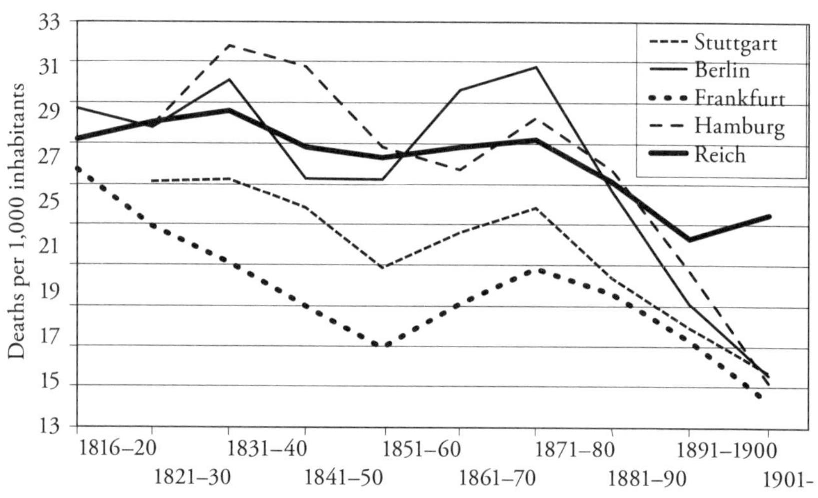

Data according to Vögele 1991: 33; Reich = until 1840 Prussia, later on Deutsches Reich; Stuttgart = 1820–29; 1830–39; 1840–49.

The Stuttgart database provides more detailed information on the development of mortality with respect to sex, age, and social position. As was the case in the *Reich* as a whole, the decline of the mortality rate was above all due to the decline in infant mortality and the decline in fertility. It was not before the turn of the century that the average life expectancy of adult inhabitants increased gradually, with women profiting earlier than men.

The Development of Infant Mortality and its Assessment by Contemporaries

In the course of the nineteenth century infant mortality became one of the pivotal health issues the interested public was intensely concerned with. Infant mortality rates increased continuously from the start of industrialisation until the 1860s and 1870s. In German states with traditionally a relatively low level of infant mortality such as Prussia, it was not until the twentieth century that infant mortality dropped to the level of the early nineteenth century. In states where infant mortality was traditionally above average first improvements became visible in the 1880s.[4] In Württemberg, infant mortality rose to a peak in the 1850s and 1860s, when almost four out of ten infants died before their first birthday; in the following decades it visibly declined (1915–1918: 15 percent).

Contemporary observers already noticed an inversion of the usual town-countryside difference in infant mortality, especially in the southern and south-western parts of the *Deutsche Bund* and the future *Deutsche Reich* which were regions with infant mortality rates above average. In Bavaria, Württemberg, and Baden – areas in which, as a rule, there was no or little breast-feeding – survival chances of infants were higher in urban areas than in the rural hinterland. This observation also applied to Stuttgart where in the 1830s only every fourth infant under the age of one died. Until the 1850s infant mortality continued to decline. The relatively high survival chances of infants in Stuttgart decreased in the 1860s during the town's first big period of population growth. Infant mortality rose dramatically by 20 percent to a level comparable to the one at the beginning of the 1830s. The rising level of infant mortality in Württemberg's capital mobilised its medical professionals. In the following decades they committed themselves to reducing infant mortality (Cless, 1868). Both explanations for and the means to remedy the situation as offered by the city's physicians are quite interesting. An admonishing call to the people of Württemberg, issued in 1868, claimed that the high rates of infant mortality did not have natural causes. The call rather blamed 'the

4 The rate of infant mortality is calculated as the percentage of children who did not reach their first birthday in relation to all live births in that same period. As for infant mortality in the towns of the Deutsche Reich see Vögele, 1994 and Vögele, 2001: 130–161 and the references mentioned there.

Figure 2. Infant Mortality in Württemberg and Stuttgart

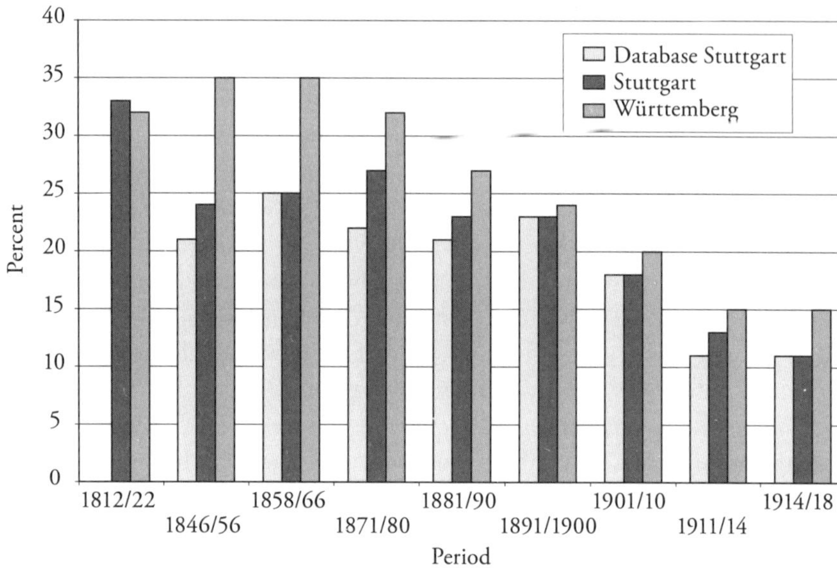

Source: Database Stuttgart

actions and the failures of people, that is, a wrong treatment of infants, foolish habits, superstitions, a lack of understanding and willingness for sacrifice, in short: the lack of sensible, careful, and conscientious care' of infants (Cless, 1868: 4). In accordance with contemporary medical discussions, the author of the call declared that the high rate of intestinal diseases of infants, which occurred especially in summer, was due to the fact that in Württemberg breast-feeding was rare or uncommon.[5] However, he explicitly did not put down these shortcomings to the social position of the mothers.[6] He interpreted them as

5 Already at the beginning of the nineteenth century women in Stuttgart were criticised because of their missing willingness to breast-feed. On the other hand, prolonged breast-feeding was also criticised (see Cleß, Schübler, 1815: 39f.).

6 The pattern of explanation which referred to social position was not unusual. In midnineteenth-century Berlin, for example, infant mortality – though regarded as unalterable – was regarded as caused by social conditions (see Helfft, 1858: 2).

characteristic of gender-specific working conditions, and an organisation of work which apparently did not allow breast-feeding women to be relieved by servants. 'The peasant women reject breast-feeding as inconvenient and a disruption of work and trade, [...] but he who has hands shall work and he (sic) who has breasts shall breast-feed, that is the reason why nature has provided them' (Cless, 1868: 6). He appealed to the mothers: 'As long as breast-feeding does not become the country's habit again the reproach weighs heavily on its motherly population that it is their own fault that their children suffer harm, that there is lack of motherly love which reveals itself only in the breast-feeding mother' (Cless, 1868: 7). In case of a conflict between mother's love and work, the mother had to decide for the former. 'Surely, under all circumstances, the mother must do without a part of the work she is used to for the sake of her child, if she does not want to neglect it irresponsibly; when breast-feeding it, she is ever-more bound to it' (Cless, 1868: 7). It may be due to the urban and upper-class origin of this physician that he believed that the re-organisation of the work of women was left to the free will of the families concerned. He further recommended a joint campaign for breast-feeding by physicians, midwives, pastors and women's associations as a service to the fatherland.

Is the Stuttgart database suitable to verify the observations of the local physicians? Which causes are held to be responsible for infant mortality in the nineteenth century by current research? Which findings are confirmed by the Stuttgart data? A number of factors appear to have had an impact on nineteenth century infant mortality which is understood as a good 'indicator for essential dimensions of survival chances in a given social milieu' (Spree, 1981b: 49–98; Imhof, 1981; Spree, 1995; Vögele, 2001: 138ff.). Regarded as important factors are: the legitimacy of the infant, nutritional habits, dwelling conditions and the 'value' of the child; further factors are the climate, the development of the hygienic infra-structure, or the public health service, and finally the income, the educational status of the parents, and the workload of the mother. Last, but not least, a connection between fertility and infant mortality is stated.

Many of these determinants cannot be checked with the information contained in the database; individual nutrition habits or concrete dwelling conditions elude statistical analysis. It is however possible to correlate the social position of the parents with infant mortality. Thus, we can at least indirectly draw conclusions on the impact of education, profession, material conditions, and of the organisation of work and family. The class-specific development of infant mortality in Stuttgart between 1830 and 1920, which can be established by means of the Stuttgart database, may serve as an example.[7]

Already before the era of industrialisation infants from upper-class families had significantly better chances than children from the middle and lower classes to survive the critical first year. But, while the mortality of infants from the upper and middle classes declined continuously after the especially 'dangerous' 1860s (apart from the sharp increase after the turn of the century which was probably caused by a wave of influenza) the mortality of infants from working-class families increased massively towards the end of the century. The development of infant mortality in Württemberg's capital – where industrial growth was modest and where a medical network existed which offered relatively good access to medical care for all social classes – therefore follows the trend Spree characterised as being typical for infant mortality in the *Kaiserreich*: an increase of infant mortality in the lower classes and a simultaneous class-specific differentiation of infant mortality.[8]

Whereas in the 1830s about twice as many infants born to lower-class families died than did infants born to upper-class parents (1,8:1), in the 1890s 3.3 lower-class infants died in comparison to only one upper-class infant. Moreover, the gap between middle-class infants and lower-class infants increased as well in this period.

Infant mortality and social class are thus clearly linked. There is also a relation between family income and infant mortality which can be shown by a comparison of the taxed income of parents in 1913 and the survival chances of their children born between 1890 and 1919. However, the effects of financial conditions cannot be interpreted as a simple equation: the better the material conditions, the lower the level of infant mortality.

That the extent of infant mortality indeed depended on the organisation of work within the family shows the comparison of the mortality rate with the occupational status of the father. The case of Stuttgart confirms the well-known phenomenon of better survival chances for children born into families headed by civil servants or white-collar workers. As early as the 1830s infant mortality in these groups – irrespective of household income – dropped to a

7 As for the class model used see Müller, 2000: 381–385.

8 See Spree, 1981b, as for infant mortality see especially 49–93. The chart is based on live births only.

Figure 3. Infant Mortality in Stuttgart and Social Class

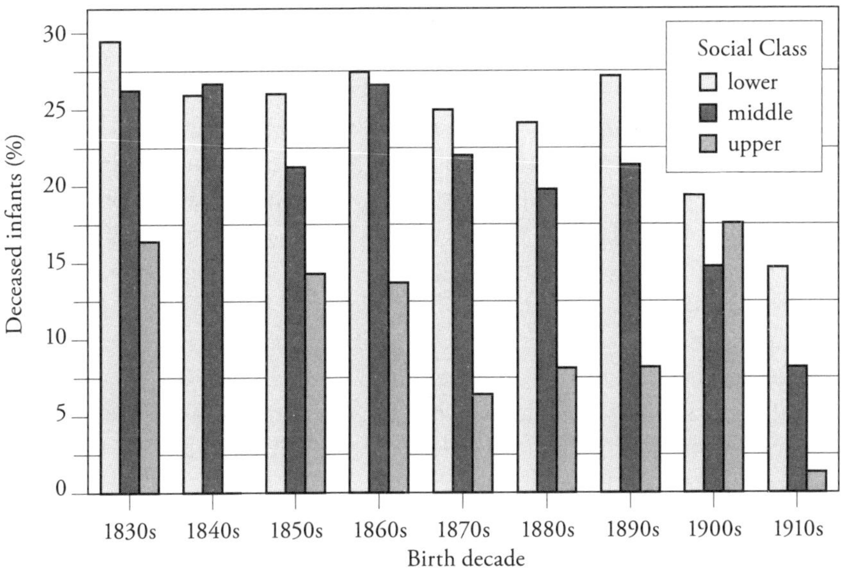

Source: Database Stuttgart

Figure 4. Taxed Income 1913 and Infant Mortality

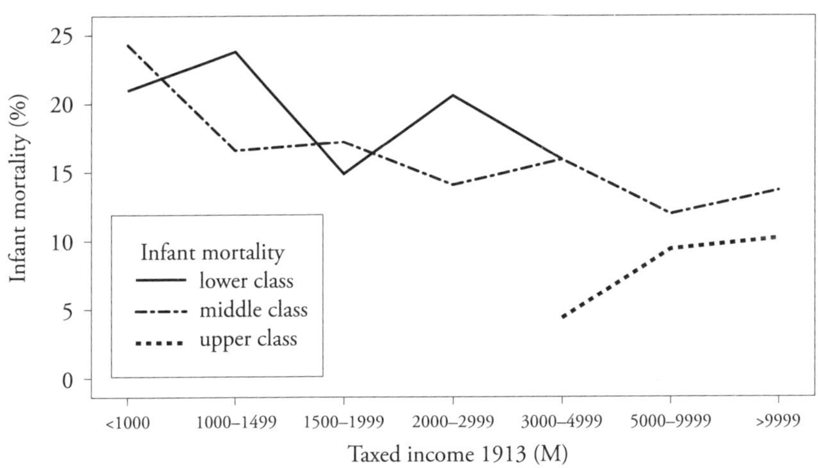

Births 1890-1919, source: Database Stuttgart

level which was so low that for the society as a whole it was not reached until the years of the Weimar Republic. As already mentioned, the occupation of the wives in these social groups was traditionally restricted to domestic family tasks, irrespective of differences in income. The new bourgeois ideal of femininity was quite early acclaimed by civil servants and white-collar workers. On the other hand, compared to other social groups the families of the educated middle classes experienced an exorbitantly high increase in infant mortality in the initial phase of industrialisation in Stuttgart and the accompanying demographic crisis of the 1850s and 1860s. At this point in time they began to search for the individual and social causes of this deplorable state of affairs. It is from their ranks that the physicians originated who were to deal conscientiously with the problem of the survival of infants. They not only began to analyse the effects of urban industrial growth but they also began to build a critical municipal public audience, which, in the second half of the nineteenth century, was increasingly and strongly concerned with health issues in general and infant mortality in particular.

In pre-industrial Stuttgart infant mortality was especially high in families of self-employed heads of household in contrast to families headed by civil servants and white-collar workers. Small wine-growers or small commercial entrepreneurs needed their wives as helpers in their businesses even when infants or toddlers had to be taken care of. The intensive breast-feeding campaigns by Stuttgart's medical profession and members of the reform-oriented upper class could not change the economic requirements of the households of the self-employed. It was only after the turn of the century that in these circles infant mortality began to decline as well. It may be assumed that at that point in time women in these social groups could or did devote more time to the care of their infants. Their changing behaviour might be the result of the declining number of children ever born to them, of rising incomes and the development of the bourgeois gender model.

The example of working-class households shows that infant mortality in pre-industrial Stuttgart did not only depend on the income of the family. It was also clearly determined by the employment status of the mothers. Despite the widespread assumption that working-class wives were not gainfully employed, the majority of them contributed to the family income. Nevertheless, jobs such as carrying newspapers, cleaning, laundering, etc., were easier to reconcile with breast-feeding than the business tasks of wives of commercial entrepreneurs or farmers which, at least on market days, forced them to be absent from home

Figure 5. Infant Mortality in Stuttgart and Occupational Category of the Father

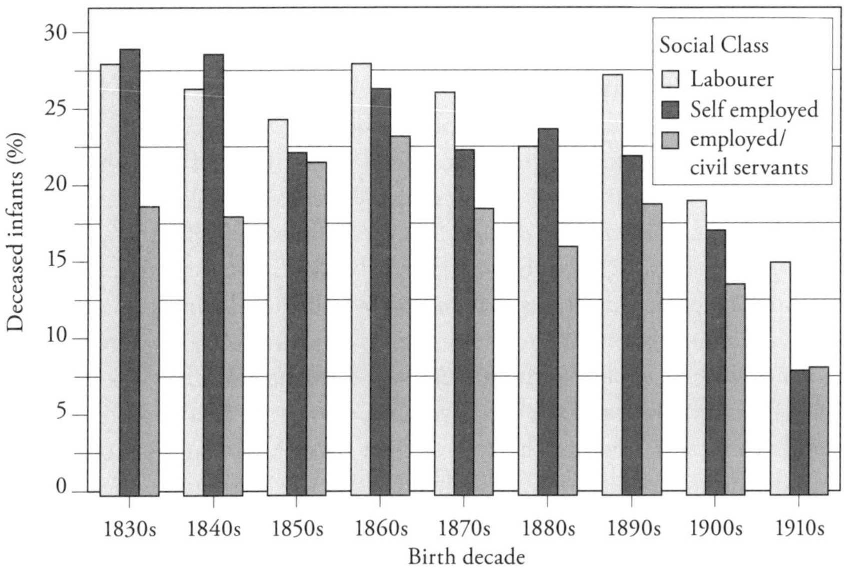

Source: Database Stuttgart

for half a day or even all day long. Correspondingly, until about the middle of the nineteenth century infant mortality in working-class households was lower than infant mortality in households of the self-employed. It was only when industrialisation gained further pace in Stuttgart, when social problems increased and population growth led to an overcrowding of unsanitary and ill-equipped working-class quarters, that infant mortality in working-class families increased rapidly and began to outnumber infant mortality in households of the self-employed. In the 1850s and 1860s the situation reached a critical climax. A long-term comparison of infant mortality rates in working-class households and households of the self-employed which spans the nineteenth century thus proves to be a suitable means to show two contrary trends which evidently intersected in the last decades of that century. Young mothers in middle- and upper-class families headed by white-collar workers, civil servants, and the self-employed were increasingly relieved from non-domestic occupations. This improved the survival chances of their children. Simultaneously, the worsening sanitary and living conditions, due to the increasing industrialisation of the town, deteriorated the survival chances of working-class children for a long time. Only the thorough improvement of the hygienic and sanitary living conditions in urban areas could bring relief.

Even the substantial decline in infant mortality after the turn of the century can only be explained by a combination of factors: i.e. source of family income, level of income, and corresponding family life style. This can be illustrated by the relationships between taxed income (1913), the occupational position of the father, and the level of infant mortality (figure 6). Despite the fluctuations which can be observed it becomes apparent that even very favourable income conditions did not lead to a further rise in the already high survival chances of infants from households of white-collar workers and civil servants. In households of the self-employed infant mortality only declined when their income reached a high level, and, as must be assumed, the mothers could spare more time for the care of their infants. But survival chances of working-class children continually increased with rising family incomes and related improvements in living conditions.

Figure 6. Taxed Income 1913, Occupational Category, and Infant Mortality

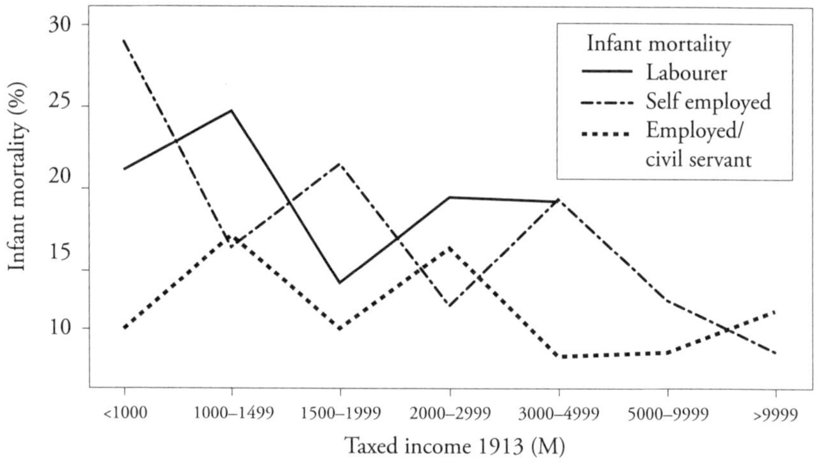

Births 1890-1919, source: Database Stuttgart

That the income level as such is not the single determining factor for the survival chances of infants, but that the organisation of work within the family plays a decisive role as well, can be shown by a comparison between working-class families and families of the self-employed with similar incomes. An annual income between 1,599 Marks and 2,000 Marks – a middle income for workers – contributed to a decline in infant mortality amongst the working classes when compared to workers with lower income. Self-employed heads of household with a similar income – a low income for self-employed – however still needed their wives to help in business, so that it must be assumed that in these households children could not expect the degree of care which became possible when the family income rose beyond that level.[9] It is thus clear that the specific organisation of work and family and suitable notions of femininity and maternity as developed by civil servants and white-collar workers proved to be the driving force behind the demographic process of modernisation (see for example Spree, 1981a).

The Development of Fertility in Stuttgart

The 'demographic transition' is marked by a decline in the number of births. This also applies to the city of Stuttgart. Whereas women who had married during the 1820s were giving birth to an average of seven children, that number decreased to 2.7 children for couples who married in 1910.[10]

9 In 1913 the average annual income for workers was 1,991 Marks, for self-employed 6,705 Marks. Only a third of all workers were earning more than 2,000 Marks. Two thirds of the self-employed were earning more than 2,000 Marks. Of all self-employed only 17 percent were earning less than 1,500 Marks. In the latter group families were running only a small business. We assume that the group of self-employed family heads with incomes between 1,500 and 2,000 Marks were not earning enough to finance additional labour but were strongly dependent upon the labour of their wives.

10 Only complete first marriages entered all calculations in connection with reproductive behaviour. This means that only those couples were taken into account of which both partners had married for a first time, of which the wife survived until the age of 45, and the husband did not die before the end of his wife's reproductive period. About 40 percent

Figure 7. Number of Children by Decade of Marriage

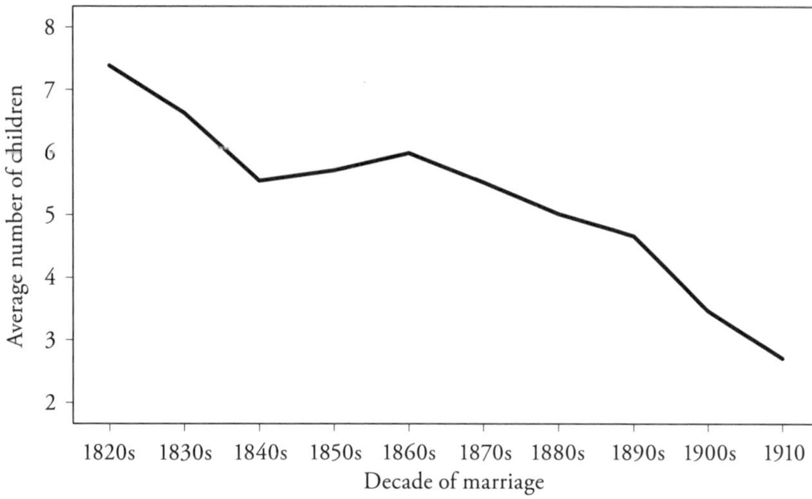

Source: Database Stuttgart

This development decisively altered the life courses of the women concerned. An increase in life expectancy, a decrease in infant mortality and changes in reproductive behaviour are all mirrored in the biographies of Stuttgart women. The life expectancy of women born in the nineteenth century increased by an average of five years. The period in life in which they concentrated on their role as mothers shrunk drastically. A new phase, the so-called post-marital partnership evolved, a phase which women had a chance to shape and define themselves. Women reduced active motherhood to only a few years as the date of their last birth came at ever younger ages during the nineteenth and early twentieth century. They also reduced the number of offspring by preventing further pregnancies when the desired number of children was reached and by lengthening the intervals between births.

of these women married while having an illegitimate child or being pregnant (prenuptial pregnancies were calculated as births occurring within seven months after marriage). Prenuptial pregnancies and births in detail 1820/29 36.0%; 1830/39 30.5%; 1840/49: 34.0%; 1850/59: 42.5%; 1860/69: 46.3%; 1870/79: 43.1%; 1880/89: 45.8%; 1890/99: 44.5%; 1900/09: 38.6%; 1910: 44,1%

Figure 8. Age at Marriage, at First and at Last Birth by Marriage Cohorts

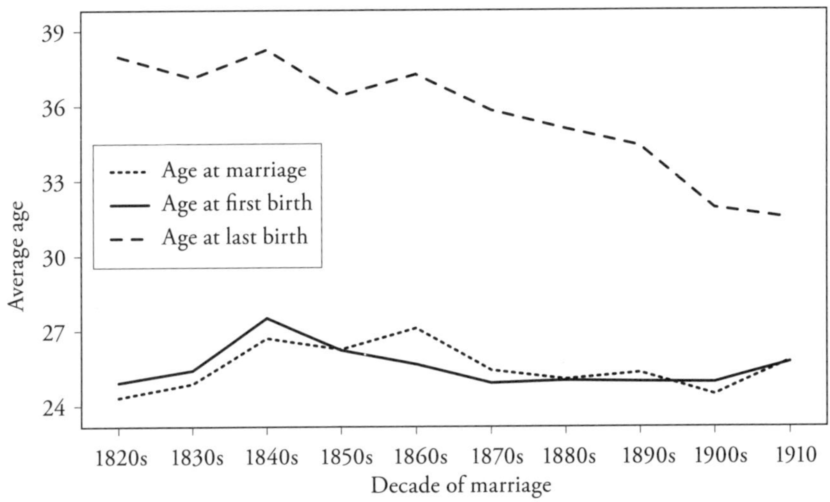

Source: Database Stuttgart

Figure 9. Average Birth Interval (in Months)

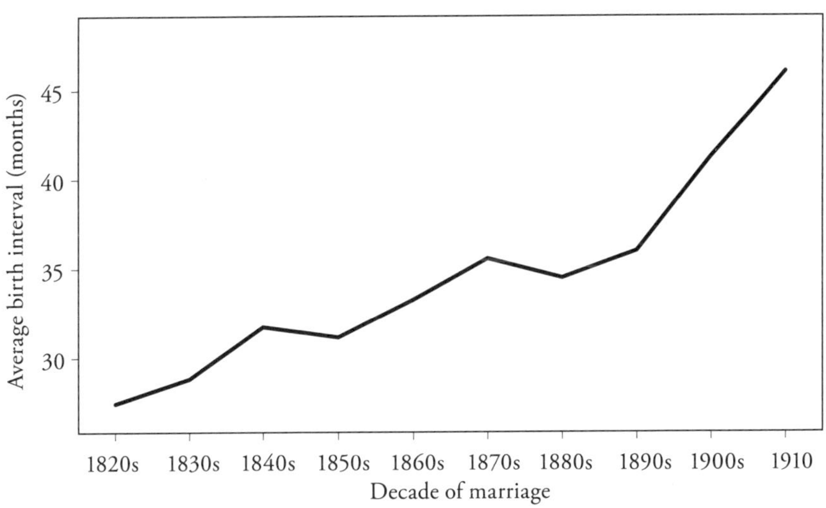

Source: Database Stuttgart

The Demographic Role of Women

The above mentioned changes cannot be explained without reference to the use of contraceptive practices and family planning intentions. But who was responsible for the adoption of birth control? Who 'controlled' the time span between births? What role did women play in the transition to a more modern type of reproductive behaviour?

Regarding the nineteenth century, we have only few narrative sources available. Among the most important contemporary German sources regarding contraceptive practices and family planning intentions are surveys by doctors who had become aware of the spread of birth control among their patients at the beginning of the twentieth century (also Dienel, 1995). One of these surveys was carried out by Oskar Polano, a doctor and professor working at Würzburg hospital. He questioned about 500 women who visited his practice as patients. Of this group of female patients 339 women (67.4 percent) were actively using contraceptive methods. Max Marcuse, a doctor, sexologist and editor of the journal *Zeitung für Sexualwissenschaften* had also been querying patients in his Berlin practice before and during World War I. He asked his female patients for example: 'How do you or your husband prevent having (further) children?'.[11] Out of the 100 women he interviewed, a similar percentage (64 percent) as in Lower Franconia had prevented a conception at least once (Polano, 1916). Marcuse furthermore interviewed 300 married men (most of them suffering from venereal diseases) who were treated in a field hospital during the war (Marcuse, 1913 and Marcuse, 1917). The answers given by Marcuse's patients show that the use of contraceptive measures was initiated by either the husband or the wife, but that the woman had probably been the driving force in most of the cases.[12] Therefore, this topic often led to conflicts between the partners. As one woman stated: 'There is always a war with my husband about this thing. But then, he is not the one who has to have the baby'. Many women had even tolerated unfaithfulness of their husbands in order to prevent further pregnancies.

11 'Wie haben Sie oder Ihr Mann sich denn geschützt, damit Sie keine (nicht noch mehr) Kinder bekamen?'

12 In her study of birth refusal (Gebärstreik) Inka Haas also states that, in most cases, the women took the initiative to have fewer children (Haas, 1998: 50f.).

Indicators for Changes in Reproductive Behaviour

Birth control by contraception was not the only option to influence the (desired) number of children. On which further factors did fertility and family size depend? How and where did women's influence on her own fertility work? Related science presents us with a number of important demographically relevant factors, which are to be measured against the Stuttgart data.

The first factor to discuss is age at first marriage. Although state and local authorities tried to control birth rates and population growth by marriage laws,[13] changes in the age at first marriage do not seem to have been relevant in the dramatic alterations in reproductive behaviour in Stuttgart and other communities. This is especially true since in some cases first children were born before marriage (see figure 8). The following part will therefore not explicitly refer to age at marriage.

Another indicator of reproductive behaviour is the timing of the first birth. That the latter is not solely dependent on marriage is clearly demonstrated in figure 8.[14] A new tendency to postpone the birth of the first child was emerging at the beginning of the twentieth century. It can only be speculated on which of the partners in a relationship had decided on the timing of the first pregnancy. But mental and social circumstances, for example longer periods of training or higher standards of living, surely played a role in the timing of the arrival of the first child. Postponing the first pregnancy may have been aimed at controlling ultimate family size. It is however just as likely that this postponement was motivated by the couple's decision to enjoy a number of years without children.

An important indicator for declining fertility is the age of the mother at the birth of her last child. The choice to refrain from further pregnancies at an early point in time clearly demonstrates the intention of families to limit

13 For laws concerning marriage in Württemberg, see Müller, 2000: 205ff. and 275ff. These laws allowed marriage only when based on sufficient property. It is important to know that in our research area these marriage laws did not have any influence on fertility.

14 There is a substantial period during the 1850s and 1860s that first births came earlier than marriage. This is the period with the highest illegitimacy rates in nineteenth-century Württemberg. In addition, in the late fifties and early sixties the restriction of trade in combination with the restriction of marriage were eased off. That is why we can find couples with some prenuptial born children which are now allowed to marry.

the abundance of children once the desired number was reached. Compared to nearby and relatively rural Feuerbach, the women in the governmental city of Stuttgart started relatively early not to make use of the full length of their reproductive phase anymore.[15] The age at last birth decreased significantly towards the end of the examined period of time. A use of contraceptives is likely. It is assumed that the agreement of both partners was required to successfully implement this strategy (Jütte, 2003; Gehrmann, 1979: 463).

Finally, the extention of birth intervals may be regarded as a clear prove of planned family limitation. Many signs point towards a dominant influence of women in this respect. By extending the duration of breast-feeding women were able to increase the time span between individual births. The relationship between breast-feeding and contraception was sufficiently well-known at that time.

Were Stuttgart Women Controlling their Fertility?

Based on the Stuttgart data, the above mentioned indicators allow a more detailed analysis, e.g. regarding social and chronological aspects. The information registered in the database about the women's social background shows how social and family experiences of the women influenced outcomes in terms of family planning and numbers of children.[16] This will be shown in the following part:

We begin by looking at the average number of children born to women in different marital cohorts and different social groups, which is the most significant sign of social change. Tables 1 and 2 show that, much as expected, massive social differences existed in family size. Upper-class families were the trendsetters of family limitation in the twentieth century, together with civil

15 Müller, 2000: 277ff. This finding confirms the thesis that family planning started in the upper social classes and in cities, and subsequently spread to other parts of the population and the country.

16 Another criterion for social background is religious denomination. About 80 percent of the analysed women were Protestants, only 10 percent were Catholics. The demographic behaviour of the 13.8 percent of Catholic women in the 1890,1910 cohorts was not significantly different from the Protestant part of the population.

servants and white-collar workers, the latter two according to the social position within their profession. The educated middle classes on the one hand, and the newly emerged group of white-collar employees on the other, were paving the way.[17] This finding is also supported by other studies. The German historian Nell, for instance, confirmed the trendsetting role of these social groups (Nell, 1973: 119).

In Stuttgart, upper-class families with heads in civil servant and white-collar occupations were reducing the number of children born to them from an average of 5.0 in the first marriage cohort to 3.1 in the second cohort and further down to 2.9 in the final cohort under study.[18] By contrast, among middle-class families in those same occupational groups the average number of children in the second marriage cohort was as high as 5.1. This also applied to self-employed families. Here, traditional fertility behaviour stayed on longer.

The behaviour of merchants and shopkeepers[20], mostly belonging to the middle classes, was however remarkable. Couples married in the 1890s and

17 The average number of children for all couples married in 1905 was 3.09 children for white-collar employees, 3.15 children for middle-grade civil servants, 4.14 children for self-employed artisans, 4.67 children for blue-collar workers and 5.40 children for farmers and 6.05 children for agricultural workers. See Jütte, 2003: 180.

18 All figures mentioned in the text which cannot be found in the tables or graphs result from further calculations of the database.

19 Distribution of so-called complete first marriages by marriage cohorts

Marriage cohort	Frequency	%	Valid %	Cumulative %
1830,1850	402	20.9	25.0	25.0
1860,1870,1880	490	25.5	30.4	55.4
1890,1910	719	37.4	44.6	100.0
Total	1611	83.8	100.0	

Source: Database Stuttgart.
Note: 1830 = 1828, 1831; 1850 = 1849–1851; 1870 = 1869–1870; 1880 = 1879–1880; 1890 = 1889–1890; 1910 = 1909–1910.

This somewhat unusual grouping of marriage cohorts derives from the project's method of data selection. There is always a concentration at around 1830, 1850 and so forth. This pecularity was taken into account here.

20 The group of merchants and shopkeepers consists of both self-employed and employed persons.

Table 1. Age at Marriage, Age at First and at Last Birth, Birth Intervals and Number of Children by Marriage Cohort and Occupational Class of the Husband[19]

Marriage cohort / Social class		Age at marriage mean	Age at first birth mean	Age at last birth mean	Aver. birth interval (months) mean	Number of children mean
1830,1850	Lower classes	26.5	26.0	38.4	28.3	7.1
	Middle classes	26.3	26.3	36.9	30.3	6.0
	Upper classes	23.5	23.3	34.4	34.2	5.3
1860,1870 1880	Lower classes	28.0	25.7	36.5	33.3	5.4
	Middle classes	25.9	25.1	35.7	34.1	5.6
	Upper classes	24.9	25.4	33.6	48.2	3.3
1890,1910	Lower classes	26.2	25.0	33.5	39.2	4.2
	Middle classes	25.4	25.5	33.1	38.9	3.7
	Upper classes	24.4	25.2	32.2	44.1	3.1

Source: Database Stuttgart

1910s were reducing the size of their family to 2.6 children. What motivation lay behind their family model? In the social sciences, merchants are often perceived as the bearers of bourgeois modernisation processes. Together with civil servants and white-collar workers, they are regarded as the core group in the development of the bourgeoisie. The family-based organisation of work among the self-employed members of this group is of course not sufficient on its own to explain a transition process such as the adoption of bourgeois gender and family concepts. In addition, the high mobility and the easy access to information typical for this occupational group may have been important in triggering modern behaviour.[21]

21 In the first marriage cohort, almost 40 percent of all merchants (men and women) had not been born in Stuttgart. For the final cohorts, more than 60 percent of the men and women were born outside Stuttgart.

Table 2. Age at Marriage, at First and at Last Birth, Birth Intervals and Number of Children by Marriage Cohort and Occupational Class of the Husband

Marriage cohort / Occupational Category		Age at marriage mean	Age at first birth mean	Age at last birth mean	Aver. birth interval (months) mean	Number of children mean
1830,1850	Worker	27.1	26.2	38.1	31.2	6.5
	Self-employed	25.8	26.0	37.5	28.3	6.6
	Civil servant	26.2	25.9	35.6	32.5	5.1
1860,1870 1880	Worker	27.9	26.0	36.6	33.9	5.3
	Self-employed	26.1	24.9	36.0	33.2	5.9
	Civil servant	25.8	25.5	35.0	37.2	4.7
1890,1910	Worker	26.3	25.0	33.7	39.7	4.3
	Self-employed	25.1	25.2	33.6	39.6	4.0
	Civil servant	25.4	25.5	32.3	38.7	3.3

Source: Database Stuttgart

Regardless whether the family head was self-employed or in paid employment elsewhere, there seems to have been a prevailing inclination within the upper classes to spend the first part of marriage without children, to enjoy life and to limit the total number of children. As the nineteenth century progressed, Stuttgart's high-society couples were allowing more and more time between marriage and the beginning of first pregnancy, e.g. upper-class self-employed women were having intervals of 20 months on average. The length of the time span between marriage and first pregnancy is longer for members with an entrepreneurial background than for civil servants or white-collar employees. The women in the latter group apparently found themselves more often deeply routed in the role of housewife and mother and less so in a socially prominent position as was common among entrepreneurial families.

More significant than the postponement of the first birth were the changes in the age of the mother at which her last child was born. In Stuttgart, upper-class women in the first marriage cohort in particular had reached the end of their reproductive life at the age of 34. They managed to give birth to their last child at an average age of 32.2 in the final cohort under study (see table 1).

If 'occupational status' is taken as the decisive criterion, it becomes clear that again civil-servant and white-collar families were leading the way in the modernisation of reproductive behaviour.[22] Upper-class women, who married after 1890, had their last child at the undoubtedly very early average age of 31.8 years. And again, merchants' wives were setting the trend. On the whole, however, women of all classes were following this development as is demonstrated by the following tables.

As the nineteenth century progressed, the proportion of women who had their last child before the age of 40 was increasing steadily. In the final marriage cohort, eight out of ten women were under 40 years of age at the time of their last birth. Whereas 38.2 percent of the women who had married around 1830 or 1850, had their last birth between the ages of 40 and 44, this distribution changed for the final cohorts, when 27.2 percent of the women were giving birth to their last child between 30 and 34 years of age (see table 3).

These findings confirm again the leading role of white-collar and civil servants' families. More than 85 percent of wives in these social groups was under 40 years of age at their last birth. Women who had their last child at higher ages were clearly an exception. In lower-class families, however, about a third of the women had already passed the age of 40 when their last child was born (see table 4). One should bear in mind that, at least in the first half of the nineteenth century, winegrowers were considered to be rather rustic and to belong to the lower classes. Now let us again have a look at the trendsetters. More than 60 percent of the women in the first marriage cohort who had

22 Age at last birth for wives married to self-employed, civil servants/white-collar workers of upper- or middle-class status and merchants:

Period	Self-employed MC	Self-employed UC	Civ. serv./ white collar UC.	Civ. serv./ white collar UC	Merchants
1830,1850	37.1	35.6	36.0	33.5	33.4
1860,1870,1880	36.0	32.4	35.1	35.2	33.9
1890,1910	33.9	32.5	32.2	31.8	31.3

Source: Database Stuttgart

Table 3. Age at Last Birth for Various Marriage Cohorts

Age at last birth	Marriage cohorts 1830,1850		1860,1870,1880		1890,1910	
	Number	%	Number	%	Number	%
15–19	2	.6	1	.2	4	.6
20–24	8	2.3	19	4.4	60	9.3
25–29	28	7.9	53	12.3	128	19.9
30–34	61	17.3	87	20.1	175	27.2
35–39	102	28.9	124	28.7	152	23.6
40–44	135	38.2	128	29.6	117	18.2
45–49	17	4.8	20	4.6	8	1.2
Total	353	100.0	432	100.0	644	100.0

Source: Database Stuttgart

Table 4. Age at Last Birth by Social Class

Age at last birth	Social class Lower class		Middle class		Upper class	
	Number	%	Number	%	Number	%
15–19	3	.5	4	.4		
20–24	44	6.8	56	5.9	5	4.6
25–29	74	11.5	150	15.7	26	24.1
30–34	126	19.5	217	22.7	31	28.7
35–39	185	28.7	248	26.0	30	27.8
40–44	189	29.3	257	26.9	14	13.0
45–49	24	3.7	22	2.3	2	1.9
Total	645	100.0	954	100.0	108	100.0

Source: Database Stuttgart

married a merchant gave birth to their last child between the ages of 30 and 34, which figure eventually increased to two-thirds.

Whether successful entrepreneur or high-ranking civil servant, they were all practising family limitation together with their wives. Already in the first marriage cohort, upper-class birth intervals had been longest, with 34.2 months on average (see table 1), as compared to other social groups. Historical demographers assume that birth intervals of more than 31.5 months indicate the use of birth control methods (Wrigley, 1969: 92; Müller, 2000: 280f.). Whereas 30 percent of upper-class self-employed wives married around 1830 or 1850 were giving birth with an average interval of 31–48 months, this was the case for 36 percent of the wives of civil servants and white collar employees. Clearly, women in these latter social groups had all been practising active birth control. In the cohorts married towards the end of the nineteenth century, seven out of fifteen women (46.7 percent) were prolonging the interval between births to over 48 months. This means that on average four years passed between any two births in upper-class families headed by civil servants or white collar employees. The very length of the intervals renders it likely that conception had not, or at least not exclusively, been influenced by prolonged breast-feeding, but by Stuttgart women's increasing use of modern contraceptives.

So far, the analysis has been moving on well-known terrain. It has shown transitions in female life courses and family forms. We have made likely suggestions but have not proven the influence that women had on different family models. It may be helpful to look at the family of origin of the women in our cohorts in order to focus more clearly on women's role in the adoption of family limitation, as it integrates her upbringing, education and experience before her marriage. The Stuttgart Database allows for the so far hardly ever studied interpretation of the women's social and family background, as measured by their fathers' occupation.

For the first marriage cohort the analysis shows that in particular women from an entrepreneurial upper-class background, but also women with fathers occupied in the category 'trade, catering and services', had a willingness to start a family at a comparatively early age. Nevertheless, they also tried to limit the size of their family once the desired number of children was reached. In principal, these finding also apply to daughters of white-collar employees and civil servants, who did not, however, limit fertility to the same extent as did daughters from entrepreneurial families.

Table 5. Age at Marriage, at First and at Last Birth, Birth Intervals and Number of Children by Marriage Cohorts and Selected Occupational Groups of the Wife's Father[23]

Marriage cohort / Occupational category		Age at marriage	Age at first birth	Age at last birth	Average birth interval (months)	Number of children
		mean	mean	mean	mean	mean
1830,1850	Winegrower/farmer	25.0	25.2	38.6	26.4	7.8
	White collar/civil servant	26.8	26.0	35.8	34.0	5.1
	Artisan lower/middle class	26.1	26.0	37.1	29.1	6.3
	Merchant/caterer/service Middle class	25.0	24.1	37.5	32.2	6.5
	Entrepren. upper class	23.2	24.4	35.3	30.9	6.0
1860,1870	Blue collar worker, lower class	27.9	23.2	35.9	39.7	6.1
1880	Winegrower/farmer	26.0	25.4	37.2	31.6	6.2
	White collar/civil servant	25.6	25.4	36.0	34.8	5.2
	Artisan lower/middle class	27.8	26.2	36.8	32.6	5.6
	Merchant/caterer/service Middle class	24.3	24.3	32.6	33.5	4.4
	Entrepren. upper class	25.3	24.9	35.1	41.0	4.8
1890,1910	Blue collar worker, lower class	25.6	24.4	33.3	38.9	4.2
	Winegrower/farmer	26.5	25.7	34.1	37.1	3.9
	White collar/civil servant	25.2	25.5	32.4	41.1	3.5
	Artisan lower/middle class	25.4	25.0	33.2	38.7	4.1
	Merchant/caterer/service Middle class	25.1	25.5	32.5	43.1	3.2
	Entrepren. Upper class	26.5	25.8	30.7	34.5	2.7

Source: Database Stuttgart

23 The occupational status of the woman's father was based on occupations recorded in family records and registry office documents. These entries only allowed a rough categorisation which differs from the here otherwise applied system of social classes.

Table 6. Age at First and at Last Birth, Birth Intervals and Number of Children by the Husband's and the Father's Occupational Status

Husband's occupational status	Father's occupational status	Age at first birth	Age at last birth	Average birth interval (month)	Number of children
		mean	mean	mean	mean
Worker	Winegrower/farmer	25.3	35.2	34.41	5.0
	White collar/civil servant	26.2	35.7	40.00	4.3
	Artisan lower/middle class	25.7	35.5	33.13	5.3
	Merchant/caterer/ service middle class	24.8	35.1	33.68	4.9
	Entrepren. upper class	25.9	35.4	34.60	4.9
Self-employed	Blue collar worker, lower class	23.7	36.4	45.84	5.5
	Winegrower/farmer	26.2	37.1	34.35	5.6
	White collar/civil servant	25.5	34.5	36.05	4.8
	Artisan lower/middle class	25.4	35.6	33.68	5.3
	Merchant/caterer/ service middle class	24.9	33.8	36.43	4.6
	Entrepren. upper class	24.7	34.5	38.29	4.7
White collar / civil servant	Blue collar worker, lower class	25.4	32.8	31.99	4.2
	Winegrower/farmer	25.8	35.0	31.39	4.7
	White collar/civil servant	25.1	32.9	37.54	4.0
	Artisan lower/middle class	25.9	34.4	38.51	4.2
	Merchant/caterer/ service middle class	25.0	34.0	37.67	4.2
	Entrepren. upper class	24.1	33.0	36.96	4.2

Source: Database Stuttgart

Decisive, in many cases, was not only the women's social background but also the social environment they had married into. If a blue-collar worker started a family with a white-collar or civil servant's daughter, they had only 4.3 children as compared to the average of 5.1 children per family. But if a self-employed male married a winegrower's or a farmer's daughter, the family would keep more strongly to the tradition of natural fertility behaviour. In these marriages 5.6 children were born on average. The social background of the woman was the decisive factor for the size of her family which is demonstrated by the following example involving women from white-collar and civil servant families. Whenever they started a family with a blue-collar husband, they clearly began to control their birth intervals. The average intervals of 40 months for this group of women clearly speaks the language of birth control. But if the husband was self-employed, the woman's influence apparently waned as the birth intervals shortened by an average of four to five months in comparison. Corresponding social backgrounds of marriage partners seem to have intensified the according family model. Marriage within the social group of civil servants and white-collar employees in particular resulted in a reduced number of children, which figure fell as low as 4.0 children per couple. The same effect may be observed for the rural proportion of the population. In this case however, chances were that the number of children increased rather than decreased as traditional customs and forms of employment in rural families were followed more closely. Summing up, the reproductive behaviour of young couples was determined by the family model taken over from the woman's family background, and by the form of paid employment in the newly started family.

Infant Mortality as Postnatal Birth Control?

When considering which role women played in the demographic transition not only fertility or pregnancy prevention provide a suitable basis for reflections on women's scope for action. Women were responsible for birth control and, to a much higher degree, for the care of their newborn children. We already analysed the effect of the family organisation on the chances of children's survival. Even contemporaries noticed that high rates of infant mortality often corresponded with high numbers of children. They wondered if neglect of infants should be interpreted as a form of postnatal 'birth control'. By detailed analyses of the connection between the birth rank of siblings and infant mortality researchers try to clarify this problem (Imhof, 1981; Shorter, 1986).

What information can we gain from the Stuttgart database? In Stuttgart the same phenomena can be observed as in other German regions (Schraut, 1989: 148–155; Müller, 2000: 289–297). The more children were born into a family, the lower were the chances of infants to survive the critical first year of life. But which factor should be regarded as the cause and which one as the consequence? Were infants in large families neglected, or did the early death of many children result in many 'new attempts' to make sure that at least some children survived beyond the critical first years? An examination of birth rank may provide first hints for the solution of this question. The more siblings were born before the birth of a given infant, the lower were his/her survival chances during his/her first year. But the position in the sequence of siblings only reveals part of the picture because in view of the high infant mortality the birth position of the infant alone did not say very much about survival prospects. More often than not a third-born child took over the place of the second-born child.

If one not only considers the number of preceding births but also takes into account the number of older siblings still alive, then a well-known phenomenon becomes clearly visible. A child's chances at survival depended primarily on the number of older siblings with which it competed for nutrition, care, and attention (Knodel, 1988: 84–101). Until the fifth living child there is an observable increase in infant mortality in relation to the position in the sequence of siblings. For children in higher birth orders, the scope of variation in the family situation prevents us to draw clear conclusions. Nevertheless, it is evident that the certainly still welcome second- and third-born children had higher mortality rates than the first-born child.

Table 7 shows that the relationships described above could be observed throughout the nineteenth and until the early twentieth century. Therefore it must be assumed that deliberate postnatal 'birth control' was not exercised. It was presumably easier to organise the care for one infant only within the extended family than to organise the care for several small children at the same time. Often older siblings or individuals who did not directly belong to the family may have been deployed in the care of younger siblings, thus allowing the mothers to work in the family's business or to contribute to the

Table 7. Development of Infant Mortality by Position in the Birth Rank of Living Siblings

Infant mortality by birth cohorts		Birth rank (living children) 1	2	3	4	5	6–10	Sum
1830/1859	%	18.9	25.1	27.2	29.1	31.3	22.4	24.7
	Number	174	222	188	138	92	79	893
1860/1889	%	19.2	23.0	24.8	27.6	28.9	25.0	23.4
	Number	334	325	270	202	128	131	1390
1890/1919	%	13.8	18.6	22.1	22.4	24.3	25.1	18.9
	Number	266	308	238	140	93	107	1152
Sum	%	16.9	21.6	24.4	26.2	28.0	24.3	22.0
	Number	774	855	696	480	313	317	3435

Source: Database Stuttgart

Figure 10. Infant Mortality, Occupational Category of the Father and Birth Rank (Living Children)

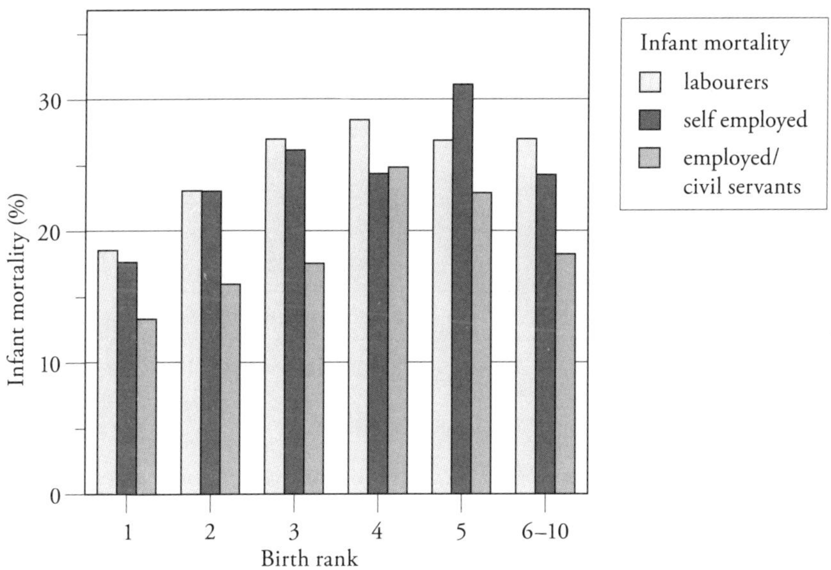

Source: Database Stuttgart

family income through non-domestic jobs. We may safely assume that the care provided by older siblings did not always meet the necessary hygienic standards, especially, when the mother's job prevented her from breast-feeding. The supposed failures of older siblings taking care of their younger brothers and sisters may be observed for all social classes. Although the social position of the family remained decisive for chances of infants to survive, it is nevertheless clear that infant mortality increased with the child's higher position in the birth ranking of living brothers and sisters.

Table 8. Infant Mortality for Selected Social Groups by Birth Rank

	Proportion of infants' deaths (%)							
	Birth rank						Sum	
Social groups	1	2	3	4	5	6–10	Number	%
Labourer LC	18.6	23.1	27.0	28.5	26.9	27.0	1223	23.6
Self empl. LC	20.2	32.1	34.3	25.0	29.5	24.4	266	27.5
Employed/civil servants LC	16.8	22.2	17.4	31.0	32.5	16.7	135	21.2
Self empl. MC	17.9	22.5	25.6	24.9	31.8	24.9	1161	23.1
Employed/civil servants MC	13.2	15.5	18.5	24.5	23.1	19.9	518	17.1
Self empl. UC	7.9	8.0	12.1	13.2	26.3	5.9	34	10.4
Employed/civil servants UC	8.8	9.8	10.3	14.6	4.3	5.0	36	9.5
Sum	16.7	21.1	24.3	25.8	27.8	23.9	3373	21.7

Source: Database Stuttgart, LC = lower classes, MC = middle classes, UC = upper classes

Comparing the effects on infant mortality of the occupational category of the father and the organisation of the family and the household, it is evident that chances to survive for children of white-collar workers and civil servants in particular were influenced least of all by the question of birth ranking. This indicates that the chances of infants to survive the critical first year were not the result of deliberate postnatal birth control but depended on the economic situation of the family. Once again the question is important, to what extent the organisation of family, work and gender roles set mothers free to nurse their children or to prepare adequate nursing by others.

Conclusions

When answering the question *Were women present at the demographic transition?* the following might be said regarding infant mortality and the development of fertility. The particular organisation of work and family life in bourgeois households of civil servants and white-collar employees allowed mothers to be exempted from other duties earlier than in any other social group. The extra time mothers in these social groups could devote to child and infant care decisively influenced their children's chances at survival. The earliest successful strategies to limit the number of children ever born can also be traced to these same social groups which were, moreover, continuously growing in importance as the nineteenth century progressed. The life styles and gender roles of bourgeois or middle-class families offered women a meaningful enhancement of their roles and tasks based on newly defined concepts of femininity and motherliness. And finally, this group vehemently and successfully used the public debate on infant mortality to transfer their own family and gender concepts to other social classes. This bourgeois concept of child care and birth control certainly depended on the agreement of both partners regarding a specific family size. However, the demographic analysis presented in this study suggests that the input by women of family ideals and contraceptive knowledge which originated from their own family background played an important role.

This gendered perspective is not only relevant to the study of declining fertility. The consequences of the decline in both infant mortality and fertility also concerned women in particular. Women's lives were fundamentally altered by what might be labelled as the 'retreat of the death experience from the nursery'. As the database shows, on average, every ninth mother suffered at least one stillbirth in her life, almost every second mother lost at least one child in its first year of life and every fourth mother even lost two or more of her infant children in the period under study. In addition, there must have been a considerable number of miscarriages which were, however, not recorded in the Württemberg registration offices.[24] The changes over time though have been remarkable. Almost every second mother born between 1800 and 1829 had been affected by the death of at least one infant. By contrast, only one third of mothers born after 1860 had to share that experience.

Furthermore, there is the issue of the increased period of life women spend as widows without the support of the family as a provision for old age. The Stuttgart database shows that on average six out of ten women survived their husband in the period under study. They had to face the uncertainty of income support in a society narrowly confining female gainful employment and poorly remunerating the work of women. The number of women concerned by this problem was rising during the nineteenth century (born 1810/19: 50 percent, born 1880/89: 64 percent). The number of years that women had to get by on their own, with or without children was increasing as well. The prolonged time span without parenting tasks may have presented women with new demands in their efforts to shape their lives in sensible ways. Since at the same time the number of children was decreasing, it further reduced the pool of family members that widows could rely on for support in old age.

It is in the light of these findings that not only the model of the demographic transition requires a gendered perspective, but so do the historical and current debates on the future of the welfare state in general and pension schemes in particular.

24 The national law at that time (Reichsgesetz) does not mention the necessity to report immature stillbirths. For the city of Magdeburg Landsberg reported 1,458 miscarriages out of 6,447 births that were recorded by midwives, doctors and hospitals in 1912. Those miscarriages must at least have been pregnancies recorded beyond the necessities of the law. If the Magdeburg figures were representative, we then have to calculate with one immature stillbirth for every 4.4 births (see Landsberg 1907).

References

Cless (1868), *Die Kindersterblichkeit in Württemberg. Ein Mahnruf an das Volk*, Stuttgart.

Cleß, G. and Schübler, G. (1815), *Versuch einer medizinischen Topographie der Königlichen Haupt- und Residenzstadt*, Stuttgart.

Davidoff, Leonore and Hall, Catherine (1987), *Family Fortunes, Men and Women of the English Middle Class, 1780–1850*, London, Hutchinson.

Dienel, Christiane (1995), *Kinderzahl und Staatraison: Empfängnisverhütung und Bevölkerungspolitik in Deutschland und Frankreich bis 1918*, Münster, Westfälisches Dampfboot (Theorie und Geschichte der bürgerlichen Gesellschaft, vol. 11).

Frevert, Ute (1988), 'Bürgerliche Meisterdenker und das Geschlechterverhältnis. Konzepte, Erfahrungen, Visionen an der Wende vom 18. zum 19. Jahrhundert', in ibid. (ed.), *Bürgerinnen und Bürger im 19. Jahrhundert*, Göttingen, Vandenhoeck & Ruprecht, 17–48.

Gehrmann, Rolf (1979), 'Einsichten und Konsequenzen aus neueren Forschungen zum generativen Verhalten im demographischen Ancien Régime und in der Transitionsphase', *Zeitschrift für Bevölkerungswissenschaft*, 5, 445–485.

Gillis, John, Tilly, Louise A. and Levine, David (eds) (1992), *The European Experience of Declining Fertility, 1850–1970. A Quiet Revolution*, Cambridge, Blackwell.

Haas, Inka (1998), *Gebärstreik: Frauen gegen den staatlich verordneten Muttermythos*, Frankfurt a. M. dipa.

Habermas, Rebekka (2000), *Frauen und Männer des Bürgertums: eine Familiengeschichte*, Göttingen, Vandenhoeck & Ruprecht.

Hausen, Karin (1976), 'Die Polarisierung der "Geschlechtscharaktere" – Eine Spiegelung der Dissoziation von Erwerbs- und Familienleben', in Rosenbaum, Heidi (ed.), *Seminar: Familie und Gesellschaftsstruktur*, Frankfurt, Suhrkamp, 161–191.

Helfft (1858), 'Über die Sterblichkeit der lebend geborenen Kinder in Berlin innerhalb des ersten Lebensjahres', *Monatsblatt für medicinische Statistik und öffentliche Gesundheitspflege.*

Imhof, Arthur E. (1981), 'Unterschiedliche Säuglingssterblichkeit in Deutschland, 18.–20. Jahrhundert – Warum?', *Zeitschrift für Bevölkerungswissenschaft*, 343–382.

Jütte, Robert (2003), *Lust ohne Last. Geschichte der Empfängnisverhütung*, München, Beck.

Khalatbari, Parviz (1999), 'Demographische Transition – der Prozeß der Unterbrechung der Kontinuität in der Bevölkerungsbewegung', *Zeitschrift für Bevölkerungswissenschaft*, 24, 29–45.

Knodel, John (1988), *Demographic Behaviour in the Past. A Study of Fourteen Village Populations in the Eighteenth and Nineteenth Century*, Cambridge, Cambridge University Press.

Landsberg, Otto (1907), 'Statistik der Fehlgeburten', *Allgemeines statistisches Archiv*, 7/2, 53–62.

Livi-Bacci, Massimo (1999), *Europa und seine Menschen. Eine Bevölkerungsgeschichte*, München, Beck.

Mackensen, Rainer (1999), 'Theoretische Notizen zum Konzept der Transition', *Zeitschrift für Bevölkerungswissenschaft*, 24, 5–28.

Mackinnon, Alison (1995), 'Were Women Present at the Demographic Transition? Questions from a Feminist Historian to Historical Demographers', *Gender & History*, 7, 222–240.

Marcuse, Max (1913), 'Zur Verbreitung und Methodik der willkürlichen Geburtenbeschränkung in Berliner Proletarierkreisen', *Sexualprobleme*, 9, 752–781.

Marcuse, Max (1917), *Der eheliche Präventivverkehr, seine Verbreitung, Verursachung und Methodik*, Stuttgart, Ferdinand Enke.

Mitterauer, Michael (1992a), 'Geschlechtsspezifische Arbeitsteilung und Geschlechterrollen in ländlichen Gesellschaften Mitteleuropas', in Mitterauer, Michael, *Familie und Arbeitsteilung*, Wien, Böhlau, 58–148.

Mitterauer, Michael (1992b), 'Familie und Arbeitsorganisation in städtischen Gesellschaften des späten Mittelalters und der frühen Neuzeit', in Mitterauer, Michael, *Familie und Arbeitsteilung*, Wien, Böhlau, 256–300.

Müller, Rita (2000), *Von der Wiege zur Bahre, Weibliche und männliche Lebensläufe im 19. und frühen 20. Jahrhundert am Beispiel Stuttgart-Feuerbach*, (Veröffentlichungen des Archivs der Stadt Stuttgart; vol. 85), Stuttgart, Hohenheim Verlag.

Nell, Adelheid von (1973), *Die Entwicklung der generativen Strukturen bürgerlicher und bäuerlicher Familien von 1750 bis zur Gegenwart,* Diss. Bochum, Hochschulschrift.

Opitz, Claudia (1998), 'Von der "querelle des femmes" in den Salons zur Frauen-Volksbewegung. Überlegungen zur Politisierung von Frauen während der französischen Revolution', in Frauen & Geschichte, Baden-Württemberg (eds), *Frauen und Revolution. Strategien weiblicher Emanzipation 1789 bis 1848,* Tübingen, Silberburg, 14–32.

Polano, Otto (1916), 'Beitrag zur Frage der Geburtenbeschränkung', *Zeitschrift für Geburtshilfe und Gynäkologie*, 79, 567–578.

Schmid, Pia (1992), 'Rousseau revisited', *Zeitschrift für Pädagogik*, 38, 839–854.

Schmid, Pia (2000), '"O, wie süss lohnt das Muttergefühl!" Die Bestimmung zur Mutter in Almanachen für das weibliche Publikum um 1800', in Opitz, Claudia, Weckel, Ulrike and Kleinau, Elke (eds), *Tugend, Vernunft und Gefühl, Geschlechterdiskurse der Aufklärung und weibliche Lebenswelten*, Münster, Waxmann, 107–125.

Schraut, Sylvia (1989), *Sozialer Wandel im Industrialisierungsprozeß. Esslingen 1800–1870*, Esslingen, Thorbecke.

Scott, Joan W. and Tilly, Louise A. (1984), 'Familienökonomie und Industrialisierung in Europa', in Honegger, Claudia and Heintz, Bettina (eds), *Listen der Ohnmacht*, Frankfurt, EVA, 99–137.

Shorter, Edward (1986), 'Die große Umwälzung der Mutter – Kind – Beziehungen vom 18. bis zum 20. Jahrhundert', in Martin, Jochen and Nitschke, August (eds), *Zur Sozialgeschichte der Kindheit*, Freiburg, Alber.

Spree, Reinhard (1981), 'Angestellte als Modernisierungsagenten, Indikatoren und Thesen zum reproduktiven Verhalten von Angestellten im späten 19. und frühen 20. Jahrhundert', in Kocka, Jürgen (ed.), *Angestellte im europäischen Vergleich*, Göttingen, Vandenhoeck & Ruprecht, 279–308.

Spree, Reinhard (1981), *Soziale Ungleichheit vor Krankheit und Tod*, Göttingen, Vandenhoeck & Ruprecht.

Spree, Reinhard (1995), *On Infant Mortality Change in Germany since the Early 19th Century*, München, Mimeo.

Vögele, Jörg (1991), 'Die Entwicklung der (großstädtischen) Gesundheitsverhältnisse in der Epoche des Demographischen und Epidemiologischen Übergangs', in Reulecke, Jürgen and Castell Rüdenhausen Adelheid zu (eds), *Stadt und Gesellschaft*, Stuttgart, Franz Steiner Verlag.

Vögele, Jörg (1994), 'Urban Infant Mortality in Imperial Germany', *Social History of Medicine*, 7, 401–425.

Vögele, Jörg (2001), *Sozialgeschichte städtischer Gesundheitsverhältnisse während der Urbanisierung*, Berlin, Duncker & Humblot.

Wrigley, E. A. (1969), *Bevölkerungsstruktur im Wandel*, München, Kindler.

Wunder, Heide (1992), *"Er ist die Sonn', sie ist der Mond". Frauen in der Frühen Neuzeit*, München, Beck.

Gender and Religion Shaping the Pace of the Fertility Decline

A Comparative Analysis of two Swiss Cantons (1860–1930)

Anne-Françoise Praz

'Were women present at the demographic transition?' was the provocative question addressed in 1995 by Alison Mackinnon to historical demographers, reproaching them for their 'inability to envisage women as active agents in social change' (Mackinnon, 1995: 222). Ten years later, the question to what extent women were active agents of the first fertility transition is still controversial; but whatever scholars assume to be historically true, there is a growing acceptance of the importance of focusing on women, and more specifically on gender, in explanations of the first demographic transition.

The first part of this paper emphasizes some theoretical and methodological developments in research on the fertility decline. On the one hand, scientists take methodological individualism more seriously: they are aware of the problems aggregation causes and seek to produce as much individual data as possible. On the other hand, studies try to go beyond simple correlations between supposedly causal factors and corresponding fertility outcomes and set out to identify mechanisms through which structures on the macro-level influence private decisions. As a result of these methodological improvements the focus on gender appears as a natural development.

To substantiate these theoretical and methodological remarks, the second part of this article provides some results produced by such an integration of gender into the explanatory mechanisms. More precisely, thanks to this gender perspective, we propose a new interpretation of the well-known Coale conditions for the adoption of fertility control. Subsequently, we focus on the difficulties in finding, constructing and interpreting indicators of gender. In spite of these problems, we hope to be able to show that the integration of gender into the analysis of fertility decline is a scientifically fruitful move.

Gender and the Focus on Individuals

As many contributions to this volume put forward, research on the European fertility decline has to a large extent relied on macro-theoretical analysis, linking the reproductive behaviour to structural changes such as industrialisation and secularisation. This tendency obscures the fact that all reproductive decisions are made at the individual level; nations, provinces, communities, and even households do not decide to procreate and to rear children.

We will not dwell on models that use aggregates only; their shortcomings are well-known. It is more interesting to analyse models that do not seem to use any 'decision-aggregate' and yet fail to take the last step of disaggregation down to individuals. In historical demography, a prominent example is Ansley Coale's model that enumerates three preconditions for the adoption of fertility control. As a reminder, according to this model, fertility control must be 'an acceptable mode of thought and form of behaviour', reduced fertility must be perceived as advantageous, and contraceptive techniques must be known and available (Coale, 1973: 65). Coale's model is consistent with a methodologically individualist approach, as the behaviour under study is considered from the perspective of the individual. Yet Coale, like many scholars before and after him, departs from this consistency when he identifies this *individual*, the basic unit of study, as the *parents*, the *couple* or the *household*. Such a simplification overlooks the fact that the individuals in this unit – husband and wife for example – are endowed with different rights and resources and are, consequently, differently positioned regarding Coale's conditions.

More consistent with methodological individualism, institutional economics provides adequate models that show how property rights, contractual obligations and social norms, shape the distribution of resources inside the household, the bargaining power and the decision-making processes (Pollack, 1985; Folbre, 1996: 135). As husband and wife may not have the same interests and constraints with respect to fertility control, changes in the bargaining power between men and women can be crucial for the adoption and success of contraception. First of all however, such a change in marital bargaining power has to be demonstrated, and the contribution of Alison Mackinnon in this volume points in this direction: 'Did women's bargaining power within partnerships increase in the latter part of the nineteenth century', she asks, 'and if so, what factors made a difference?'.

However, the attention to differing interests of husbands and wives and to their bargaining power in fertility decisions is not shared by all theorists of the first fertility transition. Ron Lesthaeghe for example, who produced influential studies especially on Belgian fertility (compare the contribution by Eric Vanhaute and Christa Matthys in this volume), underlines the correlation between fertility decline and the diffusion of the bourgeois model of asymmetrical sexual roles within marriage (Lesthaeghe, 1995: 136). Nevertheless, this finding does not lead him to examine the differing interests and the bargaining power of the spouses. Geoffrey McNicoll in contrast asserts that the more distinctive the roles of husband and wife, the greater the scope for differences in fertility interests, with power relations within the family deciding which interest will prevail (McNicholl, 1994: 207).

The familiar interpretation of the first fertility transition that views this change as a shift from a social to an individual control of reproduction fits in with a consistent disaggregation only at first glance. Before the transition (Lestheaghe, 1980), fertility control is considered to have been essentially based on the control of marriage, through patriarchal power and community rules, and also on habits and traditions like breastfeeding and cultural norms restraining coital frequency. During the transition, the prevalence of these community and patriarchal rules was eroded by various institutional and economic changes, and the young gained more autonomy regarding marriage and fertility decisions.[1]

This model of the emergence of an individual control of reproduction during the first fertility transition does not follow up on its individualistic stand as this *individual*, gender neutral, is again the *couple* and the decision is assumed to be in a hypothetical common, or even consensual, interest. Thus, the differing interests and constraints of men and women regarding birth control during that period remain hidden and scholars do not investigate

1 Recent research discusses this model by criticizing the focus on parity-specific family planning as the single modern form of controlled fertility and by examining other forms of control such as spacing or starting (Van Bavel, 2004). A late age at first marriage for example, generally conceptualized as an institutionalized social constraint, might also reflect a process of individual, conscious choice; therefore the timing of the first transition ought to be reconsidered (Szreter, Garrett, 2000: 52). However, this discussion solely concerns the concept of social control itself. The idea of a shift from a social to an individual control of reproduction during the first transition remains largely intact.

them. Recent research has demonstrated that given the contraceptive means usually available, husbands were able to decide unilaterally about contraception, and indeed generally acted in this way. Given the dominant gender culture, 'respectable' women had to be ignorant about sexual matters (Fisher, 2000; Fischer and Szreter, 2003). Historically, it was only during the second fertility transition (1960–1970) that every individual concerned obtained the publicly accepted rights and the technical means to control his or her fertility (Chaperon, 2004).[2]

It is not only the adult members of a household who have different interests and rights, the same is true for children, an aspect which is rarely addressed in research. Daughters and sons, or elder and younger children, were not always considered equal in respect to parental expenses, which may have influenced the motivation for fertility control.

The focus on individuals does not imply that each individual is unique, necessarily leaving the researcher bogged down in a chaos of idiosyncrasies. For each individual, the decisions can be modelled by the same mechanism that translates incentives and constraints into behaviour. These incentives and constraints do not vary arbitrarily, their distribution being highly patterned. The following section focuses on such a distribution of incentives and constraints according to sex as a crucial component in the working of mechanisms translating determinants of fertility into individual behaviour.

2 The assertion of an individual control of reproduction during the first fertility transition is also controversial regarding the intervention of the state through explicit fertility policies. This state influence only erodes in the 1950s, not because of its lack of efficiency, but more for ideological reasons. State intervention in reproductive choice was delegitimised by the traumatism of the Nazi eugenics and the political context of anti-communism and anti-totalitarianism; the idea that governments should not interfere with couples' private decisions about fertility then became widespread.

Gender and the Explanations of Fertility Decline

The controversial results of the Princeton Fertility Project[3] that aimed to explain the causes for the decline of fertility in Europe have been widely commented upon. It is by now accepted that none of the socioeconomic or demographic variables chosen correlated very well with the timing of the fertility decline. However, variation in marital fertility was often significantly related to 'culture', defined as religion, language, ethnicity or geographical region. The main criticism addressed at this project, besides the level of aggregation chosen, was the kind of explanation adopted. Commentaries put forward that correlations between convenient aggregations of micro-level data are insufficient evidence. They will tell us little or nothing about why the members of various subpopulations began to change their behaviour in order to adapt to any changing economic or cultural factor, roughly defined.

As a result of this failure, emphasis was placed on the selection of more specific indicators of determinants of fertility and the way these determinants impact on individual behaviour in different subpopulations whose environment could be described precisely. But what feature of social structure is relevant, what indicators shall be selected? Such a choice can only be legitimised by an underlying model or explanatory mechanism.

A first step in clarifying underlying mechanisms was the integration in historical demography of economic decision models proposing a general explanation of individual decision-making and permitting the transformation of all types of contextual features into the same kind of 'theoretical money', costs and benefits. Fertility behaviour can thus be considered as responding to cost-benefit incentives. These models overcome the misleading opposition between economy and culture, integrating all kinds of costs: the material costs of children as well as the moral and information costs of contraception. They are also consistent with a methodologically individualist approach, as

3 This project, initiated on the basis of modernization models linking the demographic transition to economic and social development, ended without demonstrating any necessary relationships between economic and social modernization and the onset of fertility limitation. While the project seemed to show a convergence in the timing of fertility limitation within European areas of very different levels of development, important spatial variations, shaped by differences of culture, remained to be explained (Coale and Watkins, 1986).

the costs are not considered from the perspective of an external observer, but from those of the individuals concerned. As Jane Humphries underlines in her article in this volume, the key question for individual decision-making is 'how the men and women involved perceived these costs'. The working-class autobiographies she uses permit us to capture the perceived costs of children to mothers and fathers.

A second step consists of identifying those specific features of the economic and cultural environment that could possibly represent costs and benefits. A third step is however necessary: it is only after examining the institutional context that we are able to decide if those features indeed constitute costs and benefits. The two following examples should illustrate this kind of reasoning, as well as the integration of gender into the process.

The changing economic function of children has often been put forward as an explanatory factor for the decline of fertility. To sustain this assertion, the Princeton Project proposed correlations between the level of fertility and the proportion of the labour force in agriculture or the general level of industrialisation. Unfortunately, these aggregate indicators are useless if we do not specify the features that constitute the costs and benefits of children. Certain types of agriculture rely on children's labour, others do not, so the benefit of children may be very different. Furthermore, parents may rely differently on daughters' and sons' labour. Moreover, a seemingly similar economic environment with similar material opportunities for children's work does not necessarily result in similar incentives. It is further dependent on the institutional context translating these opportunities into effective costs and benefits. For example, state laws and policies or other kinds of institutional regulations may impede parents in seizing the opportunities at hand and in relying on children's labour. The implementation of these regulations may differ in severity depending on whether boys or girls are concerned.

The second example concerns the high costs of contraception, traditionally associated with Catholic doctrine, and therefore the Princeton Project examined the impact of religious affiliation on fertility. However, an explanatory mechanism must go beyond the determination of the religious or political affiliation of individuals and specify which religious norms and values, which elements of the dominant political ideology are capable of modifying the costs under study. Here too, values and norms are often gender specific, making moral costs of contraception different for men and women. Furthermore, these religious norms or the values put forward by various discourses will not influence reproductive practices if they are not translated into institutional arrangements and enforced through religious or political institutions (McQuillan, 2004).

Recent studies on the political economy of fertility provide interesting insights into this decisive step of the enforcement of norms and values. Such studies analyse the role of the state in regulating fertility through diverse institutional means. During the second part of the nineteenth century, state institutions gained importance in regulating family life, compared to religious or other traditional institutions. The term *institutions* here, does not only refer to the administrative and political apparatus of a society, it includes the system of rights and duties of individuals, as well as the rewards and sanctions for conventional or deviant behaviour. These individual rights are crucial for the distribution of resources and the bargaining power inside the household, factors that are highly relevant for fertility behaviour. To illustrate this role of state policies, S. Ryan Johansson uses a computer metaphor: state policies are a real force able to translate the 'cultural software of fertility' – a set of abstract instructions with a strongly ethical character – into 'a set of institutionalized incentives real enough to influence the "voluntary" behaviour of the majority' (Johansson, 1991: 384).[4]

In shaping individual rights, state institutions and policies assemble individuals into categories, using categorisations already present in the 'cultural software' of each society. The categorisation by sex is historically one of the most pervasive ones. It was a prominent target for state policies during the period of the first fertility transition and an important topic in political discourse that defined suitable behaviour for men and women, leading to concrete measures delineating their respective opportunities. As a result, norms of femininity and masculinity prescribed different behaviours regarding sexuality and contraception; husbands and wives did not have the same rights and duties in marriage; women and men were not subject to the same work legislation; and girls and boys were not considered equal in school policies and in public expenses for education.

4 Interestingly, Johansson focuses not on public policies overtly planned to influence fertility – pro-natalist policies generally failed or came too late during the first fertility transition – but more on implicit policies, namely those policies that were not intended by governments to change fertility patterns but nevertheless had an important impact on the costs of children (compulsory education, exclusion of children from the labour market, admission of women into advanced levels of education).

The previous considerations allow us to render our definition of gender more precisely. Gender is not only an individual attribute, but a structuring principle of social life. It is the process as well as the result of an attribution of rights to individuals on the basis of their biological sex. In a given environment of material and technological constraints, this process associates a 'cultural software' (representations about sex differences, norms of masculinity and femininity) with a set of institutional practices that enforce it, resulting in unequal opportunities for women and men regarding the access to the commodities available.

The following part of this article proposes a demonstration of the impact of these differing rights on the pace of fertility decline. More than an ideological concern, this focus on gender inequalities refers to a central social process.

Sample and Data

The data used for this project were collected in the French-speaking cantons of Vaud (VD – Protestant) and Fribourg (FR – Catholic), two neighbouring cantons situated in the Western part of Switzerland. In each canton, two villages have been selected with respect to economic factors, in order to isolate the impact of institutional variables. The first pair of villages (Chavornay/VD and Broc/FR) experienced a similar industrialisation process (the setting up of a chocolate factory near each village) at the same time. The second pair (Chevroux/VD and Portalban-Delley/FR), two neighbouring communities situated on the shore of the same lake, maintained an economic structure based on agriculture and fishing. As the villages in each pair were almost identical with respect to economic factors, their social structure was very similar too. Before 1900, the villages were homogeneous with respect to religious affiliation. Between 1900 and 1914, a very slight religious heterogeneity occurred in the two industrialized villages because of the arrival of workers and managerial staff employed by the chocolate factories, but these all left the villages during the Great War and the post-war crisis. The districts in which the villages were situated were religiously homogeneous too.

During the period under study, the Protestant canton of Vaud was led by progressive authorities. This government resulted from a radical-democratic revolution (1845) that marginalized the liberal-conservative tendencies, mostly associated with the Church intelligentsia. The new political forces modified the institutional framework: the influence of Protestant ministers and of parochial structures was lessened and the power of political structures such as local authorities and councils was reinforced.

The institutional framework was very different in the Catholic canton of Fribourg. The conservative government – resulting from the failure of a radical-democratic revolution – based its political strategy on a tight connection with the religious organisations. To secure the conservative vote, within a population mostly dispersed in the countryside and still not reached by the rise of mass-circulation press, it had to organise a permanent and decentralised control on its potential voters. For this purpose, it was crucial to keep a close connection with the Catholic Church, thus permitting the use of the network of parishes, religious associations, and priests and nuns that were present in almost every village.

A first data base gives information about the changing quantity of children. It includes all births, deaths and marriages taken from the parochial and civil registers of our four villages as far as they relate to marriages celebrated between 1860 and 1930.[5] The actual dimension of the sample used depends on the method of data treatment and its specific selection criteria. Following classical family reconstitution methods, it is possible to use 3,501 (56 percent) of the 6,207 legitimate births collected. If we add to these 'completed families' the 'achieved' families[6], the amount of usable data climbs to 4,276 legitimate births (76 percent). Event history analysis and its more flexible rules of data selection permits us to use 86 percent of the data base, producing a total sample of 5,381 legitimate births for 1848 married and fecund women under observation.

5 In order to supplement and check these sources of information, heterogeneous and discontinuous sources were consulted, such as local population registers (continuous registers) and censuses. After linking births, marriages and deaths, the final database (all villages conflated) contains 13,076 individuals.

6 Following Leboute (Leboute, 1988: 358), we keep in the sample the 'achieved families', which are families in which one of the parents dies and/or families who leave the village before the woman has reached age 50, but for which we do know the date of the parents' marriage. Event history analysis permits us to keep in the sample even the legitimate births for which we do not know the date of the parents' marriage.

A second data base documents the changing quality of children, namely the investment in education. Administrative sources at cantonal and village levels (pupil listings, school attendance statistics and correspondence of the school authorities) provide direct information about the school career of the children in the sample. For children for whom this type of direct information was not available, the educational variable was constructed on the basis of the subsequent professions of these children at marriage or death (indirect information). Among the 5,042 legitimate children who survived until age fifteen, we managed to reconstitute the school career of 2,353 of them (1,333 boys and 1,020 girls); about one third of these school careers was reconstituted on the basis of indirect information.[7]

Besides these quantitative data, qualitative material was used to document the 'cultural software' of fertility (religious literature, political discourse, newspapers, educational periodicals and school manuals), as well as state policies and their implementation (official publications, legislations, correspondence between cantonal and local authorities).

Re-interpreting Coale's Conditions: The Motivation for Fertility Control

Coale's model demands that research on fertility first ascertains the existence of a motivation (economic advantage) for fertility control, and secondly, the 'thinkability' or moral acceptability of such behaviour. In the following, we will demonstrate that this motivation and this moral acceptability both adopt gender-specific forms and, moreover, that these forms differ according to the political and religious context.

Our first hypothesis specifies Coale's condition of economic advantage by using Caldwell's model of the effect of mass education as the primary deter-

7 The comparison of the direct with the indirect information has given a good fit. The few professions for which this fit was unstable have not been taken into consideration. Fortunately, missing data (children for which direct or reliable indirect information are missing) are concentrated in the generations born before 1880, when both the processes of fertility decline and implementation of compulsory schooling were in their initial phase.

minant of the onset of the fertility transition. Education not only increases the costs of children in reducing a child's potential for work in the labour market or in the household, it also speeds up changes in norms and values regarding the child as a future rather than a present producer (Caldwell, 1980: 225). However, the norms and values regarding the quality and quantity of children, able to shape the motivation for birth control, can be very different, as attested by our Swiss cantons.

In the Protestant canton of Vaud, the government was keen to weaken the influence of religious institutions. Nonetheless, religious ideologies did not vanish: analysis of the dominant political discourse shows that the government adopted the Protestant values regarding fertility, giving them a political varnish. The education of children, intended to enlighten the spirit and promote individual autonomy in Protestant thought, was seen as a necessary condition for prosperity and democracy. Human co-responsibility in God's creation, in particular parental responsibility for child care and education (Perrenoud, 1974: 983–987), became a civic commitment of parents. According to educational periodicals, both men and women had to develop the intellectual capacities God had given them. Knowledge was considered important for women, the mothers of future citizens.

The importance of education in Protestant culture, and moreover its relevance for women, is attested for in other studies. In Norway for example, according to Ida Blom elsewhere in this volume, girls' education was seen as increasingly important by middle-class parents, and they consented to pay high fees for private schools, the public system being considered less reputable. In our Protestant setting by contrast, the public system was considered efficient. As primary schools were free and post-primary education was relatively affordable even for working-class parents, the class differential in access to education was less pronounced.

In the canton of Vaud, the Protestant views on education were efficiently implemented by a school policy that strictly enforced school attendance for both boys and girls. Parents were not allowed to take their children out of school before they reached the legal age of sixteen. Co-education was the rule until that age, and post-primary education for girls and boys was fostered by decentralisation of secondary or professional schools. This school policy constitutes a perfect example of the implicit fertility policies described by Johansson (see footnote 3). In defending the rights to education of all children, daughters and sons, the state significantly increased their costs for parents and, following the second of Coale's conditions, these growing costs constituted an important incentive to practice birth control.

To investigate why the integration of gender in such an explanatory mechanism can be crucial for an understanding of the pace of the fertility decline, we compared the 'cultural software of fertility' of both cantons, as well as their respective school policies. In the conservative Catholic culture of Fribourg, knowledge was considered as potentially dangerous, a source of the sin of pride or of rebellion against the established authorities. The opinion voiced in the Catholic educational periodicals was clear-cut: education for girls was necessary to prepare them for their task as skilled and pious housekeepers, but the two deterring figures of the coquettish female and the learned woman underlined the idea that knowledge was vanity for women and a danger to family and society. The girls' school programme, according to their social destiny, had to make ample room for housekeeping and needlework, but limiting the study of other disciplines to the most basic skills. School policies in Fribourg were sharply gender biased. The control and repression of school absenteeism did not follow a regular and determinate path, particularly not for girls. Educational structures were mostly segregated by sex; the cantonal state provided post-primary public – and free – schools for boys only, whilst leaving girls' post-primary education to religious and private educational institutes that only rich families could afford. Above all, the school system permitted many exceptions in school attendance for teenagers, especially for girls, whom parents often took out of school before the legal school-leaving age.[8]

Finally, what was the impact of these different discourses and policies on actual parental investment in education? We will only give here the final results of an analysis developed elsewhere.[9] Through a multivariate analysis of children's educational careers, we were able to demonstrate the importance of the religious and political context for the level of parental investment in education according to the sex of the child. Using a logistic regression, we first measured the factors that modify a child's chance of attending post-primary school or

8 In the canton of Vaud, according to the cantonal school laws of 1865 and 1889, the legal school-leaving age for girls and boys was 16. In Fribourg, the cantonal school law of 1884 stipulated the same school-leaving age, but when parents wanted to take a child out of school one year earlier, a special request had to be made for boys only.

9 Praz, 2003 and 2006.

not, which signified important monetary costs for the parents. The variable *sex male* multiplies this chance 'only' by 2.45 in the Protestant canton of Vaud, compared to 4.75 in the Catholic canton of Fribourg (see table 1). Second, we constituted a file of time sequences of children's educational careers between the ages of thirteen and eighteen. Using a Cox-regression, we then measured the impact of the same factors on the risk of leaving school. The time spent at school indicates the opportunity costs parents incurred, because the longer the child attends school, the later he or she contributes to the family budget. The same result emerges: for Catholic boys, the risk of leaving school earlier is reduced by 62 percent, compared to Catholic girls; for Protestant children, the relative risk difference between girls and boys goes down to 16 percent (see table 2).

Table 1. The Relative Risk of Attending Post-primary School for the Children of Broc and Delley-Portalban (Fribourg), Chavornay and Chevroux (Vaud)

Variables	All children N = 2353 Prob > chi2 = 0		Catholic children N = 1193 Prob > chi2 = 0		Protestant children N = 1160 Prob > chi2 = 0	
	Relative risk	P > |z|	Relative risk	P > |z|	Relative risk	P > |z|
Sex male	**3.29**	0.00	**4.75**	0.00	**2.45**	0.00
(reference: female)	*1.00*	*ref.*	*1.00*	*ref.*	*1.00*	*ref.*
Religion Catholic	0.76	0.01				
(reference: Protestant)	*1.00*	*ref.*				
Father's occupation						
(ref. farmer – land owner)	*1.00*	*ref.*	*1.00*	*ref.*	*1.00*	*ref.*
day-labourer, unskilled worker	1.17	0.33	**1.47**	0.06	0.84	0.51
factory worker	**1.95**	0.00	**2.37**	0.00	1.43	0.24
Trade-craftsman, civil servant	**2.80**	0.00	**2.75**	0.00	**2.82**	0.00
skilled occupation	**12.30**	0.00	**20.68**	0.00	**7.95**	0.00
occupation unknown	1.51	0.20	0.50	0.52	1.72	0.12
Birth order						
eldest of 4 children or more	0.77	0.06	0.76	0.17	0.78	0.17
Death of either parent	1.08	0.55	1.21	0.37	1.01	0.95

Note: bold printed rates are significant at minimum 90%.

Table 2. The Relative Risk of Leaving School Earlier for the Children of Broc and Delley-Portalban (Fribourg), Chavornay and Chevroux (Vaud)

Variables	All children N = 6940 Prob > chi2 = 0		Catholic children N = 3156 Prob > chi2 = 0.01		Protestant children N = 3784 Prob > chi2 = 0	
	Relative risk	P > |z|	Relative risk	P > |z|	Relative risk	P > |z|
Sex male	**0.51**	0.00	**0.38**	0.00	**0.84**	0.01
(reference: female)	*1.00*	*ref.*	*1.00*	*ref.*	*1.00*	*ref.*
Religion Catholic	1.67	0.00				
(reference: Protestant)	*1.00*	*ref.*				
Father's occupation						
(ref. farmer – land owner)	*1.00*	*ref.*	*1.00*	*ref.*	*1.00*	*ref.*
day-labourer, unskilled worker	0.93	0.27	0.89	0.13	1.02	0.87
Factory worker	0.93	0.35	0.94	0.49	0.94	0.66
trade-craftsman, civil servant	**0.84**	0.00	**0.84**	0.05	**0.81**	0.01
skilled occupation	**0.61**	0.00	**0.63**	0.05	**0.66**	0.07
occupation unknown	0.92	0.58	1.15	0.66	0.89	0.46
Birth order						
eldest of 4 children or more	1.10	0.07	1.12	0.11	1.04	0.61
Death of either parent	1.02	0.68	1.02	0.83	1.01	0.85

Note: bold printed rates are significant at minimum 90%.

These two regressions show that Protestant parents incurred substantial opportunity and monetary costs for the education of their children. Following the second of Coale's conditions, we may assume that the growing costs of children in Protestant families constituted an important incentive to practice birth control. Actually, the most important decline of fertility in the Protestant villages occurred in the last twenty years of the nineteenth century, the period of the implementation of compulsory schooling in the canton. In contrast, Catholic parents avoided considerable education costs, above all by discriminating against their girls. For Catholic families birth control was thus less imperative. A further analysis – not presented here – shows that the number of sons and daughters already born into the family has a significant impact on the risk of leaving school for further children, but for Catholic girls only.

This example demonstrates that the integration of gender in the model of fertility decisions allows us to provide a new explanation for the lag in Catholic fertility, generally attributed to the doctrinal norms against contraception. This latter explanation is problematic, as the implementation of Catholic sexual morality was not effective at the period under study (1860–1930).[10] The situation is however very different from the late 1920s onwards, the period studied by Marloes Schoonheim (2005), who rightly points to the influence of Catholic pastoral care on the late fertility decline in the Netherlands. Catholic norms regarding reproduction were strongly implemented among Catholic women, not only through discourse but also through intrusive controls and dissuasive punishments.

Beside the above explanatory mechanism based on the costs of children's education, we would like to point out that there are other ways to integrate gender in explanations referring to education, as some studies in this book testify to. A classical procedure is to use the mother's educational attainment as an explanatory variable. A higher level of women's education is generally correlated with lower fertility. Angélique Janssens (see elsewhere in this volume) reminds us of the various interpretations given for this relationship. Astonishingly, in her own study she met with the opposite outcome: more educated women had higher fertility, a result very significant in the Dutch Catholic town of Tilburg. Our research in the Catholic setting of Fribourg suggests the following interpretation: the fact that most girls attended church-run Catholic schools may have placed severe limits on the impact of education in shaping modern values and aspirations.[11] The group of higher educated women in her sample includes a considerable proportion of teachers, a group quite specifically supposed to transmit Catholic norms and values, a task for which their education will have given them an ideologically charged preparation. In Alison Mackinnon's research on South

10 Indeed around 1900, the Catholic Church preferred not to recall the faithful to the proper paths of sexual morality in order to avoid conflicts that might initiate or accelerate the secularisation process (Sevegrand ,1995; Servais, 2001). In Fribourg, the Catholic Church expressed no clear warning against contraception before the late 1920s.

11 This observation is also made by Danielle Gauvreau and Peter Gossage, in their study on the fertility transition in Québec (Gauvreau and Gossage, 2001: 169).

Australia (a Protestant setting), the results match the usual interpretation, with a slight modification: rather than the woman's level of education, it is her total years in school attendance that happens to have a significant impact on the number of children she ultimately had. As a last example, the study of Spanish fertility decline by Paul Baizàn and Enriqueta Camps introduces an interesting factor in the multivariate analysis of fertility: not only the mother's educational achievement, but also the level of education attained by her own mother, and to a lesser extent also by her father, modifies the fertility outcome.

Re-interpreting Coale's Conditions: The Moral Acceptance of Birth Control

Our second hypothesis concerns Coale's condition of the moral acceptability of birth control, which we assume to have been shaped (to a large extent) by state policies. In supporting or combating traditional religious institutions, according to their political stance, state institutions and policies either enforced traditional norms on sexuality or strove to establish new rules. This process was shaped by gender, resulting in differing rights for husbands and wives regarding sexual behaviour and access to contraception and in unequal bargaining power in fertility decisions. This specific gender bias clearly differs according to a community's 'cultural software' and to its institutional setting.

Recent studies emphasize that the existence of a public debate on birth control sped up the diffusion of contraceptive practices by diminishing the weight of taboos relative to sexuality and, consequently, the moral costs of contraception (Caldwell, 1999; Szreter, 1996: 410–411). At the beginning of the twentieth century, the neo-Malthusian movement was very active in the French-speaking parts of Switzerland through conferences advocating birth-control, through the publication of books, periodicals and brochures providing contraceptive advice, and through advertisements for contraceptive devices in the mainstream press.

In Fribourg, a severe repression ensured that silence was maintained on sexual issues. For the conservative government, this repression was primarily motivated by political and electoral goals. The authorities fought neo-Malthusianism, as this ideology was thought to weaken the credibility and influence of the Catholic Church, their best ally. This policy reinforced the Catholic pastoral strategy of keeping the topic of sexuality under wraps. This strategy of silence was not at all intended by the government to influence fertility patterns, yet the implicit effects were clear. Due to state support of the Catholic Church, the traditional Catholic family morality went unchallenged. Pastoral care, as our examination of the Swiss Catholic literature of the period demonstrates, glorified families with numerous children (Praz, 2003 and 2005). The oral testimonies we collected attest to the fact that mothers of large families were congratulated by the priests who promised them heavenly rewards. The religious discourse promoted a fatalist conception of family size. In sermons, pastoral bishop's letters and edifying brochures, parents were invited to accept 'with pleasure and gratitude all the children that God might well give them' and to trust in Providence for providing the necessary means to bring them up.

This fatalism weighed heavily on women, if we take into account the concept of 'marital debt', namely the obligation of the spouses not to deny sexual gratification to their partner. As Isabel Hull put forward, this may have been one of the few elements of Catholic theology promoting coital frequency (Hull, 1996: 12; McQuillan, 2004: 29). However, Hull is not right in asserting that this obligation was surprisingly egalitarian in insisting that the debt was to be honoured by both husbands and wives. In his careful analysis of theological discourse, Flandrin underlines that norms of femininity made it impossible for a woman to express her sexual desire (Flandrin, 1981: 128–129). Consequently, to honour the marital debt, the husband had the delicate 'duty' to guess his wife's desire and 'must' take the initiative in sexual matters. Such a husband's 'duty' must have been a great burden for men in Fribourg as girls' education, according to educational periodicals, gave the highest priority to moral behaviour, stressing obedience, innocence and purity. Sexual taboos were thus particularly severe for women and our female witnesses stressed their total ignorance of sexual matters before marriage, an element that weakened their bargaining power in fertility decisions.

This analysis of qualitative material shows that the Catholic 'cultural software of fertility' in the canton of Fribourg supported the husband's right to marital sexuality and frequent sexual intercourse, thus sustaining high levels of fertility. This right was not tempered by any other element able to modify the norms of masculinity and fatherhood, for example the emphasis on the father's responsibility for the wellbeing of his family members. Fatherhood was more associated with male authority and the obedience of children and wives. These features are important, as recent research demonstrates that the husband's cooperation was crucial in the first fertility decline. In supporting Catholic doctrine through educational structures and through the repression of alternative ideologies, state policies reinforced the traditional inequality between husband and wife in sexual matters.

In the Protestant canton of Vaud, the state institutions did not follow this strategy of silence. As attested by official correspondence, the dominant political elite (Radical-democratic Party) considered neo-Malthusianism morally shocking and socially dangerous, but feared that the repression would be exploited by the socialist opposition to argue that the Radical-democratic Party was no longer the champion of democratic values. As a result of this political tolerance, an animated debate spread through the mainstream press and through religious, medical and philanthropic periodicals.

Analysis of the public debate about contraception between 1900 and 1918 in the canton of Vaud shows a redefinition of morality making clear segregations on the basis of sex and social class. While the criterion of social class remained controversial depending on the political ideology of the protagonists, the criterion of sex rallied a wide consensus. Access to and use of contraceptive means were considered unthinkable for women of all social classes, yet only problematic for certain categories of men (bachelors, workers), this latter delineation being a matter of controversy. Some examples may illustrate this process.

The public debate revealed divergences between Protestant ministers, some strongly opposed to neo-Malthusianism, others recognising the social necessity of birth control and stressing the importance of parental responsibility for the wellbeing and the education of children, a traditional feature of Protestant doctrine (Perrenoud, 1974). However, all progressive ministers shared the same conviction that this control must remain the husband's responsibility in order to preserve the wife's dignity and innocence.

> That a doctor should advise men on the methods that concern them is acceptable. But what woman would not be disgusted by these methods [...] Will the modesty of a real woman, a young married woman for example, accommodate procedures such as these? Will she not feel that it diminishes love, to lose her self-respect, her dignity as a spouse and a mother, to lower herself to such practices?[12]

Political authorities similarly strove to keep women ignorant in matters concerning sexuality and contraception. In an official report to the cantonal authorities, the President of the Council of Lausanne (the capital) expressed concerns about the presence of women in neo-Malthusian lectures, fearing that such information could pose a threat to the necessary containment of women's sexuality in marriage and therefore to the social order at large. One of these lectures was considered particularly worrying, because it was given by a woman leader of the French neo-Malthusian movement, who dealt with the subordination of women in marriage.

> In pleading the cause of the subordinate situation which married women find themselves in, Miss Roussel at the same time instructs unmarried women how to maintain intimate relations with men *which nothing obliges them to do*, and to free themselves from the natural consequences of their acts, which is an indirect way of prompting young people into debauchery.[13]

The political elites were not only afraid of women gaining access to knowledge about birth control, but they were also reluctant to spread this information to the lower classes, whose presumed lack of morality could thus be enhanced, threatening the health and morality of the whole community. Challenging this discourse, socialist newspapers campaigned for access to contraceptives for the working classes, not without implying that husbands should be in charge of birth control. The rhetoric of these articles explicitly addressed a masculine reader. Emphasis was given to the father's responsibility for the wellbeing of his children and wife, while the latter was described more as a passive victim than an active partner in fertility decisions.

12 *L'Essor*, 15 October 1905 and 12 January 1907. Original text: 'Que le médecin conseille aux hommes le moyen qui les concerne, passe encore. Mais quelle est la femme qui ne soit pas prise de dégoût devant ces moyens [...] Est-ce que la pudeur d'une femme vraiment femme, d'une jeune mariée par exemple, s'accommodera de pareils procédés? Ne sentira-t-elle pas que c'est abaisser l'amour, perdre le respect d'elle-même, sa dignité d'épouse et de mère, que de s'abaisser à de telles pratiques?'

13 Archive of the canton of Vaud, CV, K VIII b, 10 January 1907, Report written by Mr Van Muyden, the president of the Council of Lausanne, to the cantonal authorities. Original text: 'En plaidant la cause de la situation subordonnée où se trouve la femme mariée, Mlle Roussel instruit du même coup les femmes non mariées des moyens d'entretenir avec les hommes des rapports intimes *auxquels rien ne les y oblige*, et de s'affranchir des conséquences naturelles de leurs actes, ce qui est une façon indirecte d'exciter la jeunesse à la débauche.' (The italics are ours. For more developments about Nelly Roussel, see Accampo, 2003).

> Do not make any more children than your terrible state of galley-slave will allow you to feed. Do you not see that your wife is worn out and depressed by the suffering and fatigue brought on by an uninterrupted and endless series of pregnancies and breastfeeding. […] come over to neo-Malthusianism which will teach you to respect your companion, to love your household which science will teach you to people according to your means […].[14]

When Margarete Faas-Hardegger (1882–1963), the first female secretary engaged by the Swiss Federation of Trade Unions, suggested to organise informative meetings about contraception for working women, she was met with absolute refusal by the direction of the Federation. In speaking and writing about sexual issues and in advocating contraceptive rights for women, Margarete Faas-Hardegger was a rare exception. Most feminists and most women engaged in philanthropic associations either kept silent about the topic, according to the dominant norms of respectable femininity, or shared the opinion that contraceptive means were totally unsuitable for women, injuring their sensibility and threatening their dignity.

> Where does this insurmountable aversion to preventive practices experienced by so many women come from […] even those who would have need of them? […] These chaste hearts associate something inexpressible and sacred with the simultaneous and total giving of love by which two beings and two lives merge in an unreserved abandon for a higher end. To intervene in this supreme and mysterious accord, to denature that impulse, to trouble it with a conflict of contradictory interests is a profanation to their sense of intimacy.[15]

A wide consensus in this public debate about neo-Malthusianism denied women the rights to sexual and contraceptive information and thus reinforced the legitimacy of the husband's unilateral actions in these matters. However, men's rights were not unlimited. The husband had to restrict his sexual pleasure

14 *La Voix du Peuple*, No 15, 1908. Original text: 'Ne fais pas plus d'enfants que ta terrible condition de galérien ne te permet d'en nourrir. Ne vois-tu pas que ta femme se consume et se déprime dans les souffrances et les fatigues d'une suite ininterrompue de gestations et d'allaitements sans fin. […] viens au néo-malthusianisme qui t'apprendra à respecter ta compagne, à aimer ton foyer que la science t'apprendra à peupler selon tes moyens […].'

15 Emma Pieczynska, *Revue de morale sociale*, 1901. Original text: 'D'où vient l'insurmontable aversion qu'éprouvent contre les pratiques préventives tant de femmes […] même celles qui en auraient besoin? […] Quelque chose d'ineffable et de sacré s'associe pour ces coeurs chastes au don d'amour total et simultané par lequel deux êtres et deux vies se confondent dans un abandon sans réserve à des fins supérieures. Intervenir dans ce suprême et mystérieux accord, dénaturer cet élan, le troubler par un conflit d'intérêts contradictoires, c'est, à leur sens intime, une profanation.'

and practice birth control, with respect to his paternal responsibilities. These entailed the wellbeing of his children and their chances of social advancement, as well as the health of his wife, a topic particularly prominent in feminist, philanthropic and medical discourses. The argument of health, a concern that rallied a large agreement, authorized not only the mention of sexual issues in a decent and respectable way, but also allowed 'bourgeois' feminists to express an astonishingly vehement denunciation of the 'sexual exploitation of women in marriage'.[16] Moderation of masculine sexual desire appeared therefore as a public health necessity.

As in Fribourg, state policies in the canton of Vaud were important in defining the rights of women and men regarding fertility decisions: both media policies, with its emphasis on freedom of speech, and health policies, stressing the importance of information about sexual matters in order to avoid the spread of venereal diseases, had implicit effects on fertility.[17] They diminished the weight of taboos relating to sexuality and, consequently, the moral costs of contraception. They also contributed to changing norms of masculinity by challenging the husband's unlimited prerogatives in marital sexuality. Thus, the motivation of wives and husbands to use birth control gradually became more convergent.

Trying to Capture Gender

Recent research shows the importance of changing norms of masculinity and femininity, and of the social roles and power relations they involved, for the explanation of the pace of fertility decline (Fisher, 2000; Fisher and Szreter,

16 '[...] une indignation grandissante sur les prérogatives que s'arroge la sensualité masculine sur la liberté, la santé et toute la destinée de la femme. Le rôle d'instrument de plaisir auquel tout leur sexe est réduit commence à se révéler aux femmes sous son vrai caractère, odieux quel que soit son déguisement [...] le devoir conjugal, tel que l'interprète encore l'opinion courante, octroie à l'époux sur sa compagne un droit de propriétaire.' Emma Pieczynska, *Revue de morale sociale*, 1901.

17 In Fribourg, even while facing a significant increase in the incidence of venereal diseases at the end of the First World War, the authorities renounced to organize informative meetings, fearing the public evocation of such a topic.

2003). These studies highlight the increasing interest of qualitative sources for demographers. Such material is considered particularly apt to capture these gender norms, as many contributions in this volume also attest to. Based on a corpus of 500 letters sent to a Swedish organisation working for sexual enlightenment, Sofia Kling's study shows how the individual experiences of childbearing and the changing norms of motherhood and fatherhood according to social class modify the perception of the ideal family size. British working-class autobiographies are used by Jane Humphries to explore the economic roles of husbands, wives and children, and their implication for family dynamics and the gendered motivation for birth control. Ida Blom investigates a variety of women's journals to capture women's – and sometime men's – views about a range of topics related to fertility and gender roles.

While qualitative sources like publications, official reports and correspondence provide interesting insights in the gender norms diffused by the elites, personal testimonies (letters, autobiographies, oral history) give important clues to what extent these norms were shared by individual men and women of different social categories. However, the simple existence of certain norms in various discourses and testimonies is not a demonstration of their impact on fertility. The challenge consists in identifying the mechanism translating these norms into effective constraints shaping reproductive decisions, and we showed the crucial role of institutions in this process. They modify the rights and duties of individuals, formally as in the case of school legislation, or informally as in the case of implicit contracts between family members. After identifying the mechanism, the last step consists of testing this mechanism on demographic results using adequate indicators of gender.[18]

What indicator might be suitable? As gender is not simply an attribute of individuals but a social categorisation, the introduction of a variable *sex* in a statistical analysis is not sufficient when this variable is not associated with an appropriate social variable. It is only this association that permits us to capture gender. In the attempt to overcome the biological in order to capture

18 This procedure can also help us to formulate and test hypotheses about the impact of norms on reproductive behaviour, even when we lack written or oral testimonies to document the micro-social practices and the integration of norms by individuals. Since such documents are rather rare and since the last potential witnesses will shortly be leaving us, it is all the more necessary to imagine research methods using the historical material still available.

the social, the relation between sex and gender may be considered as similar to the difference made in demography between age and generation.[19]

To test the first hypothesis presented above, the impact of gendered costs of education on the pace of fertility decline, we combined the sex variable with religious appurtenance and with indicators of parental investment in education. To test the second hypothesis, namely the gendered rights in sexuality and the changing norms of masculinity that might favour the convergence of the motivation of couples to use birth control, we had to find indicators of the bargaining power of spouses, or indicators of the husband taking responsibility for contraception. These indicators could then be used as independent variables in a regression analysis.

To measure more accurately the impact of different variables on fertility, we turned to a method derived from event history analysis. For the 1848 married and fecund women under observation, we constituted a file of time sequences of their fertility histories, between the birth of the first child and the end of the mother's reproductive career (or in other case the death of her spouse or the out-migration of the family). The dependent variable is the length of the interval between births. As we computed not only the closed intervals between births, but also the final open interval (between the last observed birth and the end of observation), this method detects the adoption of stopping behaviour rather than the overall level of fertility. When married couples control their fertility and concentrate births in the first years of marriage, the final interval tends to lengthen, thereby increasing the mean of all intervals calculated for each mother. Therefore, the likelihood for another birth to occur is reduced; this tendency is indicated by values inferior to 1 in table 3. In contrast, mothers with higher fertility and consequently shorter intervals have a higher likelihood of giving another birth, attested by values superior to 1.[20]

19 Such methodological work would preclude the tendency, sometimes denounced, to reduce women to biological variables (essentially mother's age) and to assign economic and social variables to men only (Watkins, 1993: 559–60; Mackinnon, 1995: 223; Andro, 2003: 49, and Janssens in this volume).

20 For technical details on the event history approach to fertility: George Alter (Alter, 1988: 175 and 1998: 25–35), George Alter and Myron P. Gutmann (Alter and Gutmann, 1993: 160–163), George Alter and Michel Oris (Alter and Oris, 1999: 12–14).

Table 3. Hazard Model of the Determinants of Fertility by Religion and Period of Observation (All Villages)

Catholics	1860–1898 N = 1489 Prob > chi2 = 0		1899–1930 N = 2705 Prob > chi2 = 0	
	Relative risk	P > |z|	Relative risk	P > |z|
Mother's age at child birth *(reference: 25–29 years)*				
15–19 years	1.04	0.87	0.99	0.96
20–24 years	0.99	0.95	1.13	0.14
30–34 years	**0.75**	0.00	**0.77**	0.00
35–39 years	**0.61**	0.00	**0.55**	0.00
40 years and more	**0.17**	0.00	**0.12**	0.00
age unknown	1.05	0.83	1.55	0.13
Mother's occupation				
Factory worker	*no factory*		**0.84**	0.02
Father's occupation *(reference: farmer, land owner)*				
day-labourer, unskilled worker	**0.82**	0.02	0.90	0.18
Factory worker	0.78	0.35	**0.72**	0.00
trade-craftsman, civil servant	**0.80**	0.05	**0.78**	0.00
skilled occupation	0.85	0.56	**0.71**	0.03
ocupation unknown	0.78	0.11	*omitted*	
Bridal pregnancy	1.08	0.50	1.14	0.21
Previous child dead	**1.59**	0.00	**1.92**	0.00
Age difference between spouses *(reference: husband 5 or more years older)*				
same age or husband less than 2 years older	1.01	0.93	0.98	0.81
husband between 2 and 5 years older	**1.20**	0.05	0.95	0.55
wife older than husband	1.07	0.52	1.13	0.11
age difference unknown	**0.72**	0.06	0.73	0.27

Table 3.
(continued)

Protestants	1860–1898 N = 2210 Prob > chi2 = 0		1899–1930 N = 2017 Prob > chi2 = 0	
	Relative risk	P > |z|	Relative risk	P > |z|
Mother's age at child birth *(reference: 25–29 years)*				
15–19 years	1.34	0.14	0.93	0.77
20–24 years	1.14	0.16	**1.20**	0.06
30–34 years	**0.77**	0.00	**0.72**	0.00
35–39 years	**0.67**	0.00	**0.55**	0.00
40 years and more	**0.21**	0.00	**0.19**	0.00
age unknown	1.43	0.03	1.53	0.12
Mother's occupation				
Factory worker	*no factory*		1.09	0.49
Father's occupation *(reference: farmer, land owner)*				
day-labourer, unskilled worker	0.98	0.82	1.02	0.88
Factory worker	1.17	0.63	**0.82**	0.05
trade-craftsman, civil servant	1.06	0.44	0.92	0.31
skilled occupation	0.83	0.44	0.77	0.13
ocupation unknown	0.74	0.02	*omitted*	
Bridal pregnancy	1.15	0.11	**1.32**	0.01
Previous child dead	**2.00**	0.00	**2.21**	0.00
Age difference between spouses *(reference: husband 5 or more years older)*				
same age or husband less than 2 years older	0.88	0.23	0.94	0.57
husband between 2 and 5 years older	0.95	0.61	0.91	0.31
wife older than husband	**1.16**	0.08	1.01	0.91
age difference unknown	0.70	0.01	0.92	0.76

Note: bold printed rates are significant at minimum 90%.

Among the usual independent variables (*mother's age*, *husband's occupation* as indicator of socioeconomic category), we integrated some variables able to capture the bargaining power of the spouses. A first idea was to observe the effect on fertility of a factor often associated with marital bargaining power in the research literature, namely the *age difference between spouses*. It is assumed that the older the husband is as compared to his wife, the more significant his bargaining power will be. We might thus suppose that women with an older husband have higher fertility levels, as in these marriages wives were less able to impose their preference for a smaller family size. Moreover, such an effect should be more perceptible in the Catholic sample than in the Protestant one, where the motivations of husband and wife to use birth control were more convergent. Unfortunately, the results do not confirm this hypothesis and the values obtained are difficult to interpret (see table 3).

We were luckier with our second indicator for women's bargaining power in fertility decisions, namely their participation in the labour market. In her contribution elsewhere in this volume, Angélique Janssens reminds us of Diana Gittins' argument, suggesting that contraceptive knowledge was acquired and exchanged on shop floors and within factory walls. Our female witnesses in the Catholic villages actually reported that contacts with other women in the factory were the only way to gather some information about contraception. Janssens also put forward that the co-working of husband and wife in industry engendered the emergence of common goals and of a common language concerning family formation and the desired number of children. Another consideration is also plausible: if women's wages were indispensable for the family budget, wives could argue that an additional child would force them to leave the labour market.

A first difficulty lies in the identification of working women in the historical source material. Based on workers' lists found in the archives of the chocolate factories and women's occupational entries at marriage in the civil registers, a certain number of mothers could be identified as being factory workers. However, we lack reliable information for other types of women's waged occupations which may have had a similar impact on their bargaining power.

We may assume that Catholic and Protestant working mothers, experiencing the same working conditions – the two factories belonged to the same company and offered similar wages and social benefits – had a similar interest in birth control, given the heavy burden of numerous children on top of paid work. Interests of Catholic and Protestant husbands may differ though, if we assume that Protestant men had integrated the changing norms of masculinity as described above. Consequently, an increase in the bargaining power of women, obtained through factory work, should only make a significant difference in the Catholic environment. In the Protestant setting, as husbands were already motivated to practice birth control, the increasing bargaining power of their wives was not necessary to convince them of the need for smaller families

To test this hypothesis, we applied the same multivariate analysis of fertility separately to the Protestant and the Catholic sample. As shown in table 3, the variable *factory worker* has no significant effect on the fertility of Protestant mothers. For Catholic mothers by contrast, a significant effect emerges: for working mothers, the likelihood of giving another birth is reduced by 16 percent, compared to non-working mothers, whatever the husband's occupation (variable under control). As differences in spousal motivation remained high in the Catholic sample, only mothers who had a leverage to better impose their interest in family size were able to reduce their fertility.

The last test concerns the differing norms of masculinity in the two cultural environments. The Protestant emphasis on masculine responsibility in sexuality, contrasting with Catholic taboos allowing masculine 'irresponsibility', is in line with longstanding norms, already perceptible before the fertility transition. In the Protestant environment, following the traditional custom of engagement, premarital sexuality was tolerated, but the groom had the moral and social obligation, well enforced by family and community, to marry his bride in case of pregnancy. In the Protestant villages under study (see the example of Chavornay/VD graph 2) about half of the women were pregnant at marriage during the period 1860–1900. In the Catholic villages, by contrast, premarital sexuality was severely prohibited by pastoral care. The custom of engagement did not exist and future spouses were not socially authorized to appear overtly as a couple until three weeks before marriage, after the bans had been published. In case of premarital sexuality resulting in pregnancy, it was consequently easier for the young man to abandon the woman if he had no intention of marrying her; this situation resulted in a high level of illegitimacy in the Catholic villages (see the example of Broc/FR graph 1).

Towards the end of the nineteenth century, the proportion of prenuptial conceptions regressed in the Protestant villages, compared to post-marriage conceptions. Attributing this phenomenon to a decrease in premarital sexual-

Graph 1. Distribution of First Births According to the Child's Status by Period of Observation – Broc, Canton of Fribourg

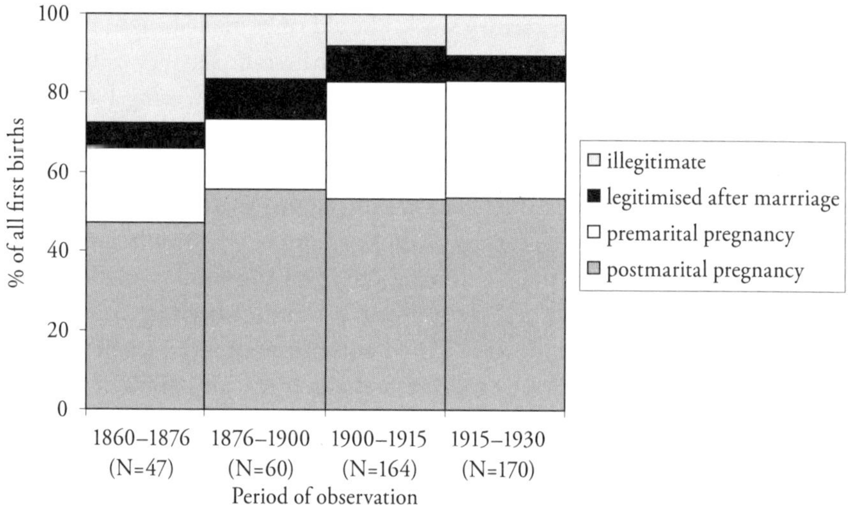

Graph 2. Distribution of First Births According to the Child's Status by Period of Observation – Chavornay, Canton of Vaud

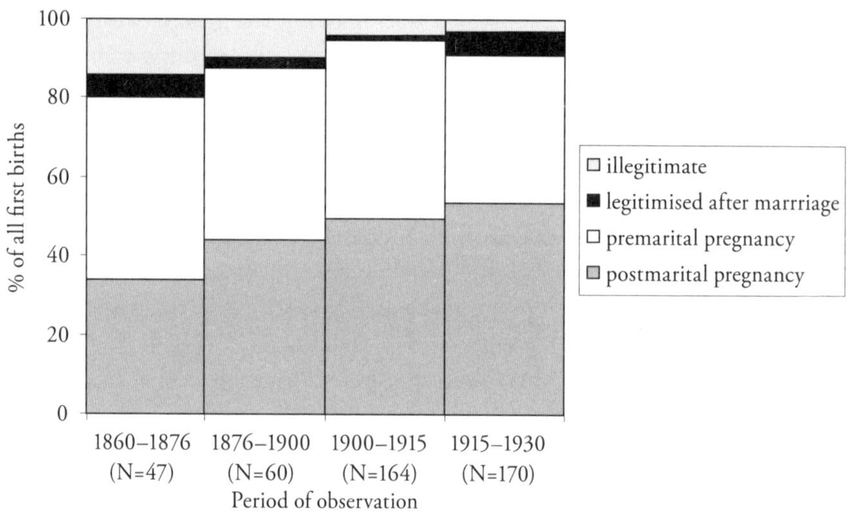

ity is less plausible than assuming a better familiarity of the young couples with contraception, especially withdrawal. In this case, the emphasis on masculine responsibility in sexual matters could have incited the grooms to practice birth control in premarital sexuality in order to achieve more autonomy for deciding about the date of marriage. We may also assume that when couples already succeeded in controlling their fertility before marriage, they were better able to control it within marriage. Consequently, for couples who did *not* experience a premarital conception – such a conception would indicate a failure of the groom's contraceptive experience or sense of responsibility – the mother will be exposed to a lower risk of giving birth. By contrast, premarital conception should be associated with higher fertility within marriage.

To test this hypothesis, we introduced a dummy variable called *bridal pregnancy*, which was set to one when the first child was conceived before marriage. However, this variable only obtained a significant result for Protestant mothers: when their first child was conceived before marriage, they had a higher likelihood of giving another birth. The result is quasi significant for the first period, more pronounced and very significant in the second, indicating a better familiarity with contraception, and/or a growing intention to reduce fertility (see table 3). The postulated correlation between premarital and marital control of fertility is thus attested.

What happened in the Catholic villages? The regression analysis does not indicate a relation between premarital and marital contraceptive practices for Catholic couples. Either these contraceptive techniques were not widespread, or the motivation to use them within marriage was lacking, because the incentives for adopting such behaviour were not strong and above all not pervasive enough to obtain a significant result. As the responsibility for contraception rests with men, the Catholic 'cultural software' that encourages a high coital frequency without stressing men's responsibility for the number of children can explain this result. However, it is obvious that this hypothesis is difficult to test rigorously.

Conclusion

There are good reasons for integrating gender as a causal factor into explanations of the demographic transition. The application of certain fundamental methodological requirements, such as the focus on individuals as decision-makers, and the emphasis on mechanisms through which structures on a macro-level influence 'private' decisions, makes this integration of gender unavoidable. When investigating the impact of social structures, of norms and values, and their implementation into incentives and constraints for individuals, we have to take into account the sex of these individuals – not only because of the biological characteristics of men and women already well examined in demography – but foremost because of their different and asymmetrical social positions.

By using different components of the gender system this article shows that it is necessary to reconsider the content of the three preconditions for the adoption of fertility control, as stated by Ansley Coale. On the one hand, the integration of gender implies looking at the way in which institutional practices attribute different rights and duties to women and men, resulting in unequal opportunities and power relations. The second of Coale's conditions stipulates that reduced fertility must be perceived as advantageous, and therefore the changing costs of children have to be considered. As the interests of mothers and fathers differ, so do their respective cost-benefit balances with respect to children; moreover, the costs and benefits of daughters and sons are not identical, as our analysis of the costs of education has demonstrated.

On the other hand, the integration of gender involves looking at the cultural software, namely the gendered norms regarding sexuality and parenthood. Following the first of Coale's conditions, fertility control must be 'an acceptable mode of thought and form of behaviour'. Beside the religious norms generally used in research as an indicator of this acceptability, the gendered norms governing sexuality and procreation have to be taken into account. In the Protestant sample analysed here, the use of contraception by women was considered unacceptable whilst the discourse stressed responsible fatherhood, thereby implicitly encouraging male control of fertility. Consequently, the still little explored impact of changing norms of masculinity and fatherhood deserves more attention. Moreover, the third of Coale's conditions asks that we specify the information available about and the access to contraceptive devices. As the initiative of contraception was quite unthinkable for women, men's access to contraceptive devices and information was decisive.

I hope that my models for the integration of gender have demonstrated that this is a fruitful enterprise. The systematic data necessary to include gender in research on the fertility decline may be difficult to produce and to interpret. However, if many researchers apply this approach, progress in operationalisation and formulation of testable hypotheses could be swift. It is furthermore easily conceivable that many already established demographic data bases could provide interesting new insights when analysed by theories that integrate a gender perspective.

References

Accampo, Elinor A. (2003), 'The Gendered Nature of Contraception in France: Neo-Malthusianism, 1900–1920', *Journal of Interdisciplinary history*, 34, 235–262.

Alter, George (1988), *Family and the Female Life Course. The Women of Verviers, Belgien 1849–1880*, Madison: The University of Wisconsin Press.

Alter, George (1992), 'Theories of Fertility Decline: A Nonspecialist's Guide to the Current Debate', in Gillis, John R., Tilly, Louise A. and Levine, David (eds), *The European Experience of Declining Fertility: A Quiet Revolution 1850–1970*, Cambridge Mass. and Oxford, Blackwell, 13–27.

Alter George and Gutmann Myron P. (1993), 'Family Reconstitution as Event History Analysis', in Reher, David S. and Schofield, Roger (eds), *Old and New Methods in Historical Demography*, Oxford, Clarendon Press, 160–163.

Alter George (1998), 'L'event history analysis en démographie historique – Difficultés et perspectives', *Annales de démographie historique* (1998) 2, 5–35.

Alter, George and Oris, Michel (1999), 'Fertility, Fecundity, and Economic Stress in the Belgian Ardennes during the 19th Century', paper presented at the Social Science History Association, Fort Worth, Texas, November 12–14, 1999.

Andro, Armelle (2003), 'Saisir les rapports de genre dans l'analyse de la fécondité', in Andro, Armelle and Condon, Stéphanie (dir.), *Questions de genre en démographie,* Paris: INED, coll. Documents de travail N° 117, 48–56.

Bocquier, Philippe (1996), *L'analyse des enquêtes biographiques à l'aide du logiciel STATA,* Documents et manuels du CEPED N° 4, Paris, Centre français sur la population et le développement.

Caldwell, John (1980), 'Mass Education as a Determinant of the Timing of Fertility Decline', *Population and Development Review*, 6, 225–255.

Caldwell, John (1999), 'The Delayed Western Fertility Decline: An Examination of English-Speaking Countries', *Population and Development Review*, 25, 479–513.

Chaperon, Sylvie (2004), 'Contester normes et savoirs sur la sexualité (France-Angleterre, 1880–1980)', in Gubin, Eliane, and others, (eds), *Le Siècle des féminismes*, Paris, Les Editions de l'atelier, 333–346.

Coale, Ansley J. (1973), 'The Demographic Transition Reconsidered', in *International Population Conference*, vol. 1, Liège, International Union for Scientific Study of Population, 53–72.

Coale, Ansley J. and Watkins, Susan C. (1986), *The Decline of Fertility in Europe. The Revised Proceedings of a Conference on the Princeton European Fertility Project*, Princeton New Jersey, Princeton University Press.

Flandrin, Jean-Louis (1981), *Le sexe et l'Occident – Evolution des attitudes et des comportements*, Paris, Seuil.

Fisher, Kate (2000), '"She was quite satisfied with the arrangements I made". Gender and Birth Control in Britain (1920–1950)', *Past and Present*, 169, 160–193.

Fisher, Kate and Szreter, Simon (2003), 'They Prefer Withdrawal: The Choice of Birth Control in Britain, 1918–1950', *Journal of Interdisciplinary History*, 34, 263–291.

Folbre, Nancy (1996), 'Engendering Economics: New Perspectives on Women, Work, and Demographic Change', *Annual World Bank Conference on Development Economics 1995*, The International Bank for Reconstruction and Development / The World Bank.

Gauvreau, Danielle and Gossage, Peter (2001), 'Canadian Fertility Transitions: Quebec and Ontario at the Turn of the Twentieth Century', *Journal of Family History*, 26, 162–188.

Hull, Isabel V. (1996), *Sexuality, State and Civil Society in Germany, 1700–1815*, Ithaca N.Y, Cornell University Press.

Johansson, S. Ryan (1991), 'Implicit Policy and Fertility during Development', *Population and Development Review*, 17, 377–414.

Kertzer, D. I. (1995), 'Political-economic and Cultural Explanations of Demographic Behaviour', in Greenhalgh, S. (ed.), *Situating fertility. Anthropology and Demographic Inquiry*, Cambridge, Cambridge University Press, 29–52.

Leboutte, René (1988), *Reconversions de la main-d'œuvre et transition démographique. Les bassins industriels en aval de Liège XVII*e*–XX*e *siècles*, Paris, Les Belles Lettres.

Lesthaeghe, Ron J. L. (1980), 'On the Social Control of Human Reproduction', *Population and Development Review*, 6, 527–548.

Lesthaeghe, Ron J. L. (1995), 'La deuxième transition démographique dans les pays occidentaux: une interprétation', in *Transitions démographiques et sociétés*, Louvain-la-Neuve, Liber amicorum Etienne Hélin, Academia, 133–180.

Mackinnon, Alison (1995), 'Were Women Present at the Demographic Transition? Questions from a Feminist Historian to Historical Demographers', *Gender & History*, 7, 222–240.

McNicoll, Geoffrey, (1994), 'Institutional Analysis of Fertility', in Lindahl-Kiessling, Kerstin and Landberg, Hans (eds), *Population, Economic Development and the Environment*, New York, Oxford University Press, 29–52.

McQuillan, Kevin (2004), 'When Does Religion Influence Fertility?' *Population and Development Review*, 30, 25–56.

Perrenoud, Alfred (1974), 'Malthusianisme et Protestantisme', *Annales ESC*, 29, 975–988.

Pollack, Robert A. (1985), 'A Transaction Cost Approach to Families and Households', *Journal of Economic Literature*, 23, 581–608.

Praz, Anne-Françoise (2003), 'Politique conservatrice et retard catholique dans la baisse de la fécondité: l'exemple du canton de Fribourg en Suisse (1860–1930)', *Annales de démographie historique*, 1, 33–55.

Praz, Anne-Françoise (2005), *De l'enfant utile à l'enfant précieux – Filles et garçons dans les cantons de Vaud et Fribourg, 1860–1930*, Lausanne, Editions Antipodes.

Praz, Anne-Françoise (2006), 'Ideologies, Gender and School Policy. A Comparative Study of Two Swiss Regions (1860–1930)', *Paedagogica Historica – International Journal of History of Education*, 42/3.

Schoonheim, Marloes (2005), *Mixing Ovaries and Rosaries. Catholic Religion and Reproduction in the Netherlands, 1870–1970*, Amsterdam, Aksant.

Servais, Paul (2001), 'The Church and the Family in Belgium', *Revue belge d'histoire contemporaine*, 21, 621–647.

Sevegrand, Martine (1995), *Les enfants du bon Dieu – Les catholiques français et la procréation au XXe siècle*, Paris, Albin Michel.

Szreter, Simon (1996), *Fertility, Class and Gender in Britain, 1860–1940*, Cambridge, Cambridge University Press.

Van Bavel, Jan (2004), 'Distinguer contraception d'arrêt et contraception d'espacement – Revue des méthodes en démographie historique', *Population*, 1, 119–132.

Van de Walle, Francine (1977), *One Hundred Years of Decline – The History of Swiss Fertility from 1860 to 1960*, Philadelphia (dactyl., Bibliothèque universitaire de Neuchâtel/Suisse).

Watkins, Susan Cotts (1993), 'If All We Knew About Women Was What We Read in *Demography*, What Would We Know?', *Demography*, 30, 551–577.

Bringing Babies into Line with Mothers' Jobs: Lancashire Cotton Weavers' Fertility Regime

JUTTA SCHWARZKOPF

Debating the Fertility Decline

In Britain, stage three of the 'demographic transition', when fertility rates followed the downward trend of mortality rates, predated the same development in most other European countries (Coleman, 2000: 33). That stage has been identified variously as having occurred between ca. 1850 and 1930 (Teitelbaum, 1984: 5), or 1860–1940 (Szreter, 1996); it has been described as 'getting under way' in the late 1870s (Seccombe, 1990: 152), or its onset has been dated precisely to 1876–77 (Levine, 1985: 191) when the crude birth rate reached a peak value. More recently, Simon Szreter and Eilidh Garrett (2000) have argued for 1816 as the onset of fertility decline as a result of their moving away from aggregate data in favour of evaluating the diverse demographic responses to economic change by different social groups and communities. Historical demographers used to concur that the decline in fertility, attributed to 'the direct application of family limitation methods' (Woods, 1987: 283), was pioneered in the middle class and subsequently diffused, though with a considerable time-lag, to the working class (J. A. Banks, 1954; J. A. & O. Banks, 1964; J. A. Banks, 1981; Gittins, 1982: 33; Teitelbaum, 1984: 5, 222). This consensus was largely based on an explanation first proposed in the British *Fertility of Marriage Report*, in which the General Register Office had analyzed the data on fertility in the census of 1911. A five-layer classification of occupations was devised to demonstrate how marital fertility declined first in the upper reaches of society, before slowly 'trickling down' to the lower classes.

First doubts were cast on this picture of uniform working-class laggardness with regard to limiting family size as early as 1938 by John Innes, whose analysis of class fertility trends demonstrated the conspicuous smallness of nineteenth-century textile workers' families, and those of Lancashire in particular. He found his class VI (textile workers) consistently less fertile than his class III (skilled workers) by over seven percent (Innes, 1938: 45). In 1986, David Levine also noted the differential rates in the decline of fertility among various groups of British workers. According to him, the fall had occurred much faster in families headed by a textile worker, a skilled worker or a semi-skilled worker than among the labouring poor (Levine, 1985: 107). Yet it was not until 1996 when Simon Szreter's study of the fertility decline in Britain appeared that the diffusionist consensus was shattered. Combining highly sophisticated methods of statistical analysis with careful assessment of the broader social and economic conditions which had a bearing on particular groups of the population, Szreter has effectively demolished the conventional image of the fertility decline as a national, socially graded, unitary process of diffusion. Instead of presenting just one fertility decline, he has broken it up into several, each the result of the intricate interplay between family-building strategies, gender and labour relations, and broader cultural and economic changes. Dismissive of any variant of modernization theory, his conclusion has been unequivocal: '... no single factor or national set of factors can explain "the" fertility decline' (Szreter, 1996: 595).

By focusing upon a particular group of workers this article builds upon and expands Szreter's argument. Not only will it become apparent that the cotton weavers of Lancashire were among the British working-class pioneers in limiting the size of their families (e.g. Coleman, 2000: 33), but by training the spotlight upon one particular group of workers and the fertility regime they evolved it also becomes possible to investigate in detail the interplay of those forces which, according to Szreter, shaped the reproductive behaviour of distinct sections of the population. The fertility regime fashioned by the Lancashire cotton weavers will be traced back to the organization of the labour process in their industry, which was characterized by an unusual degree of gender equality, leading to gender divisions in realms other than the sphere of production becoming blurred as well. Their self-perception of skilled workers whose paid employment made a vital contribution to family income gave women weavers the leverage to negotiate a more equitable gender division of power in the family. In practical terms, this translated into some degree of gender division of domestic labour as well as the limitation of family size as a result of joint decision making by husband and wife. These practices were embedded in notions of masculinity and femininity which bore little, if any, resemblance to the gender concepts current in working-class communities elsewhere. In the cotton-weaving districts of Lancashire, masculinity did not revolve around the ability to provide for one's family without recourse to any secondary income, nor was femininity centred on domesticity, the ideal widespread, though rarely attained, in the harsh realities of working-class living conditions.

Beginning with a brief statement of the way fertility rates developed in the cotton districts of Lancashire, this article will then sketch the way cotton processing mechanized. After investigating the skill content of weaving, women weavers' self-perception as skilled workers, and their attitudes to paid employment, weavers will be related to Szreter's ideal type one of couples limiting the size of their families. By way of conclusion, a brief glance will be cast at three women taking the cotton weavers' fertility regime beyond limiting family size to actually stopping to reproduce once the number of children considered ideal has been attained. Throughout, female agency will emerge as a vital, though not the only, influence on Lancashire weavers' fertility regime.

Fertility Rates in the Cotton District of Lancashire

From the early days of industrialization, pioneered in Britain by the mechanization of cotton-processing, contemporary observers suspected that the large-scale employment of women away from home must have repercussions on the size of their families. Thus in 1832, one Dr. James Blundell stated before a parliamentary committee that '... where individuals are congregated in factories, I conceive that means preventive of impregnation are more likely to be generally known and practiced by young persons ...' (quoted in McLaren, 1977: 70). With its implication of novel, and possibly undesirable, influences coming to bear on young people torn from the sheltered environment of their parental homes, this statement clearly formed part of the heated contemporary debate about the social effects produced by the relocation of production in factories in the course of industrialization. Blundell's rather impressionistic testimony was subsequently substantiated by quantitative studies relating to a later period when the relevant data became available. Thus John Innes produced the following table showing the completed fertility of wives in the census class of textile workers:

Date of Marriage	Fertility per 100 wives in textiles
1851–1861	654
1861–1871	633
1871–1881	567
1881–1886	513

Until the period 1881–1886, as Innes demonstrated, the number of children born to each hundred wives of textile families, i.e. their completed fertility, was lower than the rate for every other class except that of the skilled professionals and businessmen, and was declining (Innes, 1938: 45). More specifically, Ethel Elderton investigated the possible relation between industrial conditions and the development of fertility by registration district. She was able to show that, in Lancashire, the fall in the birthrate was greatest in districts engaged in textile industries, such as Blackburn, Haslingden, Burnley, all of which were typical weaving towns, and Oldham, the spinning capital of the world prior to 1914. Yet she also noted some degree of variation, pointing out that the near halving of the birthrate by the beginning of the twentieth century as compared to the period 1851 to 1876 was confined to 14 out of 28 districts (Elderton, 1914: 22–23). In Stockport, for instance, fertility had begun to fall significantly, though less dramatically, only in the 1880s so that, by 1911, it was ca. three-fourths of what it had been in 1861 (Lichfield, 1978).

On the basis of the Registrar General's Reports for 1901 to 1910, Elizabeth Roberts (1986: 101) has compiled the following table indicating the number of live births per thousand married women (five-year averages) in textile towns:

Place	1901–1905	1906–1910
Blackburn	197	189
Bury	177	174
Rochdale	176	169
Bolton	227	208
Preston	233	212
Burnley	193	185

While only detailed local research and complex computations would reveal the average number of children per woman weaver, the general trend is clear. Though starting from different levels and despite differences in degree, all the towns listed in the table saw a decline in the birth rate between 1901 and 1910.

The Mechanization of Cotton Processing

The reasons why couples in the Lancashire cotton district, and weaving couples in particular, limited the number of their children, and began to do so at a comparatively early stage, are closely linked with the way the cotton industry developed. The first process to mechanize and relocate in factories was spinning. The affinity claimed to exist between masculinity and the operation of intricate mechanical devices, in conjunction with the authority exerted over the ancillary workers required to operate the machines, gave mule-spinning the cachet of a prestigious and hence masculine job (Hall, 1982). Thus spinning, that archetypal female occupation, was turned into a predominantly male domain within a couple of generations, at least in Lancashire. As a result, mule spinners belonged to the best paid sections of the cotton workforce (Fowler & Wyke, 1987).

When, with a time-lag of a few decades, the first steam-looms became fully operative, the newly erected weaving sheds were staffed predominantly by women and children. Men, by contrast, were loath to enter workplaces where they would be subject to a work pace dictated by mechanical devices and a harsh discipline imposed by strangers. They preferred to eke out an increasingly precarious living by operating handlooms in their cottages, until, in the 1840s, their resistance, of near legendary status, largely collapsed and many of them reluctantly followed their wives and children into the factories. This separation of home and workplace marked the transition among the working class from the family economy to the family wage economy (Tilly & Scott, 1978), in which the family's level of consumption is based on the pooled income of all its members. For women this implied that the form and extent of their labour market participation were largely shaped by the number and ages of their children. Usually, wives were able to leave paid employment away from home only when children started earning (Anderson, 1971 for Preston; Foster, 1974 for Oldham; Lichfield, 1978 for Stockport).

On entering the weaving sheds in significant numbers, men pressed for non-gender-specific piece-rates in order to gain any foothold at all. In this endeavour they relied on the weaving unions, whose strength hinged crucially on all attempts at gender exclusiveness being eschewed (Turner, 1962). Because of the gendered sequence in which operatives were recruited, the labour process in Lancashire cotton weaving was marked by an unusual degree of gender equality. Especially in the cotton towns in the north east of the county, given over nearly entirely to weaving, such as Blackburn, Burnley, Nelson, men and women were working side by side producing the same types of cloth on roughly the same number of identical machines, and, most significantly, receiving the same piece-rates. These differed according to the class of goods produced and were laid down in price lists which minutely detailed the amount of money due for each exactly specified type of cloth. This is why workers' earnings varied from week to week under the impact of a number of variables, not least among which was individual level of skill (Schwarzkopf, 2004: 34–45). Significantly, gender did not count among them. As a result, it was perfectly possible for the earnings received by a particular woman at the end of a given week to be on a par with, or even to exceed, those of her husband. On the national level, non-gender-specific piece-rates placed women weavers among the top three groups of earners among female waged workers. In 1906, women over eighteen were able to attain better hourly earnings in only two industries as compared to 87 industries paying female workers less per hour than did cotton weaving. Men, by contrast, could earn more in 65 industries, as compared to 45, where pay per hour worked out less than in cotton weaving (Jewkes & Gray, 1935: 15). In other words, men weavers worked for a woman's wage.

Thus the family employment pattern which had evolved in the period of industrialization persisted, because no weaving family was able to subsist on the earnings of one adult alone. Factory work by women, including wives and mothers, was widespread. By 1890, there were 123,854 (ca. 62 percent) females employed in weaving as compared to 75,910 (ca. 38 percent) males (Royal Commission on Labour, 1892: 18). By 1907, the figures had risen to 218,521 (ca. 67.6 percent) females as compared to 104,696 (ca. 32.4 percent) males (Summary of Returns, 1909: 854). In 1894, 32.9 percent of the women over eighteen years of age who were employed in the cotton mills of Lancashire and Cheshire were either married or widowed (Statistics of

Employment of Women, 1894: 883). Although that proportion had fallen to 28.6 percent by 1907 (Summary of Returns, 1909: 858), it was still far in excess of the national mean of married women occupied, which had been 5.3 percent in 1901 (Savage, 1982: 10). Many of the married women employed in cotton weaving must be assumed to have been mothers of small children. This assumption cannot be quantified.

Clara Collet, the renowned political economist, who subjected the available statistics on the employment of women to close analysis in order to identify the factors accounting for the high proportion of married women employed in the cotton industry, used the category 'married women in employment' as proxy for 'mothers in employment' (Board of Trade, 1894). The need to do so is caused by the way in which data were collected and analyzed in the relevant period. Census data relating to women were classified according to age-group and marital status. In order to establish the percentage of married women weavers with children under the age of ten, one would need to refer to census enumerators' books, which record occupation, marital status as well as number and age of children per household. On the basis of this information, however, it is impossible to establish whether all women who returned themselves as weavers were actually in employment or had temporarily left their jobs with the intention of returning to them at some later stage. Detailed information of this kind is available only from local studies, which have so far been confined to the middle decades of the nineteenth century, yielding the following figures: in Blackburn, Ashton, Oldham, Burnley, Chorley, Haslingden and Preston, the proportion of married women operatives (not all of them necessarily weavers) with children under one year of age ranged in 1851 from 14.95 percent to 27.45 percent, the average being 21.03 percent (Hewitt, 1953: 136–137). In Preston more specifically, 23 percent of all wives with children worked, and 20 percent of all wives with children under the age of 10 worked away from home in 1851 (Anderson, 1971: 71). In Oldham, finally, over one-third of local women with children aged eleven or under went out to work around mid-century (Foster, 1974: 97).

The percentage of married or widowed female cotton operatives was clearly related to the preponderance of weaving in the local economy, being highest in the weaving centres of Burnley and Blackburn, much lower in the spinning towns, very low indeed in Wigan, where the labour market was fairly neatly divided between male coal-mining and female cotton processing, and virtually non-existent in the spinning town of Stockport. The majority of females took up work in the mill in their early teens, as half-timers, and many continued in employment after marriage. For them, weaving was more than just a transitory stage between leaving school and getting married.

Women Weavers' Self-perception

While the economic need for married women's paid employment persisted well beyond the period of industrialization, women's attitude to their jobs changed markedly over time. Had it been economically viable in the early period, female factory workers, especially mothers, would have much preferred abandoning paid employment away from home, their abhorrence of which they never tired of proclaiming (Schwarzkopf, 1991: ch. 4). Over time, however, employment in the weaving sheds turned into a way of life that virtually every working-class girl in the cotton districts was socialized into, not least in order to fulfil her parents' expectation of a boost to family income. Over and above meeting the financial needs of, first, their family of origin, and, subsequently, their own, paid employment became a source of pride and self-confidence for many of these women, having repercussions well beyond the immediate workplace.

From the abundance of ego-documents, both written and oral, available for cotton operatives, it is possible to piece together the requirements of the labour process in weaving, women weavers' attitudes to their paid employment as well as the strategies they employed to reconcile the exigencies of paid work in the mill with their unpaid domestic duties in the family.

The need for females to carry on in paid employment for the best part of their lives was generally acknowledged by the cotton community. Implanting in their daughters' minds the wish to become a weaver was an important objective working-class parents in the cotton district aimed at in the upbringing of their female offspring. Parental expectations were reinforced by community norms and practices, deviations from which were not condoned (Mrs. T.T. Tape 688, MSU TLSL). Practical preparation for factory work, rather than any encouragement to look forward to a life of domesticity, was part and parcel of girls' upbringing. For all children preparation for the job began in the family. Older family members would deliberately prepare younger ones for their entry in the factory, for instance by demonstrating particularly frequent and complicated processes (Roberts, 1981, respondents A1P, 7; H7P, 2). By the time youngsters entered the mill, they would already be familiar with most aspects of the labour process.

A high level of skill was necessary to deal with both the material and the machinery weavers encountered on the shopfloor. As a natural product, which is subject to nearly infinite variation, cotton requires a high degree of experience-based knowledge and ability to be processed. What is more, the many variables having an impact on cotton processing render it impossible clearly to specify each stage of the procedure. These variables relate to the widely varying character of the yarn, which in turn depends on the quality of the raw cotton used in spinning (Harig & Heap, 1994).

Apart from the yarn supplied, the machines, too, had their peculiarities, not least because Victorian machines were tailor-made rather than mass produced (Savage, 1982: 17–18). Looms were neither very sophisticated nor working at optimum efficiency. Hence it was up to the weaver to obtain the best possible results from a deficient machine by constantly readjusting it to the job in hand. Moreover, the demands made on cloth quality increased at the same time that machinery was speeded up (Ellison, 1968: 37).

The necessary weaving skills were acquired in the course of training on the job, with the learner helping, or tenting for, an experienced weaver in return for a time wage. With promotion to a set of looms of one's own began a new stage in the aspiring weaver's career, the corresponding rise in wages marking the passage to adulthood. Over time, and with experience gained, the number of looms allocated to an individual weaver increased, until after about six to seven years, four looms were mastered (Savage, 1982: 18). This included adjusting the machines to the job in hand, maintaining them in good working order as well as carrying out minor repairs. There was a strong incentive for doing so oneself rather than relying on the overlooker, because this helped reduce pay cuts through keeping machine down time low.

In weaving, the technical difficulties and hence the demands made on workers' skill increased from the production of plain, coarse cloths through fine cloths to those with complicated patterns and mixed warps. It is significant that those places specializing in the production of high-quality goods, such as Preston, Bolton, and Chorley, also had the largest proportion of females among their weaving workforce (Schwarzkopf, 2004: 29–34). None of this went unnoticed by the women concerned. Female weavers uniformly considered themselves to be performing a skilled trade that took considerable time to master (Roberts, 1981, respondents H7P, 33; T4P, 5; B1P, 7; Mrs. M.H. Tape 640, MSU TLSL). Competent weavers derived pleasure from doing their job, and doing it well (Mrs. M.H. Tape 640, MSU TLSL; Roberts, 1981, respondent B1P, 7).

The disconcertingly large number of female suicides demonstrates that failing to meet community expectations those young women saw no option but to end their lives, frequently by drowning themselves in the mill-pond. As the detailed press reports about the coroner's inquests into the young women's deaths revealed, their suicides had been caused by their failure to meet expectations. At work, overlookers drove them to increase output, while at home, parents were waiting for a larger contribution to family income. Historically, these suicides coincided with the Lancashire textile industry beginning to feel the effects of foreign competition in the closing decades of the nineteenth century. Weaving manufacturers responded with cost-cutting by means of supplying low-quality yarn, which caused a larger number of breakages when woven. Weavers were driven both by their overlookers, in order to maintain the quantity and quality of output per operative, despite the supply of inferior yarn and the continual speeding-up of looms, and by themselves, to maintain their level of pay. Within the life-course of the young women concerned, their suicides occurred at precisely that stage when they would be expected to master their first complement of looms. Failure to do so was partly the result of their period of training on the job having been curtailed by the introduction of compulsory schooling from 1880 onwards (Schwarzkopf, 2004: 85–93).

These cases demonstrate that competent tending of machines and the ability to produce faultless cloth as the prerequisites of a desired level of pay were apparently part of female weavers' identity in a way similar to that described for skill in the case of men. Precisely because women weavers' identity revolved largely around their jobs, failure to achieve such a level of competence undermined these women's self-confidence and self-esteem. Given the constraints of local labour markets, they lacked the opportunity of establishing themselves in an occupation as skilled and well paid as weaving so that some of them saw no alternative to committing suicide. Failure to become an expert weaver brought in its wake severe losses not only in financial terms, but also in terms of personal development. In fact, the two were inseparable. The more a woman excelled at weaving, the better her income, the higher her reputation, and the greater her personal satisfaction.

Female Work Culture

The factory-based organization of weaving assembled large numbers of women in one place. Thus there are indications of something approaching a female work culture (Schwarzkopf, 2004: 69–72), which revolved around female solidarity inside and outside the mill. This solidarity was ambiguous in that it not only created niches of autonomy on the shopfloor, but was also deployed to enforce conformity. As in the neighbourhood, so in the factory, the proximity and overlap of neighbours and co-workers acted as an effective means of exerting social control, especially, though not exclusively, as regards sexual mores. Yet the workplace also afforded numerous opportunities for mutual support. Women would help each other cope with the dual responsibility of caring for a family and holding down a job. They would regularly bring their family troubles to the shopfloor, seeking each other's advice.

On a lighter note, colleagues would hold parties to celebrate Christmas or birthdays. Weddings were accorded special relevance, marking as they did a status passage in the female life-cycle. These events showed women's ability to force management to back off from any interference in their celebrations of what they considered high points in a woman's life (Westwood, 1984: 89–90, 101). Furthermore, these occasions bear witness to women weavers' ability to reclaim work time and factory space for uses of their own, frustrating any attempt on the employers' part fully to regiment their workforce. These informal parties testify to female weavers' ability to reappropriate space and time designed for the generation of profit to purposes of their own, which were far removed from the exigencies of production. Finally, the organization of such informal activities focusing on the female life-cycle and the manifold ways in which women 'brought their families to work' (Lamphere, 1985) acted as strong bonding devices among groups of female weavers, empowering them to resist.

Coping with the Double Burden

Like the vast majority of working-class women, female weavers, once married, had to juggle their employment away from home and their domestic duties. The amount of time and energy spent on housework, pregnancies, births, and the rearing of children crucially determine the extent to which full-time employment away from home can be reconciled with the family commitments of a wife and mother, given a gender division of labour at societal level which makes housework and childcare female responsibilities.

Women weavers' comparatively high level of earnings enabled them to delegate some domestic tasks for payment of cash, such as washing and the minding of children, including infants, whom mothers would go and breast-feed during meal-breaks if at all possible (Tape 655, MSU TLSL). In order to relieve their domestic burden, they also relied on ready-made clothes and meals (Roberts, 1982: 51–52), causing the proliferation of fish-and-chip shops in Lancashire (Roberts, 1982: 162; Walton, 1992). Paying for domestic services was motivated by more than the search for convenience. This practice was also a matter of inclination (Statistics of Employment of Women, 1894: 881; Chew, 1912: 44; Glucksmann, 1995: 281–282). Many women weavers preferred working at the mill to the endless round of domestic drudgery. Delegation of household chores for cash was subject to the variations in weavers' income and never complete. Like other working-class women, cotton weavers relied on the help of their children, but significantly also on their husbands' assistance, who differed markedly in this respect from the majority of their working-class contemporaries.

It was the size of their contribution to family income that gave women weavers the leverage to enlist their husbands' cooperation. Although varying in extent and regularity (Roberts, 1981; Gittins, 1982; Glucksmann, 1995), men's participation in housework was accepted in the local community and taken for granted by weaving wives, who believed that they not only deserved, but were actually entitled to, help from their husbands, who, after all, benefited, too, from the extra income generated by their wives' factory labour (Roberts, 1981, respondent A1P, 52–53).

Despite all variations that undoubtedly existed, among weaving couples the degree of overlap in the experience of husbands and wives was more pronounced than among other working-class couples. Due to what Diana Gittins has dubbed their 'identical relations to the occupational system' (Gittins, 1982: 130–131), actually performing identical work, these men and women knew the ins and outs of each other's jobs, which precluded both any denigration of female paid employment and the shrouding of male jobs in any kind of mystery. The similarity of their experience at work was underpinned by the negligible or non-existent difference in the amount of wages each of them brought home. Coupled with the indispensability of the wife's earnings to family income, this enabled female weavers to be sparing of services for husbands, who, in turn, were unable to enforce such services, because they could lay no claim to being chief earners (Mark-Lawson, 1987: 320; Glucksmann, 1995: 283).

Ways of Controlling Fertility

A most important way of making family needs compatible with full-time employment while also preserving women's physical wellbeing consisted in limiting the number of children. Significantly, this also involved a major shift in weavers' masculinity away from the centrality of the capacity to inseminate. Female cotton workers derived a considerable degree of personal satisfaction from their ability to carry out a skilled job over and above their awareness of making a vital contribution to family income. They also delighted in female companionship at work. Taken together, these factors accounted for women's desire to stay on at work after marriage, rendering them averse to letting the demands made by a large family interfere with their jobs. If married weavers' continuation at the mill is accounted for in terms of the combined impact of economic need and personal inclination, then husbands' concurrence with their wives' desires appears even more significant in indicating a decisive shift in the gender distribution of power among weaving couples.

At this point, Szreter's findings and my argument about the repercussions on gender relations of the organization of the labour process in the Lancashire cotton weaving industry converge and elucidate each other. The highly sophisticated analysis to which he has subjected the *Fertility of Marriage Report* reveals that, among the working class, at least, relatively low fertility was achieved early in marriage, and often by spouses who had married comparatively late in their lives. These findings have led him to conclude that spacing the interval between births by means of low coital frequency in combination with withdrawal was the principal way of limiting family size in the concluding decades of the nineteenth century (Szreter, 1996: 432). His emphasis on abstinence and withdrawal casts serious doubt on the long prevailing view that resort to increasingly acceptable contraceptive devices – a most dubious claim with regard to working-class mores – was the chief means of controlling fertility (e.g. Tranter, 1973: 127–128). As contraceptive devices were beyond the financial reach of the majority of working-class couples, this view further underpinned the diffusionist model of the fertility decline. Szreter, by contrast, insists that the methods employed were traditional ones, embedded in a veritable 'culture of abstinence' (Szreter, 1996: 439), which had been one of the hallmarks of plebeian respectability since at least the beginning of the nineteenth century (Taylor, 1983: 76–77). Sexual restraint was part of the self-discipline cherished in plebeian culture. Thus great store was set by abstinence, failing which withdrawal was practised. If that had proved unsuccessful, abortion was resorted to (Szreter, 1996: 439). Though illegal since 1803, abortion was an accepted part of working-class life (Knight, 1977), and female cotton operatives had been known to resort to it since the early nineteenth century (Gittins, 1982: 150). Moreover, the *Cotton Factory Times*, the trade-union-friendly weekly directed at the cotton workforce, catered for its female readership's specific needs by regularly carrying thinly veiled advertisements for abortifacients.

Reasons for Controlling Fertility

Szreter has accounted for couple's resorting to birth control chiefly by their wish to maintain, defend, or enhance a specific standard of living (Szreter, 1996: 434). Hence birth control was subject to changes in the relative costs and benefits of childrearing (Elderton, 1914: 239), on which labour market negotiations between workers, employers, and the state all had a bearing. This assertion would suggest that the development of the British economy in the second half of the nineteenth century and the onset of the fertility decline in the working class were linked in quite a straightforward way. What Hobsbawm has described as 'a remarkable improvement in employment all round, and a large-scale transfer of labour from worse- to better-paid jobs' (Hobsbawm, 1975: 118) in his second phase of industrialization, taking place roughly between 1840 and 1895 and having been based on capital goods industries (ibd.: 109), meant that the value of adult men's labour rose dramatically relative to that of women and children (Levine, 1985: 189). This has led Levine to state in rather a reductionist fashion that '[t]he cost of children rose as a result of their falling industrial participation' (ibd.: 192). With particular regard to the cotton weaving industry, this way of arguing would point to the abundance of female and juvenile labour, the deployment of which was controlled and hence institutionalized by the Factory Acts (Bolin-Hort, 1989), making for a negligible gender differential in wages. As a further result of protective legislation, juvenile earnings were significantly lower than those of either parent. It therefore made most sense economically for couples to arrange their childbearing so as to maximize both spouses' ability to earn or at least not to have so many children so quickly that the wife was forced to abandon factory work before the first child reached teenage earning capacity (Lichfield, 1978; Szreter, 1996: 490–491).

Yet far from being determined by economic conditions alone, the relative costs and benefits of childrearing, Szreter asserts, are culturally variable, hinging as they do on potential parents' perception (Szreter, 1996: 464, 483). By referring to the perception of childrearing costs as shaping couples' family-building strategies, he has introduced an important cultural variable. The bearings it had on the fertility regimes evolved by different groups of workers become apparent when variations are considered more closely. In order to account for these, Szreter has constructed eight ideal types of spouse and gender relations with regard to female labour market participation. Each ideal type encapsulates a specific arrangement of the ways in which wives participated, along with their husbands, in earning the family's income as well as the meaning and significance accorded to wives' contribution. Szreter's ideal type one is characterized by

> … relatively full-scale participation by wives in the formal wage economy of factories and workshops exclusively outside the home in communities in which this was deemed thoroughly acceptable, was sanctioned by community norms and was not considered to impugn in any way the respectability of the family (ibd.: 507).

As will be apparent by now, this description fits the Lancashire cotton weaving industry perfectly.

The gender distribution of power in the family has been recognized by critics of standard theories of fertility decline as crucial in determining whether or not fertility is controlled and the methods to be used (Folbre, 1983; Seccombe, 1992: 67). Szreter has demonstrated his awareness of this issue by stressing

> […] the way in which gendered working practices in different industries could strongly influence the general pattern of associations and quality of communications between the sexes and therefore between spouses, something of great importance in determining the capacity of spouses to negotiate birth control together (Szreter, 1996: 496).

Precisely how this negotiating occurred is impossible to elucidate from the aggregate data that form the stock-in-trade of historical demography. Using oral history Kate Fisher has concluded from her research into the birth control practices of a later birth cohort from two different regions outside Lancashire that negotiating did not take the form of 'overt, consensual, and in-depth discussion' (Fisher, 2000: 309).

By emphasizing spouse collaboration both in negotiating and practising fertility control, Szreter makes a stand against the prevailing view that contraception was necessarily always the woman's responsibility alone (e.g. Levine, 1985: 198). According to him, joint decision-making in sexual matters required rather more egalitarian gender relations among couples who shared in mutually agreed family survival strategies. Central to these was both partners' engagement in paid work away from home which generated roughly the same amount of income for each (Szreter, 1996: 508). If women weavers' preference for mill-work over household drudgery is added to parents', or more precisely women's, perception of the relative costs of childrearing, then the shift in the familial distribution of power by gender involved in cotton weavers' family-building strategies becomes even more noteworthy. This shift is at least implied in Ethel Elderton's 1914 statement that '[t]he married women [in the textile districts of the north of England] have frankly told our correspondent that they make their husbands take precautions to prevent conception …' (Elderton, 1914: 61).

Mutually Agreed Family-building Strategies

Conditions conducive to joint decision-making of spouses prevailed in the cotton-weaving district of Lancashire. It is to these only that Szreter's ideal-type one is applicable. Within the county, the industry was geographically segregated, with a clear-cut north-south division emerging by the 1880s and the divide deepening further at the beginning of the twentieth century. Spinning was concentrated in a semi-circle around Manchester, while weaving predominated in the north and north-east of the county. Within the vertically segregated sections of the industry, there was internal subdivision in that virtually each district specialized in a class of goods of its own (Kenny, 1982). This made for an extraordinary degree of locational homogeneity (Burgess, 1975: 244). Under such conditions, marital homogamy was high, as born out by local testimony (Royal Commission on Labour, 1892: 163), which does not lend itself to quantification.

The homogeneity characteristic of towns given over to weaving stands out particularly clearly when contrasted with conditions outside the weaving district proper. These are instanced by Preston, situated in the west of Lancashire, on the edge of the cotton district, where the labour market was quite diverse. Engineering, mule spinning, and coal mining absorbed the bulk of male labour, while women clustered in the weaving mills which had begun to spring up in the 1840s (Savage, 1988: 207). About 60 percent of married female cotton workers had husbands in metal or cotton production, the majority of whom were well paid, such as spinners, overlookers, tapesizers and grinders (Savage, 1987: 74, 78). This made for a marked discrepancy in income between husband and wife and for spouse relations which were less egalitarian. As a result, there evolved a markedly different regime of exceptionally high fertility, the local fertility rate even exceeding the national average in 1911 (Szreter, 1996: 512).

In the weaving towns of north-east Lancashire, male and female weavers were embedded in communities with specific norms, beliefs and practices shaping people's reproductive behaviour (Szreter, 1996: 546), the transmission of which was greatly facilitated by the congregation in the weaving sheds of numerous men and women (Elderton, 1914: 236). While it has become impossible by now to replicate Fisher's investigation among the cotton weavers of Lancashire, the embeddedness of both spouses in the culture of the weaving communities may be used as a pointer. Spouses' shared cultural background would have been conducive to a joint family-building strategy being applied, not necessarily always as a result of explicit discussion, but of each spouse putting into practice the gendered precepts of sexual behaviour held by the community. These may also have been used to put pressure on reluctant spouses to conform. Deviation from community norms and sexual practices may have seriously curtailed individuals' chances to form sexual relationships.

Yet the possibility of reaching tacit agreement on fertility control represents a significant modification of Szreter's emphasis on the quality of negotiation and communication between spouses in communities with roughly equal labour market participation by men and women. For Fisher, tacit agreement on fertility control is closely bound up with her female interviewees' desire not to appear sexually knowledgeable and forward. But the coyness she has found to characterize all the women in her samples, regardless of class and place of residence and including working-class old-age pensioners with unspecified previous occupations from Blackburn (Fisher & Szreter, 2003), is conspicuously absent from the ego-documents on which much of this article is based. This may be partly attributable to the fact that, in these sources, women's accounts focus on what they see as the central experience of their lives, viz. working in a weaving shed. Sexual talk or behaviour is mentioned in order to convey the atmosphere of comradeship and conviviality they see as characteristic of workplace relationships. Consequently, their domestic life, including conjugal relations, is mentioned as a spin-off, if at all, rather than being central, as in the interviews conducted by Fisher. Even more to the point, cotton weavers were apparently quite happy to play a proactive role in relationships with men, as in the following two examples, which are admittedly embedded in a highly ritualized context. One of the methods employed in collecting money for the celebration of Christmas or birthdays involved trying to kiss male colleagues unawares, who then had to pay into the kitty (Mrs. D.W. Tape 667; Mrs. T.T. Tape 668, MSU TLSL). Sexual matters would also be broached in conversation in various ways. When the impending wedding of a female colleague was celebrated on the shopfloor, the older women would tell ribald jokes sending the younger ones giggling with embarrassment (Foley, 1973: 58). As a result, the mill was appreciated as a source of information, including on 'the facts of life', not available elsewhere (Roberts, 1981, respondent A1P, 28; respondent H7P, 24). Information was not by word of mouth alone. Occasionally, open displays of sexual behaviour could be observed. Thus a man was seen with his lover, '... fondling her, hands deep within her blouse or beneath her petticoats' (McCarthy, 1953: 45–46). This particular observer, deeeply shocked by the goings-on around her, was relieved to be protected by a change of job from what she saw as 'the rampant sexuality of factory life' (ibd.: 46). Others, less inclined to feel shocked, may have deemed displays of sexual behaviour too much of an everyday occurrence as to warrant mentioning. When sexual encounters were recounted, it was in a completely different context and because they had been unwelcome at the time and therefore resented by women who had become the targets of what today would be termed 'sexual harassment'. Women weavers were particularly vulnerable to sexual exploitation by overlookers who had the power to dismiss those unwilling to grant them sexual favours (e.g. *Cotton Factory Times*, 22.6.1888, 4; 29.11.1889, 7; 8.7.1904, 6). Yet rather than submitting to unsolicited sexual advances, women weavers were able to rely on the support of each other as well as the entire community in fending off what was seen as improper sexual behaviour and, ultimately, to ensure many an offender's dismissal (e.g. Lambertz, 1985: 34–36). Such action necessitated speaking out about sexual matters in front of men, some of them strangers, in an official capacity, such as trade-union officials, policemen or magistrates. It therefore comes as no surprise that female textile workers openly talked about '... mak[ing] (emphasis added) their husbands take precautions to prevent contraception', as the quote from Elderton (1914: 61) has already demonstrated. As this statement makes clear, such wifely behaviour was predicated upon the specific gender distribution of power in relationships which had developed in Lancashire weaving communities as a corollary of a marked degree of gender equality in the labour process. All of this formed part of the distinct culture of these communities. Yet cultural variation is curiously absent from Fisher's findings, who finds husbands and wives' contraceptive behaviour the same wherever her research takes her.

Most fundamentally, weaving communities evolved their own notions of masculinity and femininity, clearly at odds with the ideas held in the wider world of labour. Weavers' understanding of femininity involved the rejection of the centrality of domesticity in favour of competence in the workplace. Women weavers saw themselves first and foremost as skilled workers. Their self-image did not preclude wife- and motherhood, but shaped their familial functions in specific ways. Being a good wife and mother in a cotton weaving community involved bringing home earnings that significantly enhanced the family's standard of living. This version of femininity was evolved in conjunction with a notion of masculinity that did not revolve exclusively around waged work and sexual prowess. It did not preclude housework and childcare nor acknowledgement of the burden shouldered by wives and active consideration of their concerns. Here, being a weaver was no slur on a man's masculinity. Rather than making futile attempts to escape from an occupation with strong feminine overtones, these men committed themselves to trade-union activism, striving to bring weaving into the realm of skilled trades (Savage, 1988: 213). Only where the local labour market offered a variety of openings for male labour would weaving be among the less preferred options.

Socialism as Facilitator of Fertility Control

Consideration of three women whose lives are particularly well documented allows the historian to move away from the aggregate data accumulated by historical demographers and begin to explore the implications of the Lancashire weavers' fertility regime for the everyday life of women. At this level, women come clearly to the fore as crucial agents in moulding reproductive behaviour (Mackinnon, 1995). Each of the three women here considered was actively involved in contemporary socialist and feminist movements. This involvement reinforced their determination to limit the number of their offspring. As a result, couples actually 'stopped' reproducing once the family size of one child only, considered ideal by the wife, had been attained. It would therefore appear that the weavers' fertility regime created a space in which women, fortified by their political convictions, were able to shape their reproductive lives in novel ways.

Selina Cooper is a case in point. Her prominence in the suffrage movement, coupled with unusual closeness to her daughter, enabled a biography to be written of her (Liddington, 1984). She was a winder in the cotton boom town of Nelson and met her future husband, a weaver, through their mutual involvement in the local branch of the Social Democratic Federation, a socialist organization with Marxist leanings founded in 1884. On the basis of their shared interests and similar outlook on life they decided to get married. By this time, Selina was thirty-two and Robert four years her junior, thereby presenting a true case of late age at marriage. Selina's first child, who, not at all unusual by the standards of the weaving community (Roberts, 1981, respondent T5P, 17; respondent T4P, 46), had been conceived prior to marriage, died only four months old. Three years later, she had a daughter, who survived into adulthood. Selina never became pregnant again.

The Coopers thus exemplify a range of strategies in shaping the size of their family. There is late age at marriage followed by the spacing of children and, finally, stopping altogether once the second child has proved sufficiently resilient to survive. Indications are that the Coopers used contraceptives to achieve their ideal family size. They possessed a well-worn copy of *The Law of Population*, a birth control pamphlet originally published in 1877 by Annie Besant, a secularist and freethinker moving in socialist circles. The pamphlet assessed the value of various contraceptive devices and came complete with the addresses of suppliers and prices charged (Liddington, 1984: 73).

In Selina Cooper's case, three distinct, but mutually reinforcing influences meshed. Firstly, both she and her husband worked in a weaving shed and shared in the fertility regime characteristic of the weaving community. Secondly, they were both involved in the Socialist Revival, a term denoting the springing up of a whole range of bigger or smaller, long- or short-lived socialist organizations in the Britain of the 1880s. One such was the Social Democratic Federation that the Coopers had joined prior to switching their allegiance to the socialist Independent Labour Party formed in 1893 and which they found more congenial. Some strands of late nineteenth-century socialism legitimized birth control as an acceptable, albeit temporary, expedient for combating poverty (Mitchell, 1968: 89). In the legally oppressive conditions of contemporary Britain, where birth control information fell foul of the obscenity laws, some socialist organizations also facilitated the spreading of such information among the working class, as becomes apparent via Annie Besant's pamphlet. Despite the far from unequivocal stand on women's rights adopted by both the Independent Labour Party (Hannam, 1992) and the Social Democratic Federation (Hunt, 1996) the Socialist Revival did create an atmosphere in which it was possible for women both to reflect upon and to speak out about the problematic of gender.

The Women's Co-operative Guild, which Selina Cooper also belonged to, was another important channel for the spreading of relevant information. Formed in 1883 in order to give the wives of co-operators an interest in the movement, in the period prior to the First World War, it evolved into a progressive and autonomous section of the working-class movement with a sharp awareness of the specific ways in which sexual and class oppression fused in the lives of working-class wives (Scott, 1998). The North West, which had been the heartland of the Co-operative movement ever since the first shop was opened at Rochdale in 1844, also proved the strongest area of support for the Guild. Among its numerous activities geared, among other things, towards heightening women's awareness, and teaching them how best to take care, of their own physical wellbeing counted lectures on such apparently innocuous topics as 'should the poor marry?'. These may have afforded the opportunity for broaching the issue of birth control (Liddington, 1984: 56).

The important influence of involvement in the socialist movement becomes equally clear via Selina Cooper's contemporaries, Hannah Mitchell (1968) and Ada Nield Chew (1982), neither of whom was a weaver, but both of whom took up their residence in the cotton district of Lancashire. They further shared with Selina Cooper their active involvement in socialist and feminist movements. The birth of Hannah Mitchell's only son proved to be exceedingly protracted and painful so that she resolved not to undergo such torture ever again (Mitchell, 1968: 102). Each of these women had only one child, and the co-operation of the husband, which was openly acknowledged by Hannah Mitchell (ibd.), can be presumed in the other two cases. As the mother of an only child, each of these women was able to engage in political activity full-time. Their political activism was both grounded in, and taken beyond, the space the cotton community afforded women's activities away from home. Having only one child proved no hindrance to these women's employment as political organizers touring the country to further the cause of women. While these three women may well have been exceptions with regard to the degree of their political activism, and most certainly so with regard to the amount of detail known about their lives, they were not the only women moving in socialist circles. Both the Independent Labour Party and the Social Democratic Federation had one of their strongholds each in the North-West, the latter actually forming a break-away weavers' union in Burnley, which managed to win over the majority of unionized weavers in the town (Liddington, 1984: 42).

Conclusion

This article has cast some light on the reasons underlying cotton weaving couples' pioneering role in limiting fertility in the British working class. Their particular fertility regime involved timing, and thereby limiting, the number of child-births so as to make sure that they would interfere least with women's paid employment. By pointing to a combination of penury and inclination as the underlying motives, this article has highlighted women weavers' agency in shaping the fertility regime of the Lancashire weaving communities. Both their desire and their ability to do so grew out of a notion of working-class femininity, peculiar to the weaving districts of Lancashire, which revolved around competence at paid work as the precondition for making a significant contribution to family income. In conjunction with the concomitant absence of the figure of the male breadwinner this created a space in which women were able to make choices concerning their reproductive lives.

References

Anderson, Michael (1971), *Family Structure in Nineteenth-Century Lancashire*, Cambridge, Cambridge University Press.

Banks, J. A. (1954), *Prosperity and Parenthood: A Study of Family Planning among the Victorian Middle Classes*, London, Routledge.

Banks, J. A. (1981), *Victorian Values: Secularism and the Size of Families*, London, Routledge.

Banks, J. A. and O. (1964), *Feminism and Family Planning in Victorian England*, Liverpool, Liverpool University Press.

Board of Trade, Labour Department, Report by Miss Collet on the Statistics of Employment of Women and Girls, Parliamentary Papers, 1894, LXXXI.

Bolin-Hort, Per (1989), *Work, Family and the State. Child Labour and the Organization of Production in the British Cotton Industry, 1780–1920*, Lund, Lund University Press.

Burgess, Keith (1975), *The Origins of British Industrial Relations*, London, Croom Helm.

Chew, Ada Nield (1912), 'All in the Day's Work', *The Englishwoman*, 35–45.

Chew, Doris Nield (ed.) (1982), *Ada Nield Chew. The Life and Writings of a Working Woman*, London, Virago.

Coleman, David (2000), 'Population and Family', in Halsey, A. H. with Webb, Josephine (eds), *Twentieth-Century British Social Trends*, Basingstoke, Macmillan, 27–93.

Elderton, Ethel (1914), *Report on the English Birthrate*, Eugenics Laboratory Memoirs, Vols. XIX and XX, London.

Ellison, Thomas (1968), *The Cotton Trade of Great Britain*, New York, Kelly.
Fisher, Kate (2000), 'Uncertain Aims and Tacit Negotiation: Birth Control Practices in Britain, 1925–1950', *Population and Development Review*, 26, 295–317.
Fisher, Kate and Szreter, Simon (2003), '"They Prefer Withdrawal". The Choice of Birth Control in Britain, 1918–1950', *Journal of Interdisciplinary History*, 34, 263–291.
Folbre, Nancy (1983), 'Of Patriarchy Born. The Political Economy of Fertility Decisions', *Feminist Studies*, 9, 261–284.
Foley, Alice (1973), *A Bolton Childhood*, Manchester, University of Manchester Extra-Mural Department.
Foster, John (1974), *Class Struggle and the Industrial Revolution. Early Industrial Capitalism in Three English Towns*, London, Weidenfeld and Nicolson.
Fowler, Alan and Wyke, Terry (eds) (1987), *The Barefoot Aristocrats. A History of the Amalgamated Association of Operative Cotton Spinners*, Littleborough.
Gittins, Diana (1982), *Fair Sex. Family size and structure, 1900–1939*, London, Hutchinson.
Glucksmann, Miriam (1995), 'Some Do, Some Don't (But in Fact They All Do Really); Some Will, Some Won't; Some Have, Some Haven't. Women, Men, Work, and Washing Machines in Inter-War Britain', *Gender and History*, 7, 275–294.
Hall, Catherine (1982), 'The home turned upside down? The working-class family in cotton textiles, 1780–1850', in Whitelegg, Elizabeth et al. (eds), *The Changing Experience of Women*, Oxford, Blackwell, 17–29.
Hannam, June (1992), 'Women and the ILP, 1880–1914', in James, David, Jowitt, Tony and Laybourn, Keith (eds), *The Centennial History of the Independent Labour Party*, Krumlin, Ryburn Academic, 205–228.
Harig, H. and Heap, S. A. (eds) (1994), *Proceedings of the 22nd International Cotton Conference Bremen, 2–5 March, 1994*, Bremen, Faserinstitut Bremen.
Hewitt, Margaret (1953), 'The Effects of Married Women's Employment in the Cotton Textile Districts on the Organisation and Structure of the Home in Lancshire, 1840–1880', PhD London.
Hobsbawm, Eric (1975), *Industry and Empire*, The Pelican Economic History of Britain, 3, Harmondsworth, Pelican.
Hunt, Karen (1996), *Equivocal Feminists. The Social Democratic Federation and the Woman Question, 1884–1911*, Cambridge, Cambridge University Press.
Innes, J. W. (1938*), Class Fertility Trends in England and Wales, 1876–1934*, Princeton, N.J., Princeton University Press.
Jewkes, John and Gray, E. M. (1935), *Wages and Labour in the Lancashire Cotton Spinning Industry*, Manchester, Victoria University, Department of Economics and Commerce.
Kenny, Stephen (1982), 'Sub-regional Specialization in the Lancashire Cotton Industry, 1884–1914. A Study in Organizational and Locational Change', *Journal of Historical Geography*, 8, 41–63.
Knight, Patricia (1977), 'Women and Abortion in Victorian and Edwardian England', *History Workshop Journal*, 4, 57–68.
Lambertz, Jan (1985), 'Sexual Harassment in the Nineteenth Century English Cotton Industry', *History Workshop Journal*, 19, 29–61.
Lamphere, Louise (1985), 'Bringing the Family to Work. Women's Culture on the Shop Floor', *Feminist Studies*, 11, 519–540.

Levine, David (1985), 'Industrialization and the Proletarian Family in England', *Past and Present*, 107, 168–203.
Lichfield, R. Burr (1978), 'The Family and the Mill. Cotton Mill Work, Family Work Patterns, and Fertility in Mid-Victorian Stockport', in Wohl, Anthony S. (ed.), *The Victorian Family. Structure and Stresses*, London, Croom Helm, 180–196.
Liddington, Jill (1984), *The Life and Times of a Respectable Radical. Selina Cooper, 1864–1946*, London, Virago.
Mackinnon, Alison (1995), 'Were Women Present at the Demographic Transition? Questions from a Feminist Historian to Historical Demographers', *Gender and History*, 7, 222–240.
Manchester Studies Unit. Oral History Tapes, Manchester Metropolitan University, MSU TLSL.
Mark-Lawson, Jane (1987), 'Women, Welfare and Urban Politics. A Comparative Analysis of Luton and Nelson, 1917–1934', PhD Lancaster.
McCarthy, Margaret (1953), *Generation in Revolt,* London, William Heineman.
McLaren, Angus (1977), 'Women's Work and Regulation of Family Size. The question of abortion in the nineteenth century', *History Workshop Journal*, 4, 70–81.
Mitchell, Geoffrey (ed.) (1968), *The Hard Way Up. The Autobiography of Hannah Mitchell, Suffragette and Rebel*, London, Faber and Faber.
Roberts, Elizabeth (1981), *North-West Oral History Project. Social and Family Life in Preston, 1890–1940*, Lancaster University Library.
Roberts, Elizabeth (1986), *A Woman's Place. An Oral History of Working-Class Women, 1890–1940*, Oxford and New York, Blackwell.
Roberts, Elizabeth (1982), 'Working-Class Standards of Living in Three Lancashire Towns, 1890–1914', *International Review of Social History*, 27, 43–65.
Royal Commission on Labour, Parliamentary Papers.1892.XXXVII.
Savage, Michael (1982), *Control at Work. North Lancashire Cotton Weaving, 1890–1940*, Lancaster Regionalism Group, Working Paper 7.
Savage, Michael (1987), *The Dynamics of Working-Class Politics. The Labour Movement in Preston, 1880–1940*, Cambridge, Cambridge University Press.
Savage, Michael (1988), 'Women and Work in the Lancashire Cotton Industry, 1890–1939', in Jowitt, J. A. and McIvor, A. J. (eds), *Employers and Labour in the English Textile Industries, 1850–1939*, London and New York, Routledge, 203–223.
Schwarzkopf, Jutta (1991), *Women in the Chartist Movement*, London and New York, Macmillan.
Schwarzkopf, Jutta (2004), *Unpicking Gender: The Social Construction of Gender in the Lancashire Cotton Weaving Industry, 1880–1914*, Aldershot, Ashgate.
Scott, Gillian (1998), *Feminism and the Politics of Working Women. The Women's Co-operative Guild, 1880s to the Second World War*, London, UCL Press.
Seccombe, Wally (1990), 'Starting to Stop. Working-Class Fertility Decline in Britain', *Past and Present*, 126, 151–188.
Seccombe, Wally (1992), 'Men's "Marital Rights" and Women's "Wifely Duties": Changing Conjugal Relations in the Fertility Decline', in Gillis, John R., Tilly, Louise A. and Levine, David (eds), *The European Experience of Declining Fertility, 1850–1970*, Cambrdige, MA and Oxford, Blackwell.

Summary of Returns under s. 130 of the Factory and Workshop Act, 1901, of Persons Employed in 1907 in Textile Factories, Parliamentary Papers. 1909. LXXIX.

Szreter, Simon (1996), *Fertility, Class and Gender in Britain, 1860–1940*, Cambridge, Cambridge University Press.

Szreter, Simon and Garrett, Eilidh (2000), 'Reproduction, Compositional Demography, and Economic Growth: Family Planning in England Long Before the Fertility Decline', *Population and Development Review*, 26, 45–80.

Taylor, Barbara (1983), *Eve and the New Jerusalem. Socialism and Feminism in the Nineteenth Century*, London, Virago.

Teitelbaum, Michael S. (1984), *The British Fertility Decline. Demographic Transition in the Crucible of the Industrial Revolution*, Princeton, N.J., Princeton University Press.

Tilly, Louise A. and Scott, Joan W. (1978), *Women, Work and Family*, New York, Holt, Rinehart and Winston.

Tranter, N. L. (1973), *Population since the Industrial Revolution. The Case of England and Wales*, London, Croom Helm.

Turner, H. A. (1962), *Trade Union Growth, Structure and Policy. A Comparative Study of the Cotton Unions*, London, George Allen & Unwin.

Westwood, Sallie (1984), *All Day, Every Day. Factory and Family in the Making of Women's Lives*, Urbana, University of Illinois Press.

Woods, R. I. (1987), 'Approaches to the Fertility Transition in Victorian England', *Population Studies*, 41, 283–311.

A 'Silent Class' and a 'Quiet Revolution'. Female Domestics and Fertility Decline in Flanders

Eric Vanhaute and Christa Matthys*

In this article we reintroduce the hypothesis that urban female domestic servants played a significant role in the diffusion of fertility control behaviour in the last quarter of the nineteenth century. Urban female domestics were usually from a modest rural background. It is our assumption that the daily proximity with the urban upper- and middle-class pioneers in the restriction of marital fertility influenced servants' fertility behaviour in later family life, even when they returned to their villages of origin.

The regions under investigation in this article are the Belgian provinces of East and West Flanders. In the first part we confront aggregate data on the fertility decline with some results of village studies based on the technique of life course analysis. This overview makes clear that, first of all, regional and even local differences in the timing of marital fertility decline remained important until (at least) the beginning of the twentieth century. Furthermore, the generation of women born in 1880 marked a fundamental shift in rural Flemish fertility levels. Finally, the overview makes clear that individual-based research is needed to understand how a macro process such as the (European) fertility decline may be translated into individual strategies and choices.

In the second part we focus on human agency, more in particular on the rural women who served as urban domestics in the East Flemish city of Ghent. To begin with, we recapitulate the discussion about the role of domestic servants in the diffusion of 'modern' fertility behaviour, arguing that the arguments and data used so far are insufficient. Following that, we ask what kind of information we need, based on the analysis of individual life courses. We add some first data, suggesting that this kind of research could be very fruitful.

* The authors want to thank Hilde Bras, Sofie De Langhe, Jan Kok, and Angélique Janssens for their remarks and suggestions on a previous version of this text.

Figure 1. Maps of Belgium and East and West Flanders

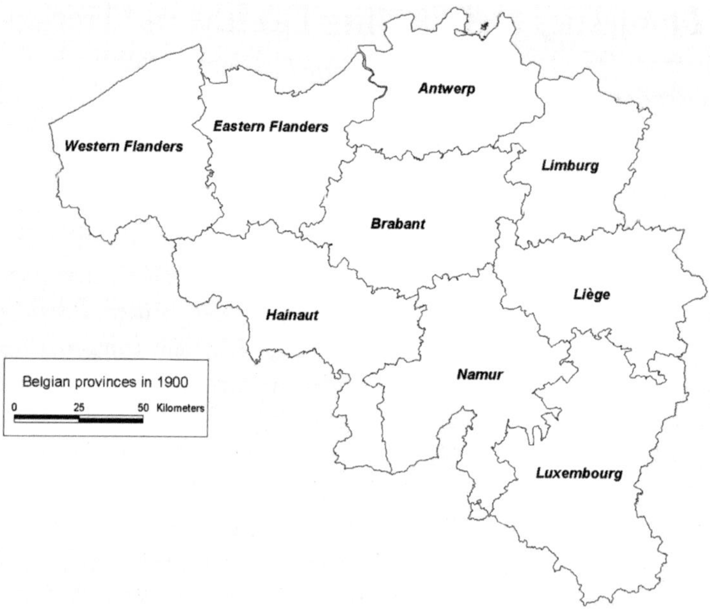

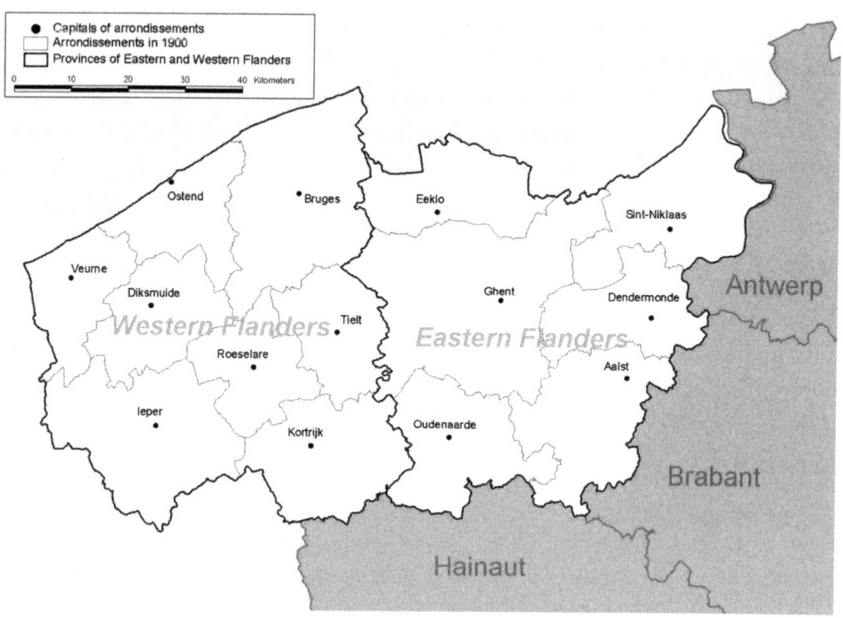

1. Fertility Decline in East and West Flanders

Regional Variation versus the Case Study

When investigating the nineteenth- and twentieth-century fertility decline in Belgium, the pioneering work by Ron Lesthaeghe is still the starting point (Lesthaeghe, 1977). The author's ambition was to test, with Belgian data, the most important explanatory hypotheses formulated within the debate on the European fertility decline. His research material consisted of aggregate data at the level of the administrative district *(arrondissement).*

Because of the congruence between the time series of marital and illegitimate birth rates, Lesthaeghe was convinced that the decline in fertility was the result of a widespread use of effective contraceptive methods. Furthermore, his figures showed a strong correlation between industrialisation and urbanisation, and the decline in marital fertility. Nevertheless, if only socioeconomic factors were taken into account, a substantial part of the regional variance remained unexplained. Other variables, such as the level of literacy or the degree of infant mortality, were integrated but did not have a clear statistical impact. Literacy was even assumed to have been a rather negative factor in the process of 'modernisation', since primary education contributed to the continuity of existing norms and values. Secularisation however – although to some extent intertwined with industrialisation and urbanisation – seemed to have played a major role in bringing down fertility levels. In the spread of a more 'modern' fertility pattern, language was another important – although not independent – factor. French speaking parts of the population were the first to make the shift away from the 'traditional' Malthusian pattern.

Around 1880 the highest rates of marital fertility were recorded in East and West Flanders. Although fertility declined after that, in 1910 it was still considerably higher than in the other Belgian provinces, with the exception of Limburg. Looking at the district figures, the indices of the regions of Roeselare and Tielt stand out, with a downward kink only after 1900, almost a generation later than in neighbouring districts.

Since Lesthaeghe's general study new methodologies and more advanced computing techniques have been developed. As a consequence, new perspectives on fertility behaviour were presented. Concerning the Walloon part of Belgium, the fertility transition was the central topic in some wide-ranging socio-demographic studies, whilst, in addition, several articles on various

Table 1. Marital Fertility in Belgium, 1880–1910 (Lesthaeghe, 1977)

	1880	1890	1900	1910
Belgium	0.751	0.678	0.596	0.443
Provinces				
Antwerp	0.837	0.761	0.661	0.508
Brabant	0.71	0.626	0.517	0.365
East Flanders	0.921	0.849	0.78	0.594
West Flanders	0.918	0.878	0.838	0.671
Hainaut	0.577	0.478	0.394	0.298
Liège	0.704	0.598	0.49	0.333
Limburg	0.881	0.872	0.877	0.822
Luxemburg	0.733	0.669	0.625	0.527
Namur	0.618	0.536	0.469	0.364
Districts East Flanders				
Aalst	0.898	0.854	0.834	0.661
Sint Niklaas	1.03	0.971	0.902	0.708
Oudenaarde	0.911	0.88	0.863	0.638
Dendermonde	1.052	0.95	0.903	0.712
Eeklo	0.945	0.875	0.821	0.629
Gent	0.845	0.764	0.651	0.466
Districts West Flanders				
Brugge	0.899	0.87	0.839	0.68
Diksmuide	0.967	0.886	0.844	0.705
Kortrijk	0.894	0.853	0.812	0.618
Oostende	0.899	0.905	0.8	0.651
Roeselare	0.987	0.949	0.945	0.743
Tielt	0.942	0.903	0.938	0.797
Veurne	0.921	0.821	0.752	0.595
Ieper	0.903	0.852	0.795	0.659

aspects and regions were published (e.g. Alter, 1978; Alter & Oris, 1999; Eggerickx, 1998; Neven, 2003; Oris, 1992). The new methods of analysis applied in these studies essentially implied the shift from aggregate information to more individual data.

Innovative research on Flanders is sparse. In 2002 Jan Van Bavel published his study on fertility control in the city of Leuven (Van Bavel, 2002). Van Bavel used individual data to challenge the conceptual distinction between 'natural' and 'controlled' fertility. Without denying the existence of a major transformation in fertility control behaviour, he questioned the opinion that stopping behaviour was a historical innovation at the start of the fertility transition and that spacing was only a temporary phenomenon. Secondly, he focused on the diffusion of 'modern' stopping behaviour among the city population. His conclusion that this behaviour first appeared within the local bourgeoisie confirms results from other studies. The significance of literacy, however, seems much more outspoken than in Lesthaeghe's study. The application of stopping behaviour within elite milieus was much more related to the level of education than to social status. Also, amongst the working classes the literate showed signs of stopping behaviour earlier in time than the non-literate. Literacy of the wife seemed especially important. Moreover, Van Bavel's study confirmed the role of language in the diffusion process. He was able to show that the woman's francophone origin was a much more decisive factor than her husband's linguistic background.

By selecting Leuven, Van Bavel examined a provincial town that was neither a pioneer nor a laggard in the fertility transition. He argued that it was more relevant to focus on a less spectacular setting in order to understand the underlying mechanisms of the overall European fertility decline. In other words, every 'average' case would show the same mechanisms, and huge socioeconomic transformations only functioned as disturbing factors in the analysis. We believe, as Lesthaeghe did, that it remains important to map and explain regional variations and to keep up a comparative perspective. Besides, the functioning of urban, semi-urban, and rural communities is determined by different social mechanisms. This remark is especially important in relation to the social diffusion of new reproductive behaviour, as we will show later.

The Girls of East and West Flanders

In the beginning of the twentieth century the Belgian statistician Camille Jacquart stressed the necessity of a comparative view in researching demographic behaviour when referring to the peculiarities of and the differences within the province of West Flanders (Jacquart, 1905). For example, birth rates in the *arrondissement* of Thielt in 1873–1894 were amongst the lowest in Belgium, while those in the neighbouring district of Ostend belonged to the highest.

Figure 2. Marital Fertility in West Flanders in 1857–1900 According to Jacquart

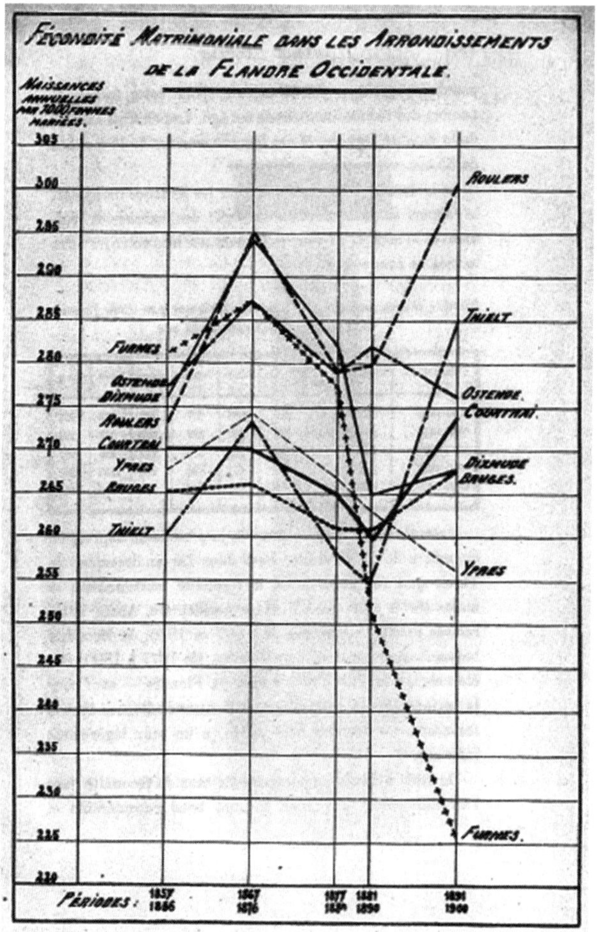

Just as Lesthaeghe did, seven decades later, Jacquart first examined changes in nuptiality before turning to marital fertility. Unlike Lesthaeghe, he was convinced that contraceptive behaviour was of minor importance. Moreover, he believed that in some regions the decline in fertility was only a temporary stage. To explain why this exceptional process took place, and why regional differences were so marked, only a longitudinal and multicausal explanation would do. For Jacquart, the regional differences in reproductive behaviour between the *arrondissements* in West Flanders were the outcomes of the different impacts of the mid nineteenth-century subsistence crisis resulting from diverging occupational structures – read: the importance of the rural flax industry. The people of the most afflicted regions, such as Tielt and Courtrai, suffered long term physical and psychological consequences of this severe hunger crisis. By the end of the nineteenth century the first post-trauma generation reached maturity. According to Jacquart, the slight amelioration of the economic situation in the 1890s had more effect on this population than on men and women living in the wealthier districts. As the figures in table 1 show, after 1900 the poor regions were able to catch up quite rapidly.

Obviously, when Jacquart wrote his book, the fertility transition was still in full progress. What makes his analysis interesting is the attention given to regional factors related to the organisation of the rural society. That is why we stress the importance of the analysis of fertility behaviour on a local level, with new data and new methods now available. So far the Ghent life course project compiled the data belonging to thirteen birth cohorts, born either around 1830, 1845, or 1880, from nine localities in East and West Flanders. In addition to that, our database contains information on three female cohorts in the city of Ghent. The total observed population consists now of 2,891 persons, 2,242 of which are women. From this dataset some information on marital fertility in nine rural villages can be compiled. In table 2 the columns B, D, and E take into account all women with children under observation in these nine villages. Column C refers only to those women who could be followed until the age of 45.

In the Flemish countryside the generation of girls born in 1880 is the one that initiated a fundamental shift away from the 'traditional' pattern of marital fertility of their parents and grandparents. They married younger, they had both their first and their last child at a younger age, and on average they had fewer children in total. However, no proof can be found that this generation was applying a strategy of birth spacing to a larger extent than earlier generations.

Data on cohorts of women who grew up in the city of Ghent illustrate the large gap between urban and rural environments. The average Ghent working-

Table 2. Parameters of Marital Fertility in nine Flemish Villages, Birth Cohorts 1830, 1847, 1880

Village	Birth Cohort	A	B	C	D	E	F
Assenede	1830	30	28.6	31.7	40.3	28	6.2
Hamme	1830	25	28	28.2	39.6	25	6.6
Koekelare	1830	38[1]	30.4	29.3	38.4		
Zwevegem	1830	13	26.6	28.4	38.8	38	6.3
Poperinge	1830	15	29.7	31.3	40.5	19	5.1
Oordegem	1830	15	29.7	29.4			4.6
Lebbeke	1847	108	30.5	29.6	37	28	6.3
Wichelen	1847	34	27.5	27.5	38.1	20	5.7
Zele	1847	39	27.7	26.9	39	21	6
Hamme	1880	62	26	24.4	34.5	27	5.3
Oordegem	1880	30	26.1	27.8			4.6
Poperinge	1880	28	25.4	24.9	36.2	28	4.7
Zwevegem	1880	35	25.7	27.3	36.8	28	4.5
Total (average number)		434	27.8	28.2	38.1	26.2	5.5

A: number of women per cohort known to have had children
B: mean age at first marriage for females (in years)
C: mean age of mother at birth of first child (in years)
D: mean age of mother at birth of last child (in years)
E: mean interval between births, excluding stillbirths[2] (in months)
F: number of births per mother

1 The figure for Koekelare includes the wives of male cohort members.

2 Stillbirths or children who lived less than three days were mostly not registered in the population registers. The latter is due to the fact that parents had a three-day period to register their newborn. A child that died within the first two days after birth had to be recorded in the death registers as a stillbirth.

class girl born in 1860 had her first child at the age of 22.6 and her last child at the age of 33, bearing a total of 4.6 children on average. The next generation born in 1880 had only 2.5 children on average, with the first child born at the age of 23 and the last at 29 years of age.

Furthermore, individual-level data provide insight in socio-professional diffusion mechanisms in the countryside. Obviously, occupational structures in the countryside differed from those in urban settings. But just as in cities, it was the local village elite, mostly active in services and trade, who were the first to apply effective birth control practices. Farmers, however, even when belonging to the local elite, turned out to be the last in adopting modern behaviour. The traditional pattern, based on restrictive nuptiality and natural fertility within marriage, remained very strong in this group until well into the twentieth century.

Existing research on the process of fertility decline in nineteenth- and twentieth-century Belgium and Flanders clarifies two things. First, a comparative analysis of regional and even sub-regional differences remains necessary to understand which variables determined the diverging patterns of marital fertility decline. However, patterns and processes only tell an aggregate story, hiding the individual actors. The notable differences in timing even on a local scale suggest that the 'channels' of individual behaviour – mutual 'bargaining' and individual and collective choices – are central in our understanding of the concrete implementation of the 'macro-process' of the fertility decline. The second conclusion is that micro research, starting from the individual life course, is indispensable to surpass the level of structural drives and constraints. The first results of life course research make clear that concerning the diffusion of fertility control, a comparison of female cohorts in big cities, provincial towns, and countryside villages may prove to be very useful in order to gain insight in the specific channels through which the 'knowledge' of fertility control was spread. We elaborate one aspect in the second part of the paper.

2. The Role of Urban Domestic Servants in the Fertility Decline: What Evidence Do We Have?

In this part we focus on the possible role of urban female domestics in the diffusion of fertility control behaviour among the lower classes in the countryside. This matter has been addressed in the literature before, as shown below, but so far research has only provided unsatisfactory results. We argue that the reason for this is the use of unsuitable data. In what follows we will indicate what information and what research model is needed to answer the question in a more satisfactory way.

To provide a definition of a 'servant' is a complicated task. There is no decisive element that unambiguously distinguishes him or her from other workers, exactly because serving was generally regarded as a 'transitional' job (Piette, 2000: 31–41). In this research we limit ourselves to a specific group: rural girls who worked as resident female servants in the city.

Historical research of domestic service touches upon different historical research fields such as migration, socialisation, social mobility, professional choice, relationships between sexes and social classes, and the influence of women on the modernisation of society (Poelstra, 1981: 47). However, until recently in European history little attention was paid to the numerous groups of domestic maids. Their non-productive tasks made them insignificant to economic history (Piete, 2000: 9–27). Unlike industrial workers, they never showed signs of collective action, which effectively eliminates them from social history. Feminist historians tended to avoid the study of domestic servants as well, since to them the subordinate role of the maid was only a symptom of patriarchal hegemony. Nevertheless, some well-known volumes were published, which provoked further discussion (e.g. McBride, 1976). In Belgium, the situation is not much better; the only exhaustive scientific work on the matter being Piette's study of domestic servants as a social class in nineteenth-century Brussels.

Indirect Arguments

The question as to whether or not young female servants moving from the countryside to the city played a significant part in the spread of contraceptive behaviour after returning to their villages, touches upon the issue of domestic servants as cultural intermediaries. The phenomenon of young working-class girls copying aspects of the private life of the urban middle and upper classes has caught the attention of several authors. As Davidoff noted:

> In any system of hierarchy expressed in rituals of deference, at a face-to-face level, there will be a continuing tension between identification with the superior and social distance. (Davidoff, 1974: 414)

Some authors focused more specifically on the ideal values and norms of the maid from the point of view of the bourgeoisie, and on the way in which servants were disciplined (Piette, 2000). Others pointed at the importance of domestic service in social mobility (Bras, 2002; McBride, 1976). Still another group of authors focused on one aspect of cultural interaction, such as language or clothing (De Metsenaere, 1996; Roche, 1978). Up to now no exhaustive research on the role of domestic servants as cultural intermediaries and transferents has been conducted.

Teresa McBride and Leonore Davidoff were the first to suggest that former maids may have played a significant role in the propagation of birth control mechanisms (Davidoff, 1974: 428; McBride, 1974). As McBride wrote:

> [...] there might have been an element of choice operating in this case as well. [...] The pattern of late marriage and family limitation might indicate no more than the result of circumstances which circumscribed servants' options, if it were not for indications that these patterns reflected more general attitudes. Servants seem to have maintained a life-style which emulated the middle classes in important respects, of which consumption is a significant example.

In Davidoff's work, the idea reached no further than a footnote, stating:

> Servants as 'cultural carriers' is an intriguing idea. It is particularly important in areas of private life, e.g. the adoption of ideal family size. The generation who were young servants in the middle- and upper-class households in the late nineteenth century, where completed family size was declining, were the generation of working-class married women whose own family size fell in the beginning of the twentieth century. Of course no *direct* connection can be drawn between these two sets of facts.

McBride brought together figures from several European areas, showing that servant couples had very small numbers of children. Because of the transitional character of the occupation, and the tiny proportion of married servants, these figures cannot be regarded as representative. McBride also pointed at 'a more general attitude', arguing that servants often tried to imitate the life style of their masters. This was especially clear in their consumption behaviour

(McBride, 1974: 72–75). Servants spent a lot of money on clothing and tried to dress as well as their masters. In the banking sector, servants were regular depositors. They seemed to be the only part of the working-class population that was able to save some money. Therefore, according to McBride, the small household size of servant couples could very well be the expression of a more general attitude of imitation. Given the link between attitudes towards consumption and attitudes on ideal family size – as formulated by Banks for the upper and middle classes (see below), a point of view that is largely supported (Szreter, 1996: 471–472) – this seems probable. Moreover, the money that former servants were able to save may have placed them in a stronger negotiation position towards their husbands, e.g. when discussing numbers of children and family size (Van Bavel, 2002: 232). However, none of these arguments *directly* confirm the author's hypothesis. Indirect arguments are supportive, but cannot suffice as evidence.

Statistical Arguments Based on Aggregate Data

In 1981 another author, writing about the Dutch case, launched a call for further examination of the subject (Poelstra, 1981: 67–68):

> New ideas about women's work and family limitation which were first gaining ground through the bourgeoisie, penetrated faster in some social groups than in others. Even if this cultural democratisation was not complete, it did take place. The question concerning the influence of the servant on this process, is by lack of research still highly speculative. It seems to me, in view of the large numbers of women who, as a servant, came in touch with another culture, worth researching. (own translation from Dutch)

Fifteen years later, Jannie Poelstra still found herself waiting for concrete evidence (Poelstra, 1996: 339).

At about the same time of Poelstra's appeal, J. A. Banks incorporated the hypothesis of female servants as diffusers of the idea of 'modern' contraception in his elaborate analysis on the fertility transition in Great Britain (Banks, 1981). According to Banks, the British fertility decline started around 1860–1870 in the upper and middle classes. In his view changes in reproductive behaviour were essentially due to new consumptive attitudes. Upper- and middle-class parents wished to secure their children's social and employment status. The necessity to raise 'high-quality children' heavily increased educational costs per child. Additionally, the 'emancipation' of middle-class women, which was above all an emancipation of 'free time', was an expensive matter, since more servants had to be hired to take over the domestic chores of the lady of the house. For both reasons, reducing the number of children served as a solution. Whilst servants played no direct role in the *take off* of the fertility decline, Banks did attribute to them a more active role in the *diffusion* of birth control behaviour. This is shown in the following figures:

Table 3. Mean Number of Births per Marriage by Marriage Dates: Selected Occupations

Occupation of the male marriage partner	Before 1861	1861–71	1871–81	1881–91
soldiers and non-commissioned officers	no cases	4.57	5.00	4.59
men of the navy and marines	1 case only	7 cases only	5.47	4.15
Coachmen, grooms	7.03	6.38	5.39	4.04
domestic gardeners	6.96	6.42	5.39	4.04
Gamekeepers	7,85	7.22	6.46	5.03
domestic indoor servants*	7.00	5.40	4.26	2.95

*other than in hotels, lodging houses, and eating houses.

The figures were taken from the 1911 fertility census which classified couples according to the husband's occupation. The figures show that the number of births was first reduced in households of domestic servants. Although the data do not provide any proof for this, Banks supposed that former female servants were for a large part responsible for the spread of fertility control behaviour. This is because between 1851 and 1901 in no occupational census did the percentage of females employed in domestic service fall below 40 percent of total employment. Moreover, Banks believed that the social diffusion and adoption of new *reproductive ideals* was much more important than the diffusion of the means to implement them.

Because of the weak statistical underpinning, Banks' hypothesis was heavily criticised. Woods rejected Banks' argument by analysing the same source used for the above table in a more sophisticated way (Woods, 1987: 287–288). Banks, for instance, did not take into account differences in the age at first marriage between occupational groups. In his analysis Woods incorporated the time of marriage, the age of the bride, and the number of surviving children. He did this for five randomly chosen individual occupations and for two occupational groups. His results did show differences in fertility levels between the various occupations, due to pre-decline levels, nuptiality patterns, and children's survival chances. However, the decline in marital fertility took place in successive cohorts in all five occupations, so *social diffusion* seemed out of the question. Looking at the graphs presented by Woods on the basis of the 1911 census figures, it is hard to understand why he did not make use of the category of 'domestic servant' in his analysis.

In his own study of the 1911 census, Szreter confirmed the untenability of Davidoff's and Bank's hypothesis (Szreter, 1996: 480–481). The author put forward three statistical arguments. First, the regions where birth control was first adopted by working-class people were areas where domestic service was lowest and industrial employment was most common. Second, in the census figures the numbers of girls in domestic service were seriously overestimated whereas female agricultural workers were under-enumerated. Third, some research suggested that large proportions of female domestic servants were employed in working-class households. Woods added some limitations of the 1911 fertility census, which may have had, as a consequence, very serious distortions (Woods, 1978: 287–288). Among them is the fact that couples were classified under the husband's occupation and that previous occupations were not taken into account. It is clear that census figures are not suited to either support or reject the hypothesis that former urban female domestic servants contributed to the diffusion of fertility control behaviour at the end of the nineteenth century. The discussion between Banks, Woods, and Szreter is based on shaky ground and must be reconsidered.

Arguments Based on Testimonial Evidence

In rejecting Banks' hypothesis, Szreter also referred to testimonial evidence. The oral histories of thirty women born between 1890 and 1914 showed that, concerning fertility control, maids were less informed than industrial workers. In addition, Szreter stressed the loneliness and the social isolation of domestic servants, and the silence between masters and servants on all private matters. Szreter's testimonial argument can be blamed for covering a population incorrectly placed in time. By the time his respondents entered domestic service, the fertility transition had already been going on for a few decades. Diane De

Keyzer's journalistic inquiry of former domestic servants in Flanders born between 1902 and 1964 revealed a more differentiated image (De Keyzer, 1995: 240–242). Chamber maids in particular came in touch with the intimate life of their masters. Young and inexperienced girls were confronted with the secrets of the bedroom:

> When I had to clean the bedrooms, there always was a glass on the Master's bedside cabinet with a strange rubber thing in it. At that time, I was still quite silly and I didn't know anything about it. Later on I understood that must have been a condom *(Pauline Verschueren).*
>
> Despite this initial naivety, soon very little could be hidden from the femme de chambre. You were confronted with all these personal things of the masters (*Zulma Delrue*). (own translation from Dutch)

The fact that employers and employees did not talk freely about fertility matters can hardly be used as an argument. Sociologists have developed the concept of 'social learning' (Van Bavel, 2004: 66–68), which should be considered as a special case of social influence, as what is sometimes called 'informational influence' in social psychology. Social learning does not imply communication; it can be based on observation-only. According to Van Bavel, the latter is the case in the process of fertility decline. The principle of observation-only social learning specifically applies to matters considered indecent to talk about and assumes that people in very different circumstances can learn from each other.

The use of testimonial data may indeed be useful to enrich the discussion. But as it became clear above, testimonial evidence cannot be used in an unambiguous way. Furthermore, the impact is limited since interviews are only available from girls who worked as maids starting in the beginning of the twentieth century. Written ego-documents on earlier periods are sparse and probably not very representative.

3. The role of Domestic Servants in the Fertility Decline: What Evidence Do We Need?

After having demonstrated that both aggregate and testimonial sources can only serve as indirect and additional evidence, we will elaborate a specific case drawing on life course information. To this end we processed the results of three case-studies that focused specifically on female domestic servants. Two of the studies take the area of origin as a starting point. The first study follows 55 female emigrants from three villages in the neighbourhood of Oudenaarde to the city of Ghent in the period 1880–1900. Information was collected in the population registers of Ghent and of the villages of origin. The second study reconstructs the life courses of the female members of the 1830 birth cohort from the village of Assenede, making a comparison between girls who had been maids in both urban and rural households and girls who had never been in domestic service at all (the total group comprised 73 girls). Information on these domestic servants was collected in the population registers in all communities of residence. The third case-study focuses on the life courses of 50 domestic servants who arrived in Ghent around 1880, irrespective of their place of birth (De Langhe, 2005; Matthys, 2003 and 2004; Van de Velde, 2002).

Domestic Servants Employed within Urban Upper- or Middle-class Households and Returning to the Countryside

Before trying to find information focussing on the (possible) role of urban female domestic servants in the diffusion of fertility control behaviour, we have to ask ourselves whether or not this group was quantitatively important enough to have had a broader impact on rural working-class society. Szreter, on the basis of British census data, argued that this was not the case. Because of the blurred appearance of domestic servants in occupational statistics, it is necessary to use both aggregate *and* individual data to get a more accurate view on the quantitative importance of returning urban maids.

First we look at the general picture of domestic employment in Belgium.[3] This is easier said than done, since before 1880 no clear distinction was made

3 The censuses do not allow a separation of Flandrian and Walloon data.

between different types of domestic employment or different types of servants. Table 4, based on the population censuses, gives the 'best aggregated guesses'.

From 1846 to 1890 the share of domestics in the total Belgian population rose considerably due to the combined effects of urbanisation, the rising numbers of middle-class households, and a lingering structural crisis in the Flemish countryside. Around 1880–1890 urban domestic service reached its summit. This is exactly the period in which fertility levels started to fall all over Belgium (see table 1). After 1910 the proportion of domestic servants in the total population gradually declined.

To estimate the possible impact of this occupational group on the members of their own generation, the share of domestics has to be recalculated in relation to the 'active' (professional) population; see table 5 (Piette, 2000: 53).

Piette's figures show that between 1880 and 1910 a considerable proportion of the active female population was indeed employed in domestic service. At the same time the table confirms the gender gap in this occupation; only a small percentage of men were employed as servants. Knowing that domestic service was a life cycle occupation tied closely to adolescence, the proportion of servants in their own generation must have been higher still, possibly amounting to 25 percent. Only the 1910 census figures allow for the calculation of such proportions.[4] The age group of 15 to 25 years contained the largest share of domestic servants. At the time of the census 73,943 girls born between 1886 up to and including 1895 were involved in 'domestic and personal service'. This makes 11.2 percent out of a total of 657,883 girls in this age group; indeed, domestic servants made up one quarter of all 305,604 girls for whom an occupational activity was recorded. In the Netherlands the percentage of domestic servants among the female unmarried population varied between 12.9 and 27 in the four age groups between 14 and 35 years. When only working unmarried females are taken into account, the proportion of domestic servants always exceeded the 50 percent limit (Poelstra, 1981: 56).

Census figures are useful to show general evolutions in domestic employment. After some recalculations they may also to some extent indicate the relative impact of this occupational category. However, to gain full insight in the quantitative importance of domestic servants we need dynamic individual-

4 *Population census 1910*, vol. IV, 502–503 and 511.

Table 4. Number of Domestic Servants in Belgium According to Censuses

Year	Male Servants	Male Belgian Population	% Male Servants	Female Servants	Female Belgian Population	% Female Servants
1846	12,790	2,163,445	0.59	33,299	2,173,603	1.53
1856	19,130	2,271,783	0.84	67,844	2,257,777	3
1866	51,625	2,419,639	2.13	87,987	2,458,194	3.58
1880	50,919	2,758,469	1.85	105,359	2,761,540	3.82
1890	55,402	3,026,954	1.83	121,048	3,042,367	3.98
1900	48,613	3,324,834	1.46	120,543	3,368,714	3.58
1910	29,591	3,680,790	0.8	131,590	3,742,994	3.52
1920	22,738	3,644,301	0.62	97,373	3,761,268	2.59
1930	18,207	4,007,418	0.45	76,678	4,084,586	1.88
1947	4,259	4,199,728	0.1	48,370	4,312,467	1.12
1961	4,889	4,496,860	0.11	45,216	4,692,881	0.96
1970	2,807	4,721,866	0.06	23,169	4,929,078	0.47
1981	2,057	4,810,349	0.04	16,977	5,038,298	0.34

Year	Total Servants	Total Belgian Population	% Servants
1846	46,089	4,337,048	1.06
1856	86,974	4,529,560	1.92
1866	139,612	4,877,833	2.86
1880	156,278	5,520,009	2.83
1890	176,450	6,069,321	2.91
1900	169,156	6,693,548	2.53
1910	161,181	7,423,784	2.17
1920	120,111	7,405,569	1.62
1930	94,885	8,092,004	1.17

Year	Total Servants	Total Belgian Population	% Servants
1947	52,629	8,512,195	0.62
1961	50,105	9,189,741	0.55
1970	25,976	9,650,944	0.27
1981	19,034	9,848,647	0.19

Table based on Buyst (1996: 115) with additional information from the censuses.

Table 5. Domestic Servants in Belgium as a Share of the Active Population

Year	% Male Active Population	% Female Active Population
1880	2.8	10.9
1890	2.6	13.7
1900	2	12.3
1910	1.2	15

level data that may give information on the life course. After all, we are interested in the number of rural women who *ever* worked as domestic servants. Statistical cross-sections tend to underestimate the weight of domestic service in the total population. Szreter claimed that the British census figures *over*estimated the number of domestic servants. We argue that the Belgian censuses tended to *under*estimate them. This became clear in the village studies based on life course analysis, e.g. Matthys' research on domestic servants from the 1830–1831 cohort of Assenede, a rural village in the north of East Flanders. Two examples may illustrate the underestimation of female domestic servants. First, reconstructing the 1830–1831 cohort by combining several sources, including the local population registers, we learned that in this cohort of 73 girls, 16 had been employed as servants in rural or urban settings. After having consulted population registers in other municipalities, we found that no less than 39 girls (of 73) had ever been employed in domestic service, more than twice as much. Second, we found, and this is worse than *bad* registration, that some employments were *not* registered at all, as was the case with three girls migrating from Assenede to Ghent. The three domestic servants, Viergenie

Dhooghe, Viergenie Van Laere, and Viergenie De Pauw, could be followed through the Ghent population registers during a very long time. All previous and subsequent addresses were carefully recorded, except their first occupational activity after arriving in the town. In all three cases there was a serious gap between the date of arrival in Ghent and the registration date of their first employment. The fact that they were still inexperienced as they got to the city may be an explanation for this administrative oblivion (no registration).

Because of the high degree of mobility among (young) servants, life course data are crucial to get a more accurate picture of the quantitative importance of domestic servants within a given cohort. As was said before, our research requires a reliable estimation of the proportion of the female population that ever worked as an urban domestic servant.

Secondly, we need to have an idea of the number of servants returning to the countryside after a period of urban employment. For this we use the same life course data. In the case of Assenede we were able to determine for 73 females born in 1830–1831 whether they ever worked as a servant (Matthys, 2004: 16). This was the case for 39 girls, or 54 percent, of whom 16, or 22 percent had ever been employed in an urban setting. Out of those 16 persons, we lost track of four girls before they reached the age of thirty. No less than 10 girls returned to the rural region where they were born, which is two thirds of all urban servants in this cohort and 14 percent of all 73 girls under observation. Nearly half (46 percent) of the 55 young females from the surrounding countryside of Oudenaarde (East Flanders) who went into service in Ghent at the end of the nineteenth century, ultimately returned to their area of birth permanently or for a longer time period (De Langhe, 2005). In a third case-study on domestic servants in Ghent, the situation is less clear because the girls were only under observation as long as they remained in Ghent. We may assume however that about 19 of the observed 50 maids (38 percent) returned to the countryside (Van de Velde, 2002). In the neighbouring Dutch province of Zeeland, between 1860 and 1940 about 34 percent (198 out of 582) of rural girls served in domestic employment at some stage (Bras, 2002: 73, 103–105, 107). Half of all first migrations from the countryside were towards the city. About 60 percent of the maids from rural origin returned to their birthplace at least once. Unfortunately, the study did not distinguish between girls who had worked in rural and those who had worked in urban households. However, we may assume that about 10 percent of all rural girls returned to their native villages after a period of domestic service in the city. Here we have a striking similarity with Flanders concerning the return of urban maids. In summary, although the number of returned servants was not massive, it seems that the mobility of young rural girls to and from the city was important enough to have had an impact on the spread of new ideas within the villages of origin.

The final argument advanced by Szreter was that a large proportion of female servants were employed not in middle-class households, but in working-class homes. This does not seem to have been the case in Ghent. The fifteen known employers of domestic servants from the Assenede study nearly all belonged to the bourgeoisie (situation around 1850, see Matthys, 2004: 33–34). None of these girls was the only servant in a family. Around 1880 the situation had changed somewhat. The number of urban domestics reached a summit. Social prestige forced the middle classes to at least employ one maid. One third of the 50 girls in Van de Velde's study of Ghent is the only servant in the household (Van de Velde, 2002: 48–56). The group of employers was very heterogeneous, but mostly middle class and lower bourgeoisie. No working-class employers were found. In the Oudenaarde cohort, the same seems to be true. Thirty percent of the employers were without income out of labour, most of them with private means, whilst 28 percent were employed in intellectual occupations, and yet another 27 percent in shopkeeping. The remaining 15 percent consisted of a heterogeneous group of middle-class occupations. According to Bras, employment periods in bourgeois households were somewhat longer than those in middle-class families (Bras, 2002: 80–82).

Life Course Data on Domestic Service and Fertility

The third step is to investigate whether or not former urban domestics who had returned to their rural villages showed a more restricted fertility pattern. This requires the identification of women from rural origins who *ever* worked as an urban domestic servant. Furthermore, to investigate fertility behaviour one needs data from several stages of the life course. As Woods correctly stated, it is impossible to talk about fertility behaviour if the age of the bride is not taken into account. The age at first marriage is one of the most important restraints on the number of children ever born. Late marriage points to more traditional behaviour. Not only the number of children, but also the timing of the births, is indispensable information in the discussion about possible stopping or spacing behaviour. To conduct the analysis accurately the duration of the period of domestic employment must also be brought into account.

As far as we know, no such detailed research concerning the role of servants in the fertility decline exists. One important exception is Van Bavel's work on Leuven in which he applied life course analysis to observe the diffusion of fertility control behaviour within this small town. What is missing in his study, however, are the dynamics between town and countryside. The Ghent research project can give some first, very provisional results.

As was mentioned earlier in the text, we have three cohorts of servants under observation. The first cohort consists of girls born in 1830–1831 in Assenede. A distinction was made between three groups: girls who had never worked as domestic servants, girls who had been in rural service only (mostly on farms), and finally, those girls who had worked in urban households.

Table 6. Fertility in the Assenede 1830/31 Cohort

Status	A	B	C	D	E[5]	F
never in domestic employment	13	26.8	28.1	42.2	–	7.4
rural maids	16	28.6	28.1	40.9	–	6.1
urban maids	7	31.3	32.1	40.3	–	2.6
Total (average number)	36	28.9	29.4	41.1	–	5.4

A: number of women known to ever have had children
B: mean age at first marriage for females (in years)
C: mean age of mother at birth of first child (in years)
D: mean age of mother at birth of last child (in years)
E: mean interval between births, excluding stillbirths (in months)
F: number of births per mother

Looking at the figures, the differences in the numbers of children between the three groups seem clear cut. However, when we take into account the age at first marriage, we must conclude that the distinction between the girls who stayed in the village and those who ever worked in a city is related to the different ages at marriage. That former urban maids did not apply stopping behaviour is also shown by the age at which their last child was born: on

5 Insufficient data.

average at the age of 40. These girls were in domestic service around the middle of the nineteenth century. Even in the urban upper-class households in which they were employed, restrictive reproductive behaviour was not systematically applied at that time.

Thirty years later, in the bigger cities of Flanders, like Ghent, the fertility decline had spread to different layers of the population. In her study Van de Velde followed a cohort of domestic servants, originally from rural backgrounds, who came to spend their later life in Ghent. On average these women had 2.4 children, while the average female textile worker raised 3.6 children (Devrieze and Vanhaute, 2001: 557–558). The former servants had their last child around the age of 34–35, which indicates stopping behaviour. This was also the case in other urban working-class populations, since the textile workers ceased childbearing at age 31–32, on average. The smaller number of children born to the former servants is again due to their older age at first marriage: 27 versus 24 years.

Around this time fertility control behaviour was still far from widespread in the rural areas. It is in this setting that former urban maids may have played a role. De Langhe's figures strongly point in this direction. A basic question in this case-study is whether the rural origins of servants or rather the settings they spent their fertile periods in, were most influential in determining fertility behaviour. The results point towards the latter explanation: 56 percent of the servants who returned to their village of origin applied stopping behaviour whilst 67 percent of the girls who stayed in the city did so. In addition, a distinction has to be made between the behaviour of girls who returned to the countryside after only a short stay in the city and those who spent several years there. In both Matthys' study (Assenede) and the one conducted by De Langhe (countryside of Oudenaarde), two groups of returning servants can be discerned. The first group consists of servants who returned to their native villages after only a short period of urban employment by one or two masters. For these girls domestic employment was probably a rather negative experience with only a minor impact on their later life. The second group consists of girls who remained in domestic service in urban households for several years and under several employers. They are likely to have been more influenced by 'city life'.

The differences are striking. The young women who stayed in urban service for several years had on average 3.8 children less than the ones who returned to the countryside within two years. In this cohort, it is clear that the small

Table 7. Fertility in the Oudenaarde cohort[6]

Maid	< 2 years	> 2 years	2–5 years	> 5 years
Number of children	5.3	1.5	1.5	1.5
Age at first marriage	27.1	26.4	26.6	26.3
Age at last child	36.3	31.1	32.8	29

number of children is not dependent upon the age at first marriage, since the girls with long urban employment even married a bit earlier than their colleagues. It is also clear that stopping behaviour was much more dominant amongst women with longer employment careers in domestic service. They had their last child five years earlier than those who returned early. This is even clearer when a further distinction is made within the group of those who stayed longer. Girls who stayed more than five years in urban domestic service stopped childbearing at younger ages than those who worked in the city between two and five years.

The only publication we know of with empirical evidence on fertility behaviour of former servants confirms these findings. Because Van Bavel's study is also based on life course data from three generations, he too was able to bring former employments into account. In his work no significant difference was noted between occupational groups within the working class. The only exception to this (in the two most recent generations born in 1850 and 1865) were servants who were showing signs of controlling behaviour earlier in time (Van Bavel, 2002: 339). The article by Angélique Janssens, in this volume, also making use of life course data, points in the same direction. The author examines the fertility control behaviour of two birth cohorts in two Dutch cities. In the earliest cohort (women born between 1881 and 1885) seamstresses and (former) domestic servants in both cities seem to be the pioneering groups in adopting fertility control, rather than other female occupational categories like weavers or teachers.

6 In total, 18 girls were domestic servants for less than two years, 16 girls between two and five years, and 20 girls for more than five years. In this table, only the girls who returned to the countryside are taken into account.

Adequate analysis should also consider the social-economic and familial background of the girls who went to the city to work as domestic servants. If it was the case that only daughters of the local elite became urban maids, the pattern of diffusion of restricted fertility behaviour in the countryside would have been very similar to the urban pattern; namely, stimulated by the local elites. However, when women in urban domestic employment were mostly lower-class girls, we may presume that the diffusion of a new fertility pattern in the countryside happened independently from the village elites. The earliest literature on domestics assumed that the urban maids mostly had a poor agrarian background (Mc Bride, 1976: 34–38). Today a more differentiated picture emerges (Piette, 2001: 286). Hilde Bras found that if all servants – that is rural and urban – were taken into account, families of unskilled workers were indeed the most important providers of maids (Bras, 2002: 71). However, when the analysis was limited to urban domestic servants it appeared that daughters with fathers who were lower civil servants, supervisors, teachers, and skilled workers had a higher statistical 'risk' to migrate as a maid to the city (Bras, 2002: 236). In both Van de Velde's and Matthys' cohorts a substantial share of the maids came from local working- and middle-class families (Matthys, 2004: 29; Van de Velde, 2002: 33). Girls from the surrounding countryside of Oudenaarde mostly had a lower-class background, but this region was very poor at the time (De Langhe, 2005: 108–112). Also noteworthy is that in all populations about two thirds of the fathers were literate.[7] This shows that girls who went to the cities to work as maids did not belong to the poorest families, but neither were they the daughters of the local elite. Bras and De Langhe also show that upper working-class (skilled workers) and rural middle-class daughters tended to have a longer 'career' in domestic service than daughters of lower working-class households (Bras, 2002: 84–85; De Langhe, 2005: 281). As a consequence they also had a smaller tendency to return to the countryside after service: only 38 percent of girls with middle- or upper working-class parents came back to their village of origin, compared to 52 percent and 50 percent of daughters from families of unskilled workers and farmers

7 De Langhe: 12/18, Matthys: 21/36, Van de Velde: 11/18. Both Van de Velde and Matthys' figures are based on the signature of the father in the birth registers. In De Langhe's cohort only marriage registers of the cohort members were used.

respectively (De Langhe, 2005: 277).[8] This implies that the diffusion of birth control behaviour in the countryside did not follow a top down pattern, and that it had different features than in the cities (cf. the role of the farmers).

International research on female domestics has also been concerned with the chances of former maids to marry a man with a higher social status. Scholars have long disagreed on this subject (e.g. Higgs, 1983; McBride, 1974). Current research assumes that women who were in domestic service, especially those employed in bourgeois households, did have a bigger chance to marry upwards into a higher social class; but this was certainly not the case for all girls (Bras, 2002: 137–138; De Langhe, 2005: 291; Mathys, 2004; Piette, 2000: 233–238). Again, the extent to which domestic servants were able to marry socially upwards is best revealed by using a life course perspective. Social mobility through marriage may also have affected our results concerning the impact of the experience of domestic service on fertility behaviour, since the adoption of the more modern demographic pattern may have been provoked by marrying a higher class husband. This question can only be answered by using the advanced statistical technique of event history analysis. This, however, requires the use of larger datasets than the ones that were used here.

4. Conclusion

The hypothesis that female urban domestic servants played a significant and very specific role in the diffusion of fertility control behaviour has existed for over thirty years. For lack of satisfying data and research methods it could never be investigated properly. In this article we argue that historical life course analysis is one of the new methods that can provide a more substantial answer to this research question. We demonstrate that we need very specific and individual data in order to carry out more thorough analyses. Based on the assumption that domestic service implies both employment and migration, we believe that it is necessary to work with well-distinguished social groups within

8 For unskilled workers' families: 11 out of 21 girls returned, for skilled workers/craftsmen 5 out of 13 and for farmers' families: 9 out of 18 daughters returned.

each female birth cohort: girls who never worked as servants, those who did but only in the countryside, urban domestic servants who stayed in the city during their fertile period, and urban domestic servants who returned to the countryside after their domestic employment (making an additional difference between those who were fast to return and those who were slow). Only by comparing these four or five groups can one fully understand whether or not domestic employment in the city had an impact on the diffusion of fertility behaviour in rural villages. A summary of the applied variables on each of the groups is shown in the scheme below.

Figure 3. Scheme for Further Analysis

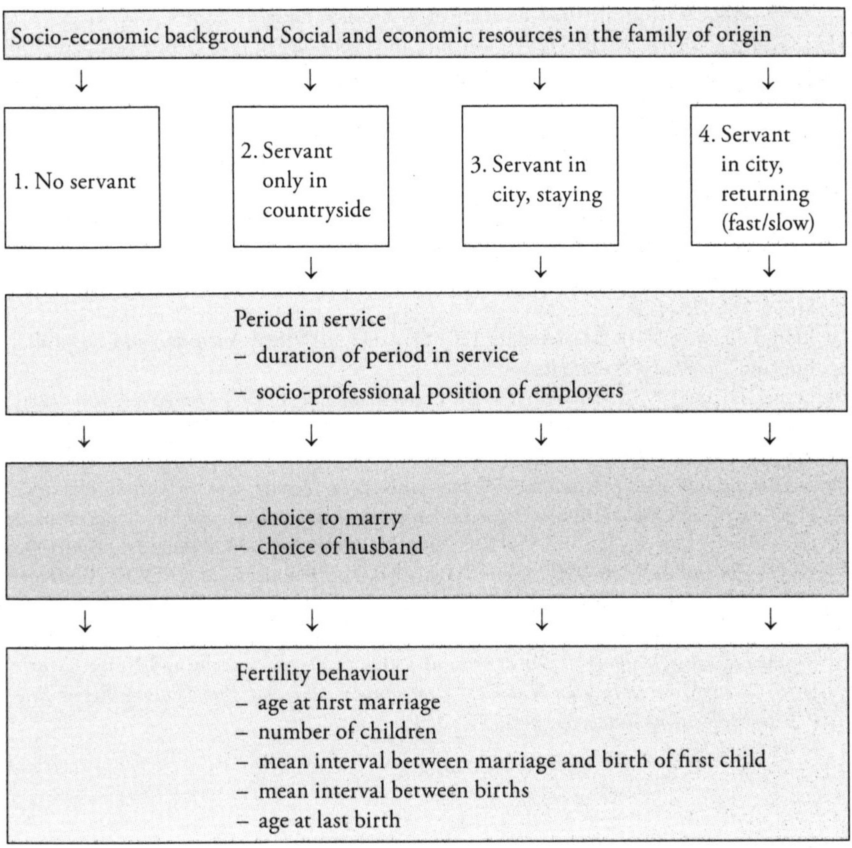

The results of the Ghent life course project are still modest, but do point in the direction of an impact of former servants on the spread of fertility control behaviour in the countryside. Moreover, patterns of diffusion do not seem to have followed the urban top down model. Future analysis, using the above scheme as a general guiding line, may lead to a more fundamental understanding of that impact.[9]

References

Alter, George (1978), *Family and the Female Life Course. The Women of Verviers, Belgium, 1849–1880,* Wisconsin, The University of Winconsin Press.

Alter, George and Oris, Michel (1999), 'Fertility and Fecundity in 19th Century Ardennes', in *Communications à la Social Science History Association,* Fort Worth, 11–15 November.

Banks, Joseph A. (1981), *Victorian Values. Secularism and the Size of Families,* London, Routledge & Kegan Paul.

Bras, Hilde (2002), *Zeeuwse meiden. Dienen in de levensloop van vrouwen, 1850–1950,* Amsterdam, Aksant.

Buyst, Erik (1996), 'De economische betekenis van het dienstpersoneel', in De Maeyer, Jan and Van Rompaey, Lies (eds), *Upstairs downstairs. Dienstpersoneel in Vlaanderen 1750–1995,* Gent, Province of East Flanders and KADOC (Bijdragen Museum van Vlaamse Sociale Strijd, 13), 113–123.

Davidoff, Leonore (1974), 'Mastered for Life: Servant and Wife in Victorian and Edwardian England', *Journal of Social History,* 8, 407–428.

De Keyzer, Diane (1995), *Madame est servie. Leven in dienst van adel en burgerij (1900–1985),* Leuven.

De Langhe, Sofie (2005), *Plattelandsmeisjes als dienstbodes in Gent 1880–1900. Een levensloopanalyse,* unpublished master thesis, Ghent University, Department of Modern History.

De Metsenaere, Machteld (1996), 'Dienstboden en taalgebruik in Brussel in de negentiende eeuw', in De Maeyer, Jan and Van Rompaey, Lies (eds), *Upstairs downstairs. Dienstpersoneel in Vlaanderen 1750–1995,* Gent, Province of East Flanders and KADOC (Bijdragen Museum van Vlaamse Sociale Strijd, 13), 177–185.

Devrieze, Anouk and Vanhaute, Eric (2001), 'Working-class Girls. The Life Courses of 33 Women Cotton Workers in Ghent around 1900', in Devos, Isabelle and Neven, Muriel (eds), *Recent Work in Belgian Historical Demography. 19th and 20th Century, Revue Belge d'Histoire Contemporaine,* 31, 3–4, 557–578.

Eggerickx, Thierry (1998), *La dynamique démographique et la transition de la fecondité dans le bassin industriel de la région de Charleroi, de 1831 à 1910*, unpublished Ph.D. thesis, Université catholique de Louvain, Département Démographie.

Higgs, Edward (1983), 'Domestic Servants and Households in Victorian England', *Social History*, 8, 201–210.

Jacquart, Camille (1905), *La dépression démographique des Flandres. Etude sur la natalité de l'arrondissement de Thielt*, Brussels, Poleunis en Geuterlinck.

Lesthaeghe, Ron (1977), *The Decline of Belgian Fertility, 1800–1970*, Princeton, Princeton University Press.

Matthys, Christa (2003), *Ondergaan of ondernemen? Levenslooponderzoek van de generatie van 1830/31 in Assenede*, unpublished master thesis, Ghent University, Department of Modern History.

Matthys, Christa (2004), *Het vagevuur op aarde. De impact van dienen en migratie van ongehuwde vrouwen op hun latere leven. Assenede, generatie 1830/31*, unpublished master thesis, University of Antwerp, Department of Women's Studies.

McBride, Teresa (1974), 'Social Mobility for the Lower Classes: Domestic Servants in France', *Journal of Social History*, 7, 63–78.

McBride, Teresa (1976), *The Domestic Revolution. The Modernisation of Household Service in England and France 1820–1920*, London.

Neven, Muriel (2003), *Individus et familles: les dynamiques d'une société rurale. Le Pays de Herve dans la seconde moitié du XIXe siècle*, Liège, Bibliothèque de la Faculté de Philosophie et Lettres de l'Université de Liège.

Piette, Valérie (1996), 'De geschiedenis van het dienen. De problematiek van bronnen en methode', in De Maeyer, Jan and Van Rompaey, Lies (eds), *Upstairs downstairs. Dienstpersoneel in Vlaanderen 1750–1995*, Province of East Flanders and KADOC (Bijdragen Museum van Vlaamse Sociale Strijd, 13), 103–113.

Piette, Valérie (2000), *Domestiques et servantes. Des vies sous condition. Essai sur le travail domestique en Belgique au 19e siècle*, Brussels, Académie royale de Bruxelles.

Piette, Valérie (2001), 'Women Going to the Cities: Migration and Stereotypes. The Example of Servants in Brussels in the Nineteenth Century', in Blondé, B., Vanhaute, E. and Galand, M. (eds), *Labour and Labour Markets between Town and Countryside (Middle Ages – 19th Century)*, Turnhout, Brepols, 278–291 (CORN Publication Series 6).

Poelstra, Jannie (1981), 'Dienstboden tussen arbeiders en burgerstand', *Tijdschrift voor vrouwenstudies*, 2, 44–68.

Poelstra, Jannie (1996), *Luiden van een andere beweging. Huishoudelijke arbeid in Nederland 1840–1920*, Amsterdam, Het Spinhuis.

Roche, D. (1978), 'Les domestiques comme intermédiaires culturels', in *Les intermédiaires culturels. Actes du Colloque du Centre Méridional d'Histoire Sociale, des Mentalités et des Cultures*, Aix-en Provence, Université de Provence, 189–202.

Szreter, Simon (1996), *Fertility, Class and Gender in Britain, 1860–1940*, Cambridge, Cambridge University Press (Cambridge Studies in Population, Economy and Society in Past Time, 27).

Van Bavel, Jan (2002), *Van natuurlijke naar gecontroleerde vruchtbaarheid? Geboortebeperking in Leuven (1846–1910)*, Leuven, Universitaire Pers Leuven.

Van Bavel, Jan (2004), 'Diffusion Effects in the European Fertility Transition: Historical Evidence from within a Belgian Town (1846–1910)', *European Journal of Population, 20*, 1, 63–85.

Van de Velde, Kathy (2002), *De lokroep van de stad. Een levensloopanalyse van 50 dienstboden in de stad Gent. 1880*, unpublished master thesis, Ghent University, Department of Modern History.

Woods, R. I. (1987), 'Approaches to the Fertility Transition in Victorian England', *Population Studies*, 41, 283–311.

Population, Family, and Society
Population, Famille et Société

Edited by / Edité par
Michel Oris

This series welcomes and encourages the dialogue between demography and family studies to revitalize social history as well as sociology and population studies. An international network of scholars based at the Laboratory of Demography and Family Studies of the University of Geneva has initiated an open-minded series that seeks to reflect the latest developments in research. The collection emphasizes comparative and international perspectives, as well as interdisciplinary approaches drawing from history, economics, statistics, sociology, geography, demography, and cultural anthropology. Innovative methodologies for both qualitative and quantitative analysis which allow authors to reformulate old problems and ask new questions are particular welcome. The series publishes both individual and collective volumes. The first group encompasses case studies or monographs coming from the Swiss or the international scientific world, including the best Ph.D. dissertations. The second group refers to collective volumes organized around a topic emerging from a scientific debate, with contributions from various disciplinary fields and/or geographic horizons.

The series accepts publications in French, English and German.

Vol. 1 Frans van Poppel, Michel Oris & James Lee (eds). *The Road to Independence. Leaving Home in Western and Eastern Societies, 16th–20th centuries.* 2004.
ISBN 3-906770-61-3 / US-ISBN 0-8204-5949-6

Vol. 2 Guy Brunet, Michel Oris & Alain Bideau (éds). *Les minorités. Une démographie culturelle et politique, XVIIIe-XXe siècles / Minorities. A Cultural and Political Demography, 18th–20th centuries.* 2004. ISBN 3-03910-220-6 / US-ISBN 0-8204-6874-6

Vol. 3 Erwin Zimmermann & Robin Tillmann (éds/Hrsg.). *Vivre en Suisse 1999-2000. Une année dans la vie des ménages et familles en Suisse / Leben in der Schweiz 1999–2000. Ein Jahr im Leben der Schweizer Familien und Haushalte.* 2004. ISBN 3-03910-370-9

Vol. 4 Jean-Marie Le Goff, Claudine Sauvain-Dugerdil, Clémentine Rossier & Josette Coenen-Huther. *Maternité et parcours de vie. L'enfant a-t-il toujours une place dans les projets des femmes en Suisse?* 2005. ISBN 3-03910-666-X

Vol. 5 Claudine Sauvain-Dugerdil, Henri Leridon & Nicholas Mascie-Taylor (eds). *Human Clocks. The Bio-Cultural Meanings of Age.*
2006. ISBN 3-03910-785-2 / US-ISBN 0-8204-7570-X

Vol. 6 Michel Oris, Guy Brunet, Eric Widmer & Alain Bideau (éds). *Les fratries. Une démographie sociale de la germanité.*
2007. ISBN 978-3-03911-255-5

Vol. 7 Angélique Janssens (ed.). *Gendering the Fertility Decline in the Western World.*
2007. ISBN 978-3-03911-311-8